Atlas of
Liposuction

Atlas of
Liposuction

Tolbert S. Wilkinson, MD
Cosmetic Surgery Center & Spa
San Antonio, Texas

Lee Ann Paradise
Medical Editor

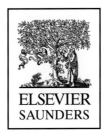

ELSEVIER
SAUNDERS

ELSEVIER
SAUNDERS

The Curtis Center
170 S Independence Mall W 300E
Philadelphia, Pennsylvania 19106

ATLAS OF LIPOSUCTION   ISBN 0–7216–9422–5
Copyright © 2005, Elsevier Inc.

Notice

Surgery is an ever-changing field. Standard safety precautions must be followed, but as new research and clinical experience broaden our knowledge, changes in treatment and drug therapy may become necessary or appropriate. Readers are advised to check the most current product information provided by the manufacturer of each drug to be administered to verify the recommended dose, the method and duration of administration, and contraindications. It is the responsibility of the licensed prescriber, relying on experience and knowledge of the patient, to determine dosages and the best treatment for each individual patient. Neither the publisher nor the author assumes any liability for any injury and/or damage to persons or property arising from this publication.

Library of Congress Cataloging-in-Publication Data
Wilkinson, Tolbert S.
    Atlas of liposuction/Tolbert S. Wilkinson.
       p. ; cm.
    ISBN 0-7216-9422-5
       1. Liposuction–Atlases. 2. Surgery, Plastic–Atlases. I. Title.
    [DNLM: 1. Lipectomy–Atlases. WO 517 W687a 2005]
    RD119.5.L55W557 2005
    617.9'52–dc22   2004049196

Acquisitions Editors: Susan Hodgson; Rolla Couchman
Developmental Editor: Peter McEllhenney
Publishing Services Manager: Tina Rebane
Project Manager: Mary Anne Folcher
Designer: Steven Stave

Printed in China
Last digit is the print number: 9   8   7   6   5   4   3   2   1

To the surgeons who are innovators
within our specialty, and to
those in all specialties who
have contributed to our
knowledge and innovations

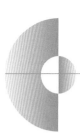

Preface

Liposuction has become an invaluable asset in the surgery of the face, breast, arms, legs, and abdomen as well as in the techniques of restoration. Yves-Gerard Illouz and Pierre Fourvier and several others of us developed fat redistribution at the time of Adrien Aiache's International Conferences in 1984 and 1985. At the 2004 Annual Conference of The American Society for Aesthetic Plastic Surgery, I was privileged to attend a teaching course by my friend Richard Ellenbogen, who reviewed the development of predictable fat grafting and showed the beautiful results that have become the standard in the past 20 years.

Readers of the *Atlas of Liposuction* will gain insights as well as learn the philosophy and the technical expertise to achieve "beauty." They will learn from my own work as well as that of others. And readers will also benefit from the advice and experience of those who agreed to contribute to the *Atlas of Liposuction*.

We certainly have come a long way since our organization dedicated to liposuction, The Lipoplasty Society of North America, was formed by Greg Hetter and other American surgeons to disseminate not only knowledge but also surgical improvements. *Atlas of Liposuction* reflects the continuing efforts of our national societies to improve the quality of our work.

As the Editor of *Technical Forum*, the bulletin of the International Society of Clinical Plastic Surgeons for over 22 years, I have access to the innovations of our specialty. Many of the ideas as well as procedures in this text were first introduced as new concepts in *Technical Forum*. Others soon found their way to the trashcan! We learned. Now we pass our experience and expertise on to you.

Courage and perseverance are required to change a procedure that seems to be working well. When one reflects upon the "acceptable results" at the time of introduction of liposuction to the United States, and upon our reluctance to learn from our South American and Canadian colleagues, it is understandable that changes within the profession would develop slowly. Those individuals quoted in the *Atlas of Liposuction* have volunteered their experience and information for all of us. There are no secrets among colleagues! Plastic surgery is unique and the same may be said for the practice of medicine in general in that with new ideas and new techniques, successes are immediately shared.

Tolbert S. Wilkinson

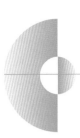

Acknowledgments

Embarking on my third and hopefully last textbook, *Atlas of Liposuction*, I must acknowledge the support of my wife Suzanne during these difficult times, and her contributions to plastic surgery in the past 22 years. Knowing of Suzanne's expertise, I encouraged her to develop a line of cosmetic products for the growing fields of liposuction and rejuvenation. The GlamouRx line was formally introduced at The American Society for Aesthetic Plastic Surgery and was the only cosmetics company in the exhibits. The response was frigid! Soon thereafter, however, other companies entered product lines.

Liposuction does not stand alone. Techniques that we initially employed in our office spa over 20 years ago are now essential to recovery. Mechanical massage post-operatively is not as effective as skilled hands, for example. Machines are impersonal and do not require the communication of staff therapist. Our estheticians, trained in lymph biology, skin repair and rejuvenation, and postoperative external ultrasound, became supportive confidants. When her company became too large, she gracefully agreed to spend more of her time with our clinic, our family, and our ranch, assuming the role of manager as well as operating room supervisor. She became a true "frontier woman" in the development of our part of Texas with tourists and longhorn cattle. My only regret is that she ruined my "warriors," turning my polo ponies into docile, happy, overweight pets.

I owe thanks to our children Scott, Noel, Theresa, and Priscilla, and to my colleagues who have generously contributed their thoughts, case reports, techniques, and philosophy as well as support. Special thanks go to Adrien Aiache, Luiz Toledo, and Alan Matarasso—friends who have worked with me in our teaching courses over the past 15 years. Adrien introduced this Texan to the good and bad of European plastic surgery. Because of his guidance and assistance in publications and teaching courses, a valuable service was provided to organize material in a presentable form.

I also have fond memories of my wife hosting my plastic surgery "idols," and her ability to charm everyone and make them feel as important to her as they were to me. Gene Courtiss, Evo Pitanguy, Greg Hetter, Simon Fredricks, Robert Ersek, Tom Biggs, Jay Anastasi, Nick Georgiade, Joe Murray, Fernando Ortiz-Monastario, and of course my old professor F. X. Paletta Sr. Simon led the society's task force that introduced modern concepts of liposuction, and Gerald published the first comprehensive textbooks. Herein, I continue their work.

I am indebted to the two plastic surgeons on the West Coast who were bold enough to embrace external ultrasound as an adjunct to liposuction—when many of us were so discouraged by internal ultrasound. Barry Silberg and Steve Hoefflin worked with the original prototypes, which led to my assignment for the Society to evaluate the first commercially available ultrasound.

Atlas of Liposuction documents for our readers that one factor of technology can contribute to patient well-being and improvement in results. When I first presented my evaluation, Ed Truppman was a guiding force of sanity and experience, along with others who are cited in the numerous articles on ultrasound.

Liposuction and the less scar-producing breast surgeries began with Onur Erol and his contribution to the circle technique. The improvements by Louis Benelli and Luiz Toledo that included liposuction are noted. All of the contributors I solicited, especially Robert Ersek, lend their experience to help readers to learn and perhaps to develop new technical improvements.

Tolbert S. Wilkinson

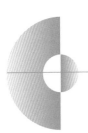

Contents

Atlas of
Liposuction

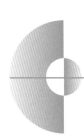

CHAPTER ONE

General Considerations

Liposuction is a medical procedure that reshapes the body through the removal of excess fat from selected areas. On the surface, liposuction appears to be a simple procedure with instant gratification; however, the decision to undergo liposuction should not be made in haste. Liposuction is, in fact, a unique operation with many issues to consider for both the patient and physician.

The liposuction technique was conceived in 1977 as an alternative to European lipocurettage procedures and was publicized in 1978. Scholarly publications appeared in 1980 and 1982, during which time the technique was refined. In December 1978, the *Midnight Globe* published a four-page article that made a splash about a new "miracle vacuum." The article, titled "Surgeon Claims Machine Vacuums Fat Away in Minutes," featured Dr. Robert Franklyn of Los Angeles, who claimed to be the inventor of the "Centurion Machine." It was somewhat crude to say the least and typical Los Angeles "hype." Franklyn predicted, "In a year or two I think the Centurion will be the most popular procedure of all plastic surgery. Plastic surgeons should keep a watch on people and their bodies the way a good mechanic does on automobiles."[1] It was at least 4 years before liposuction became a part of mainstream American medicine, thanks to Dr. Yves-Gerard Illouz and his colleagues.

In a review of the 18-year statistical evidence, as well as a personal retrospective, Dr. Mark Gorney (plastic surgeon, Napa) discussed the onset of the tidal wave that began with a 1982 presentation by Dr. Illouz. It was obvious to everyone that a completely different procedure was being introduced. Even though the slides and presentation were not standardized, the response ranged from the sublime to the ridiculous, with the formation of new societies devoted to liposuction, an attempt to patent certain words, and passionate and intemperate language among medical practitioners. This situation certainly has not abated in 22 years. Indeed, the technique of liposuction (or lipoplasty or

liposculpture as it is sometimes called) continues to be widely discussed. Certainly from an innovation standpoint the procedure is unique. As Gorney points out, "Traditionally, a procedure is conceived in a surgeon's mind, tried on experimental animals, and followed by trials in human subjects. It is then modified or improved. After that, it is performed on a limited clinical trial group and presented before an audience of peers at a surgical congress. Others then try it, refine it, and if effective, it gradually becomes a part of their bag of tricks. Not so lipoplasty; it emerged fully formed like Venus coming out of the shell."[2]

HOW IT STARTED: IT STARTED LIKE A "LOVE STORY"— YVES-GERARD ILLOUZ, M.D. (PLASTIC SURGEON, PARIS)

It was spring 1977 in Paris. My friend was very upset because of a lipoma in her back (Fig. 1-1) that was spoiling any "décolleté," and she was very fond of a large back décolleté with a low neckline. She asked me to remove it, but my answer was that I would leave a scar as long as the bump and that scars on the back are always visible. She didn't want any scar and asked me to "find something" to remove the lipoma without any visible marks.

This was my challenge, and this challenge obsessed me to such an extent that every day I thought about how to remove a fatty bump without a scar. After a few weeks I wondered whether I could suck the fat out, but it seemed impossible or very difficult because fat is solid and hard to suck. Next, I thought I could soften if not liquefy the fat mechanically by back and forth movements or by physically injecting liquid. I tried these

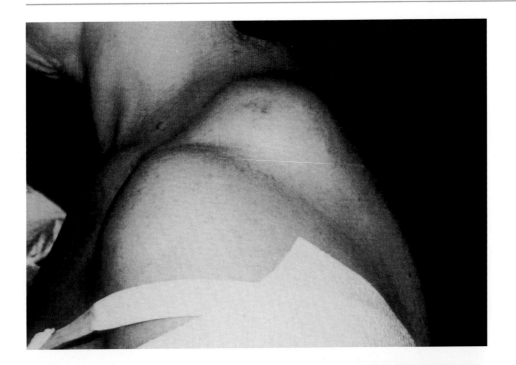

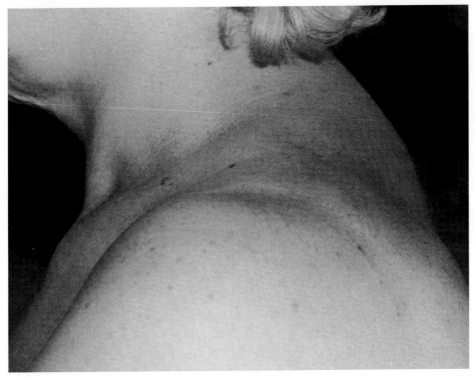

Figures 1-1 & 1-2 *Removal of lipomas and aberrant fat deposits, which once entailed unsightly skin incisions, is now accomplished by cannula extraction and "pickle fork" or cannula disruption of the fibrous capsule.*

ideas out on large pieces of animal fat and found that it worked somewhat on lamb and beef fat but produced very poor to no effect on pig fat.

I agreed to try something in June 1977, but I could not guarantee the results. My friend accepted the challenge. I used a normal aspirating cannula and motor. Surprisingly, it was working, although it was difficult and bloody.

Over the next few days I worried about the excess skin, but I observed the skin retracting slowly so that after a few more weeks, the result was nearly invisible (Fig. 1-2). At this same time, a patient consulted me because she was upset about an operation I had performed about 2 years previously. She had a riding breeches deformity procedure with classic large scars. The saddlebag had recurred, though not as extensively as before, and the scars enlarged. I agreed to do a touchup and removed the recurrent bump with an aspirating cannula and back and forth movements and then excised the scar. Thus, it was proved that the principle of discontinuous dissection was valid. On inspection, the area had a cobweb-like network that contained the still intact vessels and nerves. Suctioning of these structures produced only characteristic bleeding.

At that time, I understood all of the following:

- Fat can be sucked.
- Back and forth movements avoid destruction of large vessels or nerves and leave good nutrition for the skin. In replacing continuous dissection with discontinuous dissection, I developed the technique of tunnelization with a blunt cannula.
- Separating instead of cutting maintains connections between the superficial and deep layers.
- The skin is an elastic tissue capable of retraction; the question remained as to how much.
- Resection of a fat bump is definitive.

I believed at that point that the technique must remain simple and avoid pitfalls. With the initial positive results, I was encouraged to extend the technique to any lipodystrophy. The procedure produced some bleeding, with 20% of the aspirated material being blood. It was also physically exhausting to perform this technique. Although no surgical complications occurred, the cosmetic results were not perfect; some dimpling and wave-like deformities developed. To study and analyze the technique further, I offered free suction to my first 100 patients. Based on my analysis, the technique has been refined and its application extended, with the following observations:

- The physically exhausting and hemorrhagic aspect of the method led to the impression that smaller blunt cannulas (5, 6, and 8 mm) could be used instead of the 10-mm one used for the first cases. A stronger pump would be needed with a cannula whose diameter was smaller. This change in technique also made the dissection less traumatic by reducing the number of passages and thus the risk of bleeding.
- As a plastic surgeon, I was used to performing extensive infiltration for surgery of various types, and at first, I was infiltrating a normal saline solution. Because of the physical laws that govern cellular osmosis, a slightly hypotonic solution containing hyaluronidase permitted more even diffusion into fatty tissues. Epinephrine at a dose of 1 mg/L was used occasionally during this period, specifically, when the patient chose local anesthesia or when halothane was not used as a general anesthetic.
- The irregularities that had been observed led to the guideline that a minimum of 5 mm, sometimes more, of subcutaneous fat had to be maintained. Consequently, other cannulas were designed that could respect this thickness. Some cannulas with the opening half an inch from the end were used. The opening was always pointed down and away from the skin.
- These refinements reduced bleeding and made the procedure safer and easier to perform, with the hope of improving results. Other areas of the body were then treated, such as the hips, knees, and buttocks (steering clear of the Bermuda triangle to avoid flat buttocks). When a groove developed unexpectedly, the technique was extended to create a subgluteal crease.

Summary

Liposuction has been applied in many areas and is now accepted throughout the world. The study, research, and clinical trials about fat that have been conducted have opened new doors for plastic surgery. It is hoped that its applications will lead to new discoveries in the years to come.

My greatest ambition is to reuse the fat, not just as a filling, but after some genetic manipulations to transform these cells into other cells—cardiac, bone, cartilage, and nervous and other cells—and then use them in treating severe disease. That would be the ultimate glory of the fat cell. *It is still a love story.*

> **CLINICAL PEARL**
>
> Noncosmetic indications for liposuction, such as lymphedema, axillary hyperhidrosis, or hydradenitis, have had limited success. Removal of lipomas, however, has been successful if the surgeon understands that a "pickle fork" or other device must be used to break the fibrous banding around the lipoma to allow complete evacuation without leaving a shell in which a seroma may form.

> **CLINICAL PEARL**
>
> Pre-tunneling was advocated in the initial phases of liposuction, particularly in thicker areas such as the chest and back. It made sense to use a blunt cannula without suction to break up the adhesions and also to spare the surgeon the extra effort. Pre-tunneling is also advised for internal ultrasound-assisted liposuction procedures, even if one is using the small "Contour Genesis" probe.

HISTORY

Fat grafting was the only alternative to soft tissue augmentation, which before 1926 involved rubber, purified latex, and paraffin. By 1985, Chajchir, Illouz, Ellenbogen, Teimourian, Aiache, Toledo, and I were presenting and publishing reports on successful fat grafting. The principles included nontraumatic harvesting of small packets of fat, separation of the fat from anesthetic and oil from ruptured cells, and nontraumatic regrafting. Though widely copied in the medical community, attention was not focused on this technique until 1991, when Dr. Sydney Coleman, a plastic surgeon from New York, presented his results with alterations of the technique to make the regrafting yield "more integration and stability." He chose to use decanting and centrifuging. Others, including myself, abandoned these techniques because simpler methods of separating the oil and residua were accomplished by Telfa pad drainage.

By 2001, surgeons were using fat-grafting techniques, with variation only in the choice of a sharp injection cannula (16- or 18-gauge hypodermic needle) or blunt cannulas placed through small incisions as advocated by Coleman and Toledo. In Coleman's technique, hundreds of passes are made to infiltrate the area. Others use a "spray pattern," or multilayered injection with fewer passes, but also emphasize that fat is deposited on withdrawal into the previously created tunnels.

Unfortunately, as with any successful technique, success breeds complications. Overgrafting with difficulty removing fat is the newest challenge facing aesthetic surgeons. Abnormal contours, "beetling" eyebrows, cheek bulges, and protruding lips result from overly zealous "correction." Overgrafting is an unfortunate sequela of the disbelief in many minds of the efficacy of fat grafting. When fat was "injected" with pressure, patients could be told that the effect was transitory. The edema and dying fat cells gave temporary improvement. When surgeons began to understand that fat grafts are placed in small tunnels during withdrawal, that fat must be handled carefully and concentrated by some means, and that postoperative compression must absolutely be avoided, there was no loss of the grafts. Numerous patients are now asking for relief of overcorrection, including the "Neanderthal look" of overgrafting along the upper orbital rim and the "beetling brow" of over-grafting across the glabella area, as well as more easily correctable areas. When overgrafting occurs in the temporal fascia and the lip, a more direct approach is required for correction. Although the lip may be approached by the "reverse lip roll" procedure, as will be described later in this text, to expose and remove the excess fat under direct vision, grafts along the course of the facial nerves, either in the temporal or supermalar area, are best addressed by saline injection and dissolution via external ultrasound-assisted liposuction (XUAL). Progressing from the widely accepted method of lip augmentation and undermining of the nasolabial fold and commissure with secondary placement, Coleman's and Ellenbogen's teaching courses embraced larger areas of the face. The concept of facial beauty detailed by Steven Hoefflin emphasized that atrophy of soft tissue was not universally confined to the subnasal triangle.[3] Fat grafts are now essential in restoring a youthful contour to the entire face.

A source of debate is the contention that filling the temporal fascia and upper eyelid is an "aesthetic improvement." This technique may be appropriate in selected patients, but rethickening of the eyelid and temple area carries the risk of unacceptable elevation in an area of natural shadowing. In contrast, over-resected upper eyelid fat pads may be replaced with fat grafts in a manner similar to that often used in the "tear trough" of the lower lid adjacent to the nose.

An unexpected development was that large fluctuations in patient weight are reflected in increases or decreases in the size of the transplant. In most patients, such changes are not noticeable, but it certainly illustrates that properly placed fat grafts are autologous living transplants.

Filling of the depression adjacent to the nose and below the malar prominence has been addressed by autologous fat grafting, as well as by solid implants, as demonstrated so often by Dr. Edward Terino (plastic surgeon, Agura). Placement of silicone prostheses is beyond the scope of this atlas, but it is mentioned because a permanent contour in many individuals is better achieved with a solid material than with autologous grafts. I use a combination of the two and fill above and below chin and malar prostheses. In contrast, conversations with Sydney Coleman revealed that he prefers to do all of the filling in the mid-cheek and posterior angle of the mandible with fat grafting.

Care must be exercised in counseling patients. For many individuals, the "fatty face jowly look" is unacceptable. For others, it is a suitable alternative to more invasive procedures such as face-lifting and mid-facial deep tissue elevation.[4]

The Dark Side

Some surgeons lost sight of their professional standards, leaving ethics and decent conduct behind.

Surgeons with a knowledge of surgical physiology, long-term training in surgical technique, and familiarity with infection, wound healing, fluid balance, and management of emergencies were certain that this procedure, which was seemingly so innocuous, would be abused. They were right. Although it was a guarded secret, anecdotal reports of patient injuries and deaths soon came flooding in, with 95 confirmed.[5] Emergency room physicians in California discussed patients with lidocaine (Xylocaine) overdoses, fluid imbalance, and pulmonary failure. These cases were never tabulated.

Unfortunately, some anesthesiologists failed to recognize that large-volume intravenous infusions with massive "tumescent" infusion of fluid posed a risk to patients undergoing liposuction. In cases reported, there were often overdoses of fluid by the surgeon and corresponding overdoses by the anesthesiologist, which resulted in tragedy.[5]

Good surgeons were caught up in the hype. Unfortunately, the groundswell of tragedy soon became front and center and involved physicians from all backgrounds.

The two shining lights were the American Society for Aesthetic Plastic Surgery and the Lipoplasty Society, whose members consistently called for restraint and good common sense. They focused on the need to avoid overhydration, overdose, and risks, as well as the importance of at least some restraint in the hype and promotion of liposuction. Unfortunately, the latter has not been heeded even now. In a press release, Dr. Mark

Gorney stated, "The conflict between our duty to protect the public while simultaneously refraining from interfering with scientific progress is always a thorny one so underwriting was done (by the insurance companies) very carefully. It was based not on specialty but on proven training and the ability to recognize and respond rapidly to surgical or anesthetic emergencies or postoperative complication."[6]

> **CLINICAL PEARL**
>
> Data from the American Association for Accreditation of Ambulatory Surgery Facilities, Inc., as well as surveys of active plastic surgeons, show that intravenous sedation or general anesthesia not only does not increase the risk of complications but also reduces the pain associated with "tumescent" infusion with other types of anesthesia. The other danger in the "tumescent" approach is a toxic epinephrine, lidocaine, and/or fluid overload.

PATIENT SELECTION

Before choosing to perform a liposuction procedure, the patient must be counseled because many factors can affect the desired outcome or the surgical risk. It is helpful if the patient demonstrates a realistic attitude about the procedure and the extent to which appearance can be changed. During the consultation, the patient must be informed about "what to expect." This topic is discussed in greater detail later in this chapter. Liposuction can enhance a patient's appearance, and the ideal patient is willing to work cooperatively with the surgeon during the recovery period and understands that improvements are not always immediate.

In addition to having realistic expectations, candidates for a liposuction procedure should be in good physical and mental health. Individuals with circulatory and cardiovascular disease or diabetes and those who have recently undergone surgery in the contour area are at increased risk for complications. Patients with localized pockets of fat are preferred over those with a generalized distribution of fat. Skin elasticity and firmness are essential for the best results. Thus, it is preferable to be young and in a normal weight range; however, a wide variety of people, regardless of their age and size, have benefited from undergoing the procedure.

INDICATIONS AND LIMITATIONS

Liposuction versus Abdominoplasty with Liposuction

Though not a substitute for weight reduction, liposuction is a way to remove localized fat that is unresponsive to diet and exercise. Some patients, however, do not fit cleanly into the liposuction category. Loss of skin elasticity is a significant factor in deciding which procedure to perform; older patients, especially those with slight obesity, sometimes find abdominoplasty (commonly referred to as a "tummy tuck") with liposuction beneficial. Patients with loose abdominal skin, which can be found in women who have had multiple pregnancies, for example, sometimes fall into what can be described as an "in-between category."

When counseling patients in the "in-between category," *recommendation for a limited abdominoplasty should take precedence.* However, some may prefer a lesser degree of correction with lower cost and quicker recovery. It is important that these patients be made aware that future abdominal tightening should be considered. In many instances, an active physical exercise regimen may correct limited abnormalities in the abdominal wall. Women who have not been pregnant and have not suffered separation of the rectus abdominis muscles may or may not be able to achieve the desired flat abdomen with postoperative exercise after liposuction.

Case in point

Preoperative photographs (see Figs. 1-3 and 1-4) show an area of wrinkled skin above the umbilicus that will be excised (the "starburst" procedure). With advancement, a flap will be prepared to overhang the curve of the umbilicus in a technique to be discussed in the abdominoplasty chapter. This procedure affords a degree of skin tightening but also "opens up" the umbilicus, a choice made by the individual patient.

Her postoperative counseling has been directed toward a subsequent limited abdominoplasty with drawing of the necessary amount of skin excision and areas that will be corrected by internal muscle repair. In the case of this patient, the correction has still not been scheduled (see Figs. 1-5 and 1-6). Personal obligations as well as a sense of achievement with liposuction have made the choice of a deferred abdominoplasty the correct one for her. The addition of XUAL has produced shrinkage of the laxity in the upper portion of the abdomen that would not have occurred with standard liposuction.

Limitations of Standard Liposuction

Patients who have massive fatty deposits and distended abdominal walls can expect only limited improvement with long-scar abdominoplasty. Unfortunately, these individuals are frequently unable to modify their lifestyles despite the advantage of less weight and better posture. Reaccumulation of fat adds to the problem of limitations in fat removal in long-scar abdominoplasty and liposuction. The addition of power-assisted liposuction (PAL), ultrasound-assisted liposuction (UAL), and XUAL with skin shrinkage and reduction in surgeon fatigue has made reoperation in these individuals far less difficult.

Case in point

As shown in Figures 1-7 to 1-9, residual fat in the hips, thighs, lower part of the abdomen, upper portion of the flank, and inner aspect of the thighs remained after standard liposuction. The patient had gained weight and, because of other physical problems, was unable to carry out any exercise program. In this case the patient agreed to be one of the first volunteers to assess the effect of XUAL. Serving as her own "control," it could be seen that liposuction was far easier and skin retraction was uniform. The only surgical maneuver was removal of small lateral "dog-ears." In comparing the two procedures and addressing only the liposuction aspects, this patient reported less discomfort, earlier ambulation, and a much lesser degree of bruising that cleared far more rapidly.

To fully appreciate the effect of a secondary procedure, this patient's original photographs showed the enormity of the original procedure (see Figs. 1-10 and 1-11). The debate is whether a simple panniculectomy or panniculectomy with repair should be considered. In this patient, the repair was performed along with liposuction of the high hip and buttock area. Results at 5 months, though remarkable, were not completely

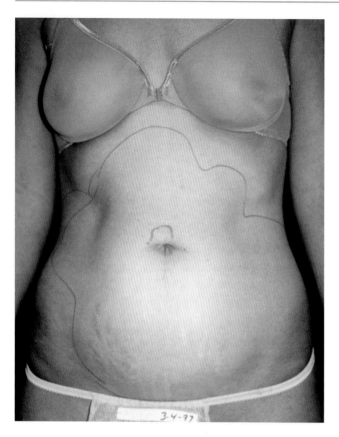
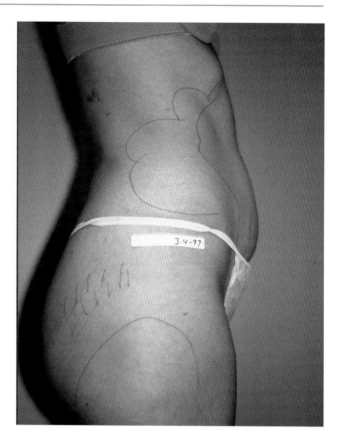

Figures 1-3 & 1-4   *A "limited" abdominoplasty in 1995 included safe liposculpture because shorter incisions, less undermining, and tension-free closure preserved the blood supply to the panniculus.*

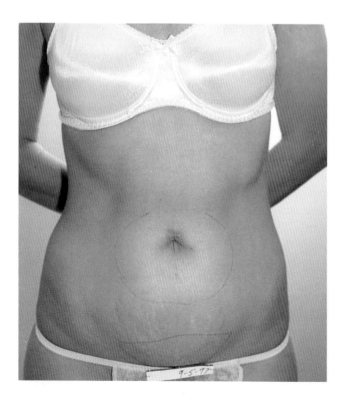
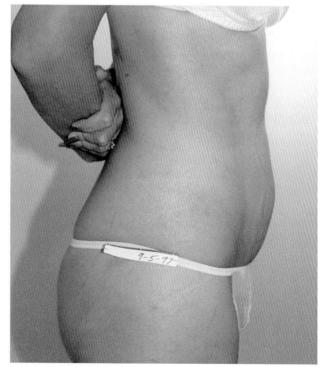

Figures 1-5 & 1-6   *Not unexpectedly, a sedentary lifestyle and weight gain require the revisions outlined, including additional skin removal and liposuction extraction. Note that fat regrafting to the mid-lateral aspect of the buttock has restored contour and has not noticeably increased with weight gain.*

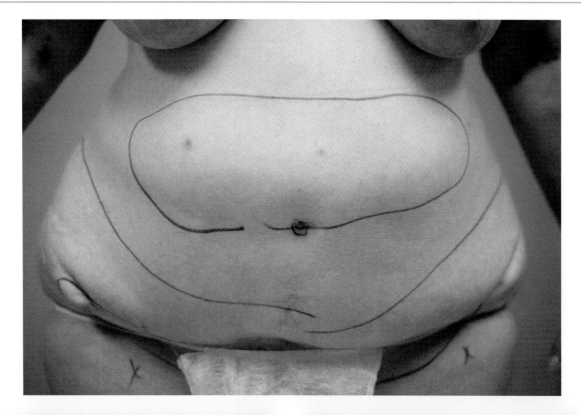

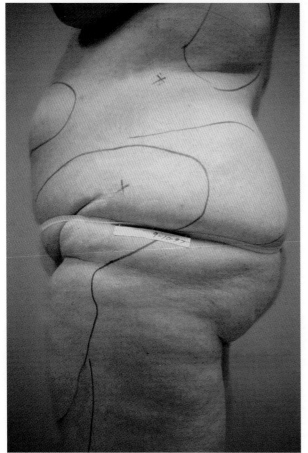
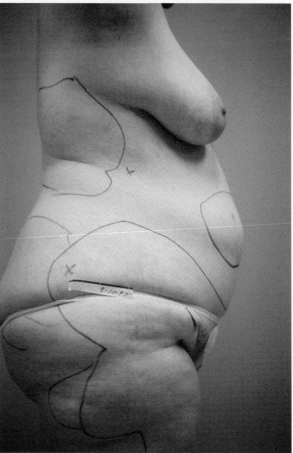

Figures 1-7 – 1-9 *The limitations of large-volume abdominoplasty are shown here in the result obtained by major panniculectomy and standard liposuction.*

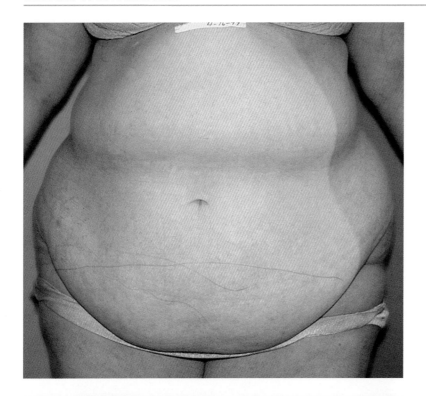

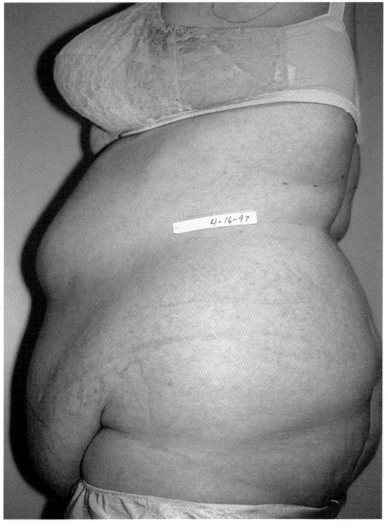

Figures 1-10 & 1-11   *The prudent approach for this category of patient is a two-stage plan: liposuction first, followed by abdominoplasty, or liposuction to a limited degree.*

satisfactory. This patient had been unable to carry out her planned exercise protocol and had gained weight in the interval. XUAL was used as a "test case." Frankly, we were skeptical that any improvement would be obtained without hanging skin folds. To our surprise, contracture of the abdominal skin was an unexpected bonus, and smoothing of the upper part of the back, high hip region, and anterior aspect of the thighs, a previously untreated area, completed a relatively short and uncomplicated procedure (see Figs. 1-12 to 1-14).

MARKING THE PATIENT

The First Interview

A candid evaluation of the areas that would be improved by liposuction and/or liposuction with abdominal repair should be made, and *illustrations from counseling books* and *"take-home" medical literature* should be provided so that the patient will be completely informed. These papers not only review the preoperative requirements for laboratory data and avoidance of hemorrhage-inducing medications but also assess the risks versus benefits of the surgery and the type of anesthesia that is chosen. A *detailed description of recovery is given in writing* before the patient makes the decision to undergo any or all of the procedures that have been suggested.

One valuable technique is to make the drawings as shown in Figures 1-15 to 1-18 with washable ink so that the patient candidate has the opportunity to stand in front of a mirror at home before washing the markings away. The candidate can assess the degree of correction that will be sought, the areas that have been included, and in this case, relocation of the umbilicus, which will be placed as a midline closure above the short-scar abdominoplasty. The posterior views show the prominence of the high hip roll and the minimal fat in the upper portion of the flanks that will be addressed with ultrasound alone. The X's are marked so that the patient is fully aware of any mid-buttock depression and dimpling in the buttocks that will be filled with autologous fat. I often do not mark the opposite side so that the patient can compare the two in the initial evaluation before making decisions.

Day of Surgery

On the day of surgery, the markings are made with surgical marking pens while the patient is standing, before any premedication is given. This period is another opportunity for an interchange of ideas and for questions to be answered, even those answered before but not fully comprehended. For abdominoplasty, the surgical markings include a line down the center of the abdomen, especially if the umbilicus is off center, and into the mons area to aid in realignment. Each side is drawn in detail after full consultation with the patient before preliminary sedation.

Case in point—Marking for fat regrafting
This patient had an unpleasant experience with liposuction across the border from Texas and was left not only with residual fullness in the high hip roll, the buttock, and the banana fold but also with an extremely long abdominal scar and residual laxity in the abdominal wall, which would be a major concern in surgery. When marking this individual, the extent of the mid-buttock depression is noted. Adjacent to this depression on the left and right hips are the entry points used by the other surgeon, which may have contributed to the natural depression by over-resection (see Figs. 1-19 and 1-20). It is virtually impossible to reach the buttock fold from this approach.

In marking the patient for fat regrafting, a new entry point is chosen anterior and 2 cm below this entry so that cross-suctioning from within the abdominoplasty and from this point can remove fat from the upper hip roll. The fat never leaves the patient's body. The syringe that performs the aspiration is then turned and used as a blunt dissector for the multilevel tunneling. Fat grafts are deposited during withdrawal. After completing the upper hip roll, the same procedure is repeated for the upper portion of the thigh, and a separate entry point is then made posteriorly to directly attack the redundancy in the "banana roll" area. When adequate fat has been obtained from syringe suction, my preference is to use the flat-bladed liposuction cannula. From the posterior entry point, this cannula is used first with the aspiration point down and then with the aspiration point up. For patients with postsurgical fibrosis, freeing the subdermal area in the buttock fold is an advantage gained by using a flat rather than a round aspiration cannula.

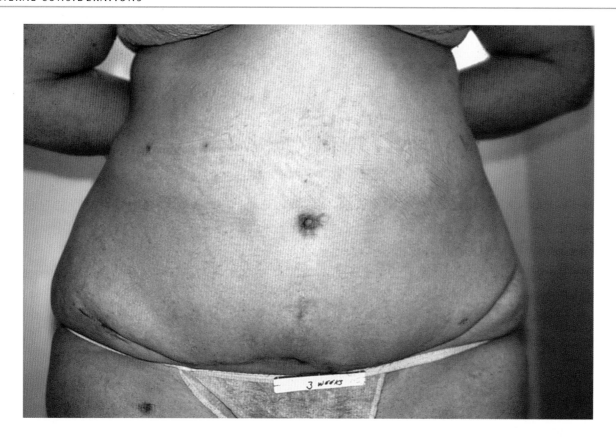

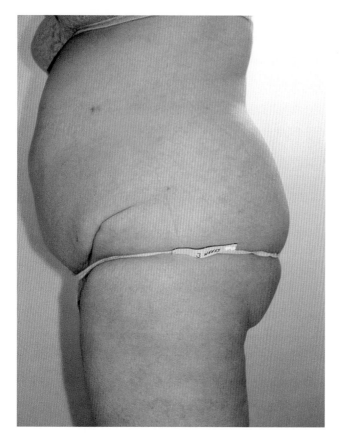
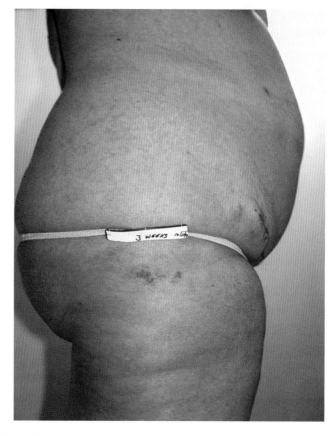

Figures 1-12 – 1-14   *This patient was the first in whom we used XUAL without skin excision, except for the lateral "dog-ears." This result indicates a greater degree of contracture with XUAL.*

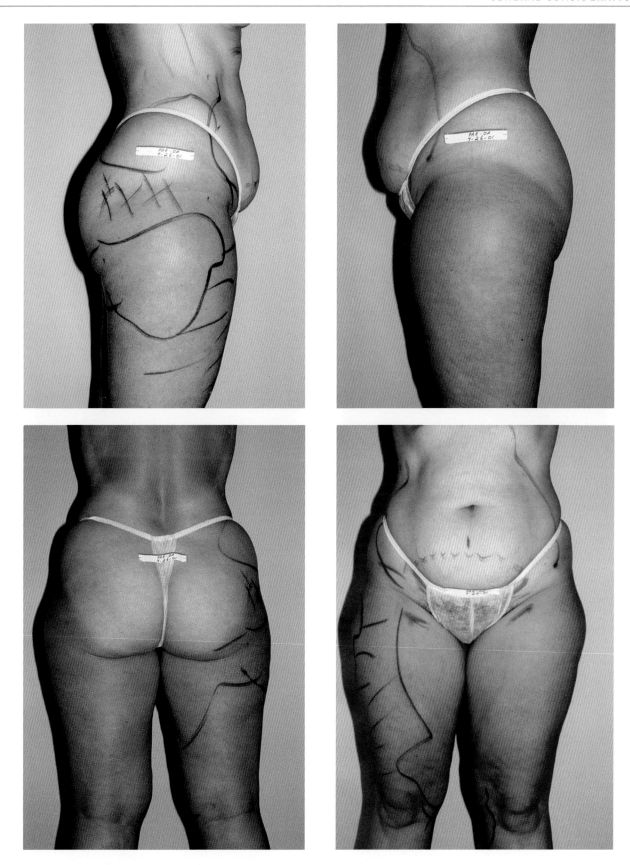

Figures 1-15 – 1-18 *Planning the procedure includes drawing on the patient's body at the first consultation with washable ink. Areas for fat removal (circles), fat regrafting (XX), and transitional area ultrasound without fat removal (vertical lines) and the extent of skin removal by abdominoplasty are a part of the photographic record.*

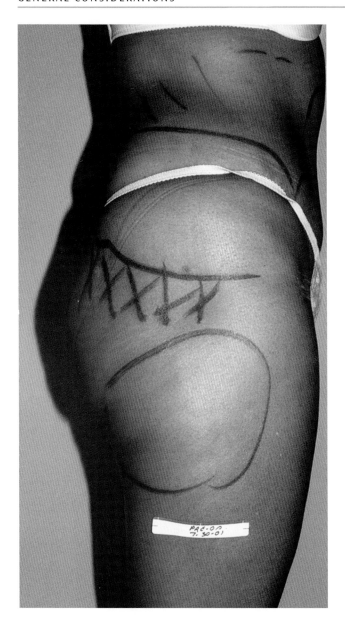
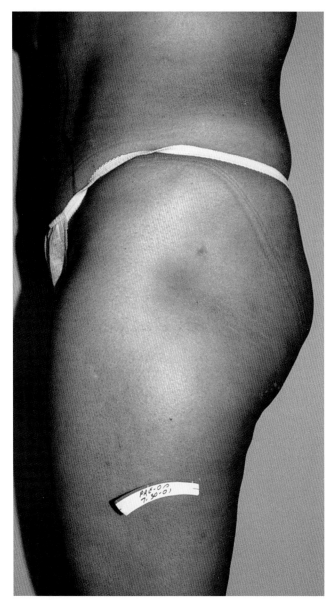

Figures 1-19 & 1-20   *Many women are not aware of slow atrophy in their mid-buttock region. Circles show her that a more favorable outcome includes liposculpture of these areas and raising the level of the area between them by multilevel fat grafting.*

ANESTHESIA

Anesthesia and Fluids

When using the tumescent technique (3:1), issues regarding fluid balance and anesthesia toxicity must be considered more than with the "super wet" technique (1:1). Office anesthesia coverage has presented new challenges for anesthesiologists. Acknowledging that the "tumescent" technique has altered the practice of lipoplasty, anesthesiologists find that the quality of intraoperative analgesia is inadequate. Patients in pain are at greater risk. Anesthesiologists who work with plastic surgeons prefer general anesthesia, sedation, or continuous epidural anesthesia for many outpatient procedures, particularly lipoplasty and especially when multiple position changes may be involved.[7] In combination with the very dilute local anesthetics used in the "super wet" solutions, fentanyl is preferred for postoperative analgesia.

Hypertension and Tachycardia as a Result of Pain

The relationship between conscious sedation and hypertension must be addressed when treating pain patients because hypertension increases the likelihood of hematomas and other complications. Standard premedications without sedation do little to avert this problem. Morphine as a premedication has the disadvantage of respiratory depression, as do other narcotics with the exception of nalbuphine (Nubain), which is our preference for intravenous analgesia and sedation. Diazepam (Valium) and midazolam (Versed), oral or intravenous, are safe premedications. In the past several years, attention has been turned to clonidine, which affects not only pain but also anxiety. Comparative studies show that the goal of decreasing anxiety, relieving the pain of local anesthesia, and stabilizing hemodynamics with premedication is best achieved with clonidine in comparison to all other commonly used premedications. Although the analysis concerned facial surgery, it was certainly referable to local anesthetics in liposuction. Clonidine produces sedation and reduces anxiety, improves hemodynamics, and decreases the need for additional sedation. It is also thought to lessen the incidence of myocardial ischemia. A reduction in postoperative nausea and improved analgesia make this choice of premedication attractive in many surgical specialties. Side effects, including bradycardia and hypotension, were reported with clonidine doses larger than 300 mg, but clinical studies report no significant decreases in heart rate. Because the peak of clonidine's effect generally occurs 60 to 120 minutes after oral administration, surgeons are advised to administer the drug 2 hours before the procedure.

Patients in whom liposuction is performed after prolonged needle injection of local anesthetics alone are at significant risk. This is quite the opposite of certain media campaigns by individuals promoting a narrow viewpoint.

On a personal note, it is important to establish whether a patient has been given clonidine for Tourette's syndrome. If the medication is continued, there is a benefit. If a patient has voluntarily discontinued the clonidine, a rebound phenomenon of hypertension will occur. Such was the case in one patient when the emergence of Tourette's syndrome sparked hyperactivity, hypertension, and violent behavior, which occurred 7 hours after an uneventful sedation/local anesthesia procedure.

Spinal Anesthesia in Liposuctioning—Dr. David Foerster (Plastic Surgeon, Oklahoma City)

Because I do not use the tumescent or "super wet" technique when I perform liposuction, I induce anesthesia for patient comfort. (I rely only on a wet technique in which I infiltrate 150 to 200 cc anteriorly and 150 to 200 cc posteriorly of a solution of 0.125% lidocaine with 1:800,000 epinephrine into the areas in which I am going to be performing liposuction.) The best way that I have found to do this is to use high spinal anesthesia. I have my own operating room and use an anesthesiologist from a nearby hospital to perform a block up to the rib cage anteriorly and up to the mid-back area posteriorly. Sometimes when we have to go a little higher than the mid-back area, such as the posterior axillary or subscapular region, we will supplement the spinal with a small amount of propofol (Diprivan) intravenously, and a small amount of local anesthetic will then be sufficient to allow us to treat such an area, which is usually a small part of the overall procedure.

By using the spinal block technique, the entire abdomen, hip rolls, waist, and lower flank region, both posteriorly and laterally, can be treated, as well as anything in the lower extremities. Because these areas constitute about 80% of the areas treated, we have very few problems with this technique when we perform liposuction. Patients have no nausea because this is not general anesthesia, and I sedate with intravenous diazepam during the procedure. We can twist patients flat on their abdomen while doing the back and side areas without worrying about the airway because they are breathing on their own throughout the procedure. I have been performing liposuction since 1983 and have had no emboli, no excessive hemorrhage, no seromas, and no venous thrombosis during this time. It appears to be the safest procedure that we do.

Is General Anesthesia Preferable to Intravenous Sedation?

Emphasizing properly functioning monitoring equipment and skilled personnel, many surgeons have reported positive experiences with general anesthesia. Steven Hoefflin (plastic surgeon, Santa Monica) and his associates report no significant complications with general anesthesia in over 23,000 "office procedures."[8] An aggressive antiembolic postoperative program includes compression units and early ambulation. This program was said to outweigh the disadvantage of a greater degree of embolism (deep vein thrombosis [DVT]) in patients undergoing general anesthesia.

Large surveys from the American Society of Plastic Surgery report that although pulmonary embolism is a rare occurrence with liposuction, a survey of facial surgery patients with DVT showed that 80% were operated on with general anesthesia.[9-11] Other surveys point to quicker recovery and return to work with intravenous sedation and, therefore, a diminished risk

> **CLINICAL PEARL**
>
> In response to a discussion among plastic surgery colleagues regarding the risks of general anesthesia versus local anesthesia, Dr. Ron Katz (anesthesiologist, University of Southern California) stated, "I am not aware of a single death associated with liposuction where anesthesia was the cause. The current mortality from anesthesia in general is 1 in 200,000." Commenting further on the wisdom of using bupivacaine as a local anesthetic, "much of the literature quoted by Dr. Klein regarding bupivacaine was not only misinterpreted but far out of date. Bupivacaine has a remarkable safety record and is the most common local anesthetic used in obstetrics. The articles from the 1970s and the 1980s concerned themselves with overdosage. The concern that bupivacaine toxicity was a danger in resuscitation was correct when the articles were written, but it is wrong today."
>
> It should be noted that one can overdose with lidocaine as well as bupivacaine, thus leading many surgeons to use bupivacaine (Marcaine) as a postsurgical nerve block after one has infiltrated "super wet" solution in other areas for simultaneous procedures.

> **CLINICAL PEARL**
>
> It is foolishness to make a statement that "intravenous fluids are contraindicated in liposuction."[13]

of DVT.[12] A few experienced surgeons perform all their procedures with patients under local anesthesia. Patients must be counseled, however, that the effect of pain from the injections carries a risk. The cardiovascular, psychological, and emotional effects of prolonged pain are well known. Patient safety must be our primary concern.

Nerve Blocks

J.W. Fletcher (plastic surgeon, Providence) is a fan of nerve blocks, particularly for abdominoplasty. The posterior rib blocks are performed with 3 cc of bupivacaine at each intercostal area, and the injection is carried down to the 12th rib. He believes that this technique gives prolonged comfort in recovery and that the issue of causing pneumothorax does not apply with experience. We would add that using the "super wet" pump to fill the subfascial spaces for the rectus as well as the oblique muscles is an added safety factor that is easy to perform during the operation.

> **CLINICAL PEARL**
>
> We are all familiar with heated intravenous solutions, blankets after surgery, and the air system called the "Bair hugger" that keeps the lower part of the body warm during extensive procedures. Joe Hunstad (plastic surgeon, Charlotte) uses the Bair hugger over the head and shoulders if he is performing circumferential reshaping in individuals who have laxity and fat literally from the chest to the knees.

FLUIDS

Dry to Wet

When Dr. Illouz introduced wetting before aspiration, plastic surgeons quickly abandoned the old technique of curettage, which often left seromas and irregularities. With greater volumes of dilute anesthetic solutions containing epinephrine, recovery was more rapid and less bruising occurred. In 1987, dermatologist Jeffrey Klein popularized office-based surgery with a catchy media name of "tumescent liposuction," a term still used today for the large-volume hyperinfusion technique. Most practicing surgeons are converts to wetting solution technology, but with smaller volumes of infusion called "super wet." A dramatic decrease in complications was seen. With the advent of UAL and XUAL, it was soon noted that "tumescent" infusion (3:1 volume of fluid to fat removal) was even less desirable. The large-volume infusion did not allow penetration of XUAL. The "super wet" technique (1:1 or 2:1 infusion) not only allowed penetration of the sound waves to "soften the fat" but also gave an unexpectedly greater degree of safety during superficial liposuction.

Rod Rohrich and Samuel Beran (Houston) modified and standardized the nomenclature of subcutaneous fluid infiltration. They also collected the data available on these techniques.[14] Their article was criticized by certain physicians who, surprisingly, claimed that patient safety would be impaired if general anesthesia was used.

The use of wetting solutions to reduce blood loss, first popularized by Dr. Illouz in 1980, was in contrast to the "dry technique," first reported to American surgeons by Fournier and Otteni. When epinephrine was added to the solution in 1984 by Gregory Hetter (plastic surgeon, Las Vegas), the "wet technique" became increasingly popular. Larger volumes were used, eventually reaching the 1:1 ratio that is called "super wet," which further reduced blood loss to less than 1% of the aspirate. Peter Fodor, Frode Samdal, Alan Matarasso, and I, as well as others, taught this technique in Lipoplasty Society instructional courses beginning in 1986.

It is important to note that the "super wet" technique, which preceded the introduction of "tumescent" procedures by Dr. Jeffrey Klein, differed in that the infiltration was not *massive* or *pressurized* and the lidocaine dosage was *reduced*. Experience soon showed that the liposuction and blood loss results were identical. "Super wet" gave the hemostatic benefits, but avoided the complications of volume and lidocaine toxicity associated with the "tumescent" technique.

Injection Formulas

Luiz Toledo (plastic surgeon, São Paulo) has changed his injection formula since 1998 by adjusting the quantity of sodium bicarbonate and substituting lactated Ringer's solution to avoid sodium overdosage. The current formula is 500 cc of lactated Ringer's solution with 20 cc of 2% lidocaine, 1 cc of 1:1000 epinephrine, and 10 cc of 3% sodium bicarbonate.

All the current formulas round out to nearly identical numbers that are similar to Toledo's: 0.076% lidocaine

with 1:526,000 epinephrine. The original hypotonic saline solutions described by Fournier have been replaced by variations of balanced-combination formulations. For example, 1000 cc of lactated Ringer's solution with 50 cc of 1% lidocaine and 1 cc of epinephrine, with or without 5 cc of an 8.4% sodium bicarbonate solution, is also effective in producing local anesthesia and prolonged postoperative analgesia.

With this formula, patients receive lidocaine doses that are well in excess of the old *Physician's Desk Reference* manufacturer's recommended maximum dose of 7 mg/kg. After considerable debate, the recommended lidocaine dosage of 35 mg/kg of body weight is now considered the safe upper limit.

For a complete analysis of safety issues related to wetting solutions, the editorial by Dr. Peter Bela Fodor (plastic surgeon, Los Angeles) in *Aesthetic Plastic Surgery* is a classic.[15] Dr. Fodor also references the Lipoplasty Society of North America teaching symposium in which more than 40 "basic courses" were given over a 10-year span and a 1:1 ratio of wetting solution to aspirate, termed "super wet," was advocated.[15]

Fodor writes, "For small volume removals and touch up procedures wetting solution can perform very adequately as an anesthetic delivery system for Xylocaine. In large volume removals, however, because of the massive amounts of fluid injected, even low concentrations of Xylocaine can result in a large total dose of anesthetic. Thus, total Xylocaine doses up to 70 milligrams per kilogram have been administered to patients who did not even have an intravenous line in place."[15] A further danger was the practice of discharging these patients from the clinic shortly after termination of the procedure and even allowing them to drive in spite of the fact that "Xylocaine is known to reach peak systemic absorption 10-14 hours after subcutaneous infiltration."[15] Reports from emergency rooms in California of patients with pulmonary edema and life-threatening overdoses of lidocaine soon became known. The consequences of ambulatory discharge, including hypovolemia, oliguria, fat embolism syndromes, and even pulmonary embolism and myocardial infarction as a result of unpredictable fluid shifts, indicate that there is no substitute for close patient monitoring with laboratory evaluation. As stated by Fodor, "The benefits of diminished blood loss and decreased ecchymosis that allow large volume removals are obtained with a more conservative amount of fluids. In other words, adapting the "super wet" technique is an approach that avoids the potential danger of fluid and Xylocaine overload and appears to be the most rational and prudent choice."[15]

Before this editorial there was confusion between the terminology, and even today the word "tumescent" is liberally applied to procedures in which lesser and safer volumes of fluids are administered.

For those brave enough to tackle large liposuction patients, Dr. Hunstad advises modifying the solution to 12.5 cc of lidocaine per liter of lactated Ringer's solution; he depends on general anesthesia for patient comfort during the procedure.

CLINICAL PEARL

Preparing the "Super Wet" Infusate

If one is treating a smaller area on an average-sized person, the simplest formula for preparing the infusate is to use 50 cc of 1% lidocaine with epinephrine per liter of infusate. Generally, this means that one chooses patients who require only 1 to 3 L. For larger patients, the "standard" preparation advocated by Dr. Hunstad is 25 cc of 1% lidocaine per liter, and the epinephrine may be added separately or included with the lidocaine mixture.

INSTRUMENTS

Curved Cannulas

To minimize the number of small openings made for liposuction, curved cannulas such as those in Figure 1-21 are used. The smaller, open-tipped cannula on the right is useful in thicker areas and for undermining directly beneath the "hip and banana" shown on the left-hand side of the illustration. The banana fold area is approached directly from the incision marked with an X at the edge of the buttock fold. Through this same

incision the longer curved cannula can be extended to the inner aspect of the thigh to the groin area to the knee. With increasing experience in liposuction, the use of 3-, 4-, and 5-mm cannulas and a variety of liposuction machines or the "syringe suction" method produces more uniform results with fewer possibilities of rippling or irregularities.

HOW I DO IT

Dr. Melvin Schiffman (Cosmetic Surgeon, Tustin)

- Liposuction of the abdomen is performed under local tumescent anesthesia or general anesthesia or under intravenous sedation with tumescence. The solution consists of 1000 cc of lactated Ringer's solution with 500 mg lidocaine, 1 mg epinephrine, and 12.5 mg sodium bicarbonate with local anesthesia or with 250 mg lidocaine without sodium bicarbonate when using general anesthesia or intravenous sedation.
- The expected amount of removal is a 1:1 ratio of injected solution to total fat and fluid removed.
- Fluid is injected with a 1.5-mm multihole cannula and removal is accomplished with 2.5- to 4-mm cannulas 29 cm in length with a release hole in the thumb groove. The larger cannula is used in deeper tissues.
- The amount of fluid removed is measured on each side and should be equal unless the patient has a preoperative discrepancy in fat mass on each side.
- Tunnels are fashioned without suction, and the suction machine is used at a vacuum of −300 mm to prevent bleeding.
- Each tunnel is suctioned back and forth four to seven times, starting from the lateral side of the abdomen to the midline in a fan shape, first in the deep layers and then in the superficial layers, followed by refining the residual areas with a 2.5-mm cannula.
- Suctioning in any tunnel is stopped if bleeding is noted in the aspirate.

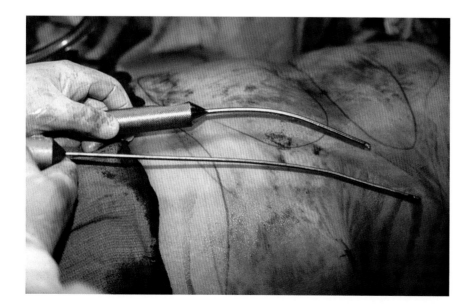

Figure 1-21 *In contrast to UAL cannulas, which are not curved, pre-softening body fat with XUAL allows the surgeon to select curved cannulas to reach difficult areas.*

Dr. Dennis Barek (Plastic Surgeon, New York)

- As liposuction became safe for large-volume removal, the areas being treated are no longer just the saddle-bags or abdomen, but now encompass the entire trunk. In fact, more and more patients are interested in sculpting the entire trunk in a single session. When this is feasible, one of the more difficult areas is the back because of its thick skin, rolls that cascade down to the flank, and iliac deposits. The entire unit is also treated along with the lateral aspect of the thorax and arm.
- Proper evaluation of the tissues is performed to avoid operating on an unfavorable patient. Those with thin, atrophic, ptotic tissues are, of course, poor candidates but are frequently satisfied with fat removal without concern about loose skin.
- Contour lines are drawn around the fat to be extracted. The patient is photographed and then administered general anesthesia in the decubitus position with the arm extended over a pad. Such positioning gives complete access to the target area.
- "Super wet" infiltration is performed through convenient stab wounds—usually three around the scapular area, two in each of the flank and hip roll areas, and one at the posterior axillary fold for the arm.
- For the flank and iliac area, I also try to remove as much fat as possible consistent with the type of skin, but preserve some fat in the area immediately below the dermis. Here, the standard "Mercedes" type of 4-mm cannula is used. In stubborn cases, I would use a "Tiger" tip cannula up to 5 mm in diameter.
- The fibrous bands separating the rolls are *aggressively lysed* with the Gram cannula.
- The arm is approached with a single 3- or 4-mm "Mercedes" type of cannula. The fat is removed in a more conservative fashion, mostly involving the dependent portion of the arm.
- The small stab wounds are left open. Compressive garments are worn for comfort for a week or two but are not necessary unless the skin is pendulous.

Case in Point—Liposuction with Etching

This man is typical of the mid-30s athlete who cannot reduce his abdominal panniculus. Formerly, he would have been considered for a limited abdominoplasty, but with determination, many of these individuals can restrengthen their abdominal musculature with exercise and dieting. Difficult areas in males include the "love handle" area extending from the rib cage to the pelvis, as in this patient (see Figs. 1-22 to 1-25). Surgeons should choose some modality to attack this area, either UAL, XUAL, or PAL. In this patient, XUAL was used, which made liposuctioning through a single entry point relatively easy and removal of the "love handle" fat no more difficult than fat from the abdominal panniculus. The 3-week postoperative photographs show that contracture of the overlying skin has already occurred to a significant degree (see Figs. 1-26 to 1-29). Also notice that "skin preparation" of entry points in the upper part of the abdomen, the groin, and the periumbilical area is accomplished with limited shaving rather than "a full-body prep," which is distasteful to most men.

Case in Point—Liposuction with Abdominoplasty

In 1983, liposuction with abdominoplasty was considered to be too risky a procedure, but results such as these were an inducement to use liposuction in a tension-free procedure (see Fig. 1-30). Note that the lateral aspect of the flanks has not been reduced and that the incision line is a straight one. The mons has not been elevated or fixed, nor has it been defatted, and there is no sculpturing of the midline, which we routinely perform with liposuction.

Revision of this patient would involve complete liposuction of the abdomen and flanks with XUAL to promote skin shrinkage, elevation of the lateral limbs of the incision to a "French line" position, and reduction of the mons.

Case in Point—Liposuction without Muscle Repair

Certain patients who have laxity of the abdominal wall will request the improvement afforded by liposuction with the intent of strengthening the abdominal muscles with exercise. Such a patient is pictured in Figures 1-31 to 1-33; this patient participated in the earliest trials of XUAL. Even at 2 weeks postoperatively, we noted skin shrinkage and rapid resolution of post-liposuction edema. At 2 weeks the bruising had completely disappeared, which would have been unusual with standard liposuction (see Fig. 1-34 to 1-36).

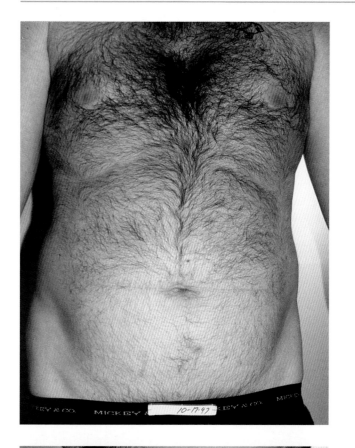
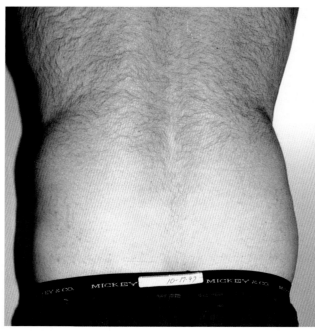
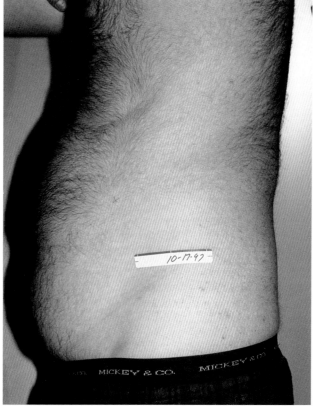
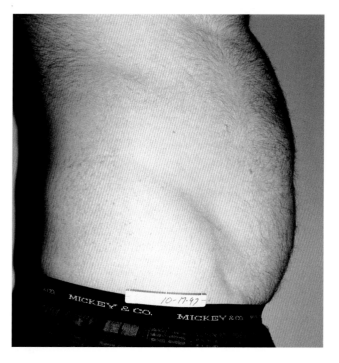

Figures 1-22 – 1-25 *Typical fat deposit area in an active male, one of the first volunteers for XUAL.*

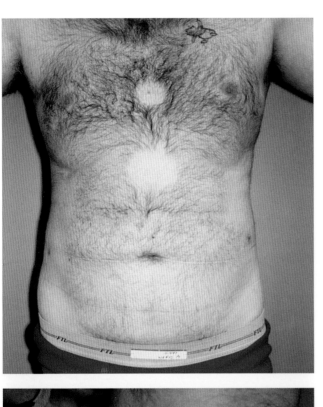
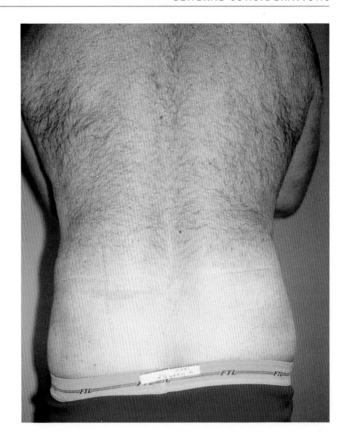
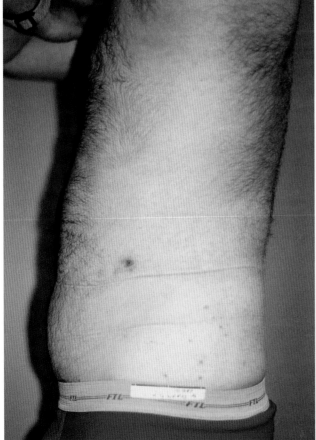
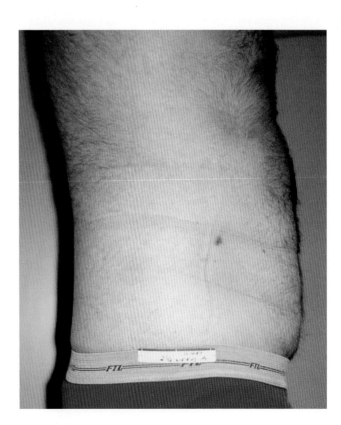

Figures 1-26 – 1-29   *A more rapid, less bruised recovery is evident 3 weeks after "etching" and superficial and deep XUAL.*

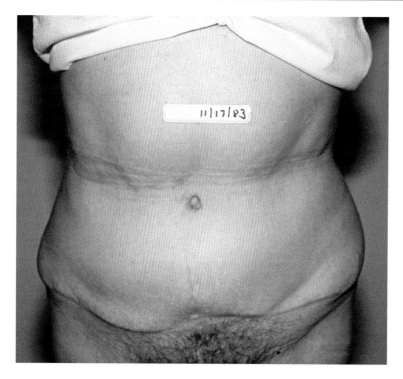

Figure 1-30 *Such irregularities were common after the extended abdominoplasty performed in 1983, before the use of liposculpture. Designing the incision as a "smile" or "French line," fixation of the mons, and other improvements are used today.*

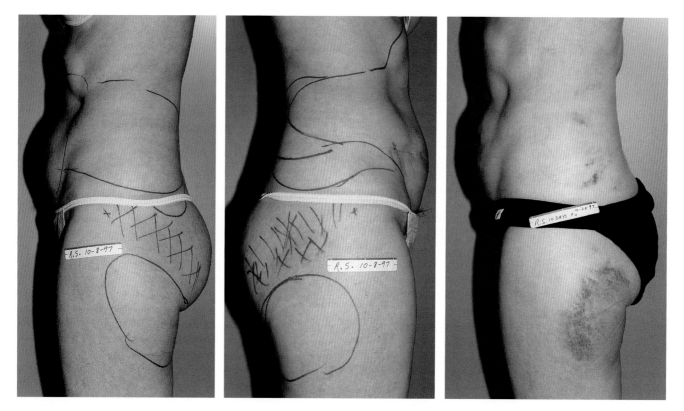

Figures 1-31 – 1-33 *Certain patients with laxity of the abdominal wall will request the improvement afforded by liposuction with the intent of strengthening the abdominal wall with exercise. This patient participated in the earliest trials of XUAL.*

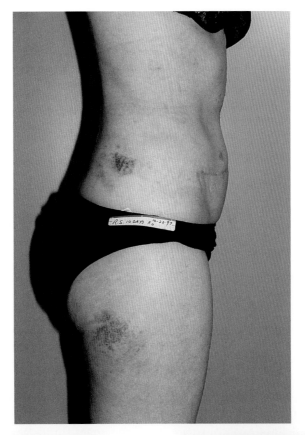

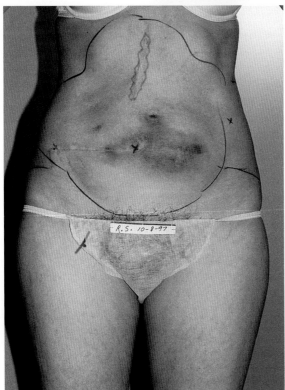

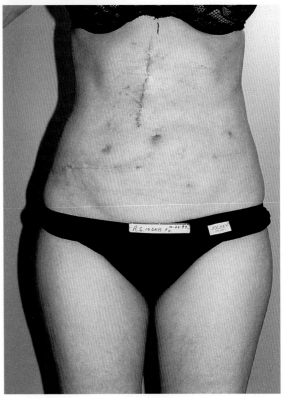

Figures 1-34 – 1-36 *Even 2 weeks postoperatively, we noted skin shrinkage and rapid resolution of post-liposuction edema. At 2 weeks, the bruising completely disappeared, which would have been unusual with standard liposuction.*

STAYING OUT OF TROUBLE

Safety Issues

In an article for *Plastic and Reconstructive Surgery* in April 2001, Drs. Rudolph de Jong (anesthesiologist) and Frederick M. Grazer (plastic surgeon) reviewed pertinent safety issues related to liposuction. Noting that extensive subsurface trauma is created and that "liposuction is by no means minor surgery," they addressed the third-space void created by removing fat that traps fluids.[13] This problem is offset to some extent by the 50% to 70% of the wetting solution that is absorbed. Therefore, "fluid replacement is more art than science."[13] This leads to the conclusion that although fluid dislocations have generally proved benign when less than 4 or 5 L of wetted fat tissue is aspirated, hypervolemic shock at one extreme and hemodilution progressing to pulmonary edema at the other extreme *are expected* complications of overdone "tumescent" infiltration. "Although lidocaine mega-dosing has been heralded as 'safe,' that inference is based solely on limited, serial blood level measurements."[13] We still do not have definitive appraisal of the cardiovascular response or the pharmacodynamics of lidocaine metabolism,[13] but guidelines established in 1985-1986 are definitive and safe.[16]

On a practical point, Drs. De Jong and Grazer noted that an obese patient has a substantial respiratory risk, especially with deep sedation, thus further emphasizing the need for patient monitoring by trained attendant personnel. They stated, "In short, intraoperative intravenous fluid replacement is a demanding balancing act in which overhydration is as undesirable as is underhydration. Tumescent anesthesia proponents, on one hand, claim that intraoperative absorption of wetting solutions all together negates the need for maintenance fluids. High volume liposuction, to the contrary, demands supplemental fluids, which are probably best titrated by periodic measurement of bladder catheter urine output," a reference to the "extensive subdermal burnlike cavity left by suction extraction."[13]

To compound the problem, one cannot measure the hematocrit for at least 48 hours after infusions.

CLINICAL PEARL

Dr. James Grotting (plastic surgeon, Alabama) simplifies his safety rules for beginning surgeons:
- Use less fluid infusion.
- Use lower suction pressures.
- Use lower UAL power.
- Use small probes and small cannulas.

According to Dr. Arthur Perry (plastic surgeon, New Brunswick), "adequate perioperative fluid management and *atraumatic* liposuction, with a minimum of banging into underlying muscle and deeper structures, are easily within the surgeon's control"[17] and are of maximum importance in the prevention of DVT. One might add early ambulation and intermittently released abdominal pressure garments.

CLINICAL PEARL

In December 1986, I noted anecdotal reports of liposuction casualties in which surgeons penetrated ventral hernias and destroyed internal organs, as well as facilitated an increase in midline abdominal sloughing from vigorous lateral suctioning.

Case in Point—Limited Upper Thigh–Lift

If at first you don't succeed—Diet and exercise

A successful businesswoman in her early forties decided that diet and exercise alone were not creating the figure that she desired (see Figs. 1-37 to 1-39). A wide-scar abdominoplasty was required with XUAL in late 1997. Surprisingly, shrinkage of her legs and back and healing of the abdominoplasty without complications were achieved quickly despite the wide scar (see Figs. 1-40 to 1-42). Her arms were treated as well, and in her face, submental repair with the application of XUAL to the cheeks was effective (see Figs. 1-43 and 1-44).

In the recovery stage, diet and exercise began to produce improvement in all areas but, as an unwanted effect, left her with loose skin in the abdomen and upper part of the thighs (see Figs. 1-45 to 1-47). Contouring of the face remained unaffected, and the 48-lb weight loss caused further recession in the arms and upper part of the body.

Subsequent photographs from July 2001 show redundancy of skin and soft tissue with very little fat in these areas (see Figs. 1-48 to 1-50). A "limited" upper thigh–lift was performed.

- An incision was made just lateral to the mons to the beginning of the buttock fold. This incision allowed for undermining and fascial fixation after the removal of 6 cm of thigh skin.
- The entire abdomen and inner aspect of the thighs were infiltrated with a "super wet" solution.
- After 10 minutes of ultrasound to the upper part of the abdomen and 10 minutes to the inner aspect of the thighs externally, liposuction was performed. As expected, little fat was obtained.

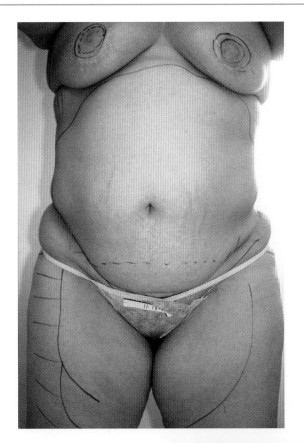
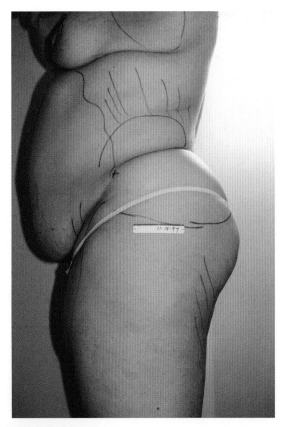
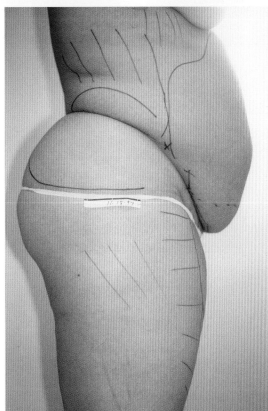

Figures 1-37 – 1-39   *The challenge of a large-framed patient with a large panniculus is in designing a staged approach. A complete diastasis repair with "floating" of the umbilicus and wide XUAL is shown for the first stage.*

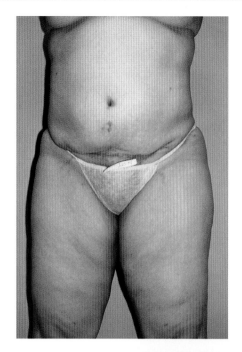
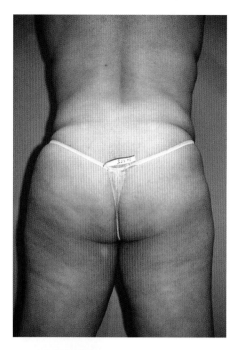
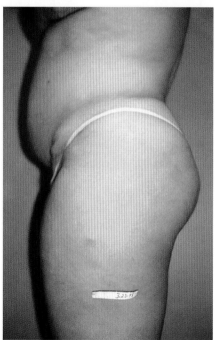

Figures 1-40 – 1-42 *A degree of skin shrinkage is apparent after the first stage and after the diet and exercise program facilitated by the restoration. The second stage will also include XUAL.*

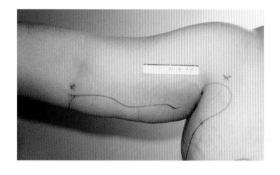
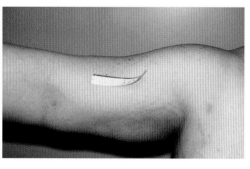

Figures 1-43 & 1-44 *Arm reduction in heavy individuals is often a two-stage fat extraction, with skin contraction by ultrasound performed during and after the procedure.*

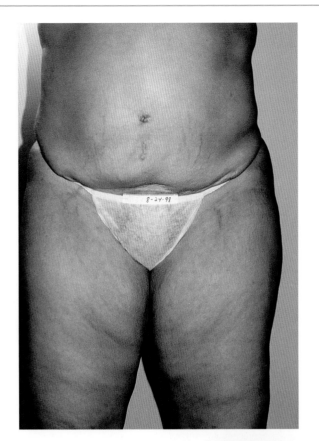
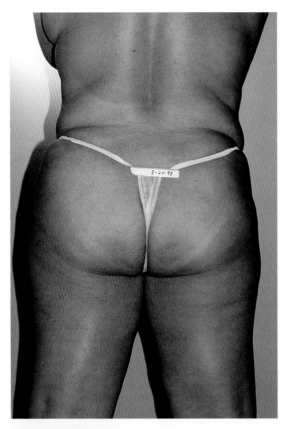
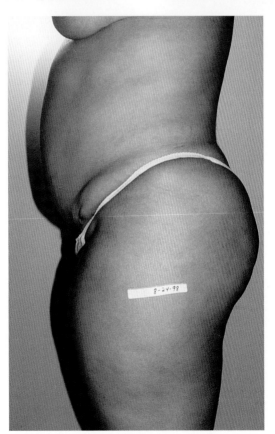

Figures 1-45 – 1-47   Results of the staged procedures with repositioning of the umbilicus and secondary abdominal wall plication plus the added skin tightening by XUAL.

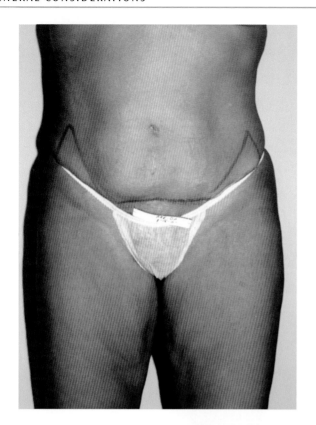
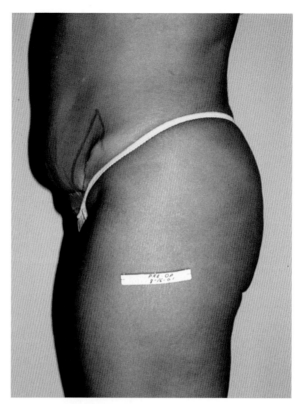
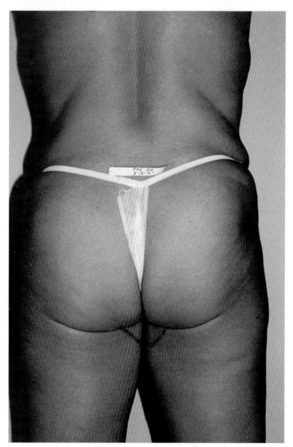

Figures 1-48 – 1-50 *Final refinements in spot areas produced this acceptable body recontouring without the necessity of extended incisions into the back ("belt lipectomy") and the added risk and scarring.*

- The entire area was then elevated in the abdomen so that the umbilicus could be reset with a full-pressure stretch of the soft tissues.
- The ends of the incision were moved upward into a favorable position, the original umbilicus was closed as a midline slit, and approximately 6 cm of excess skin was trimmed when tailoring the flap.
- A technical point of importance is fixation of the flap to the fascia and fixation of the lateral edges of the mons so that exercise does not open the vagina with air trapping after thigh-lift.
- Once these sutures are placed with heavy absorbable material, the deep de-epithelialized edge of the thigh flap is anchored into the deep fascia with non-absorbable sutures and tailored.
- Subcuticular closure completes the modified thigh-lift.

CLINICAL PEARL

In the 1983 December issue of Technical Forum, Dr. Darryl Hodgkinson noted that although the initial lip service was to use liposuction only for small isolated deposits in young females, the early teaching courses involved only older and fatter patients.[18] The 1983 warning was issued because of poor results, dissatisfied patients, and dissatisfied surgeons, who also argued that obese patients rarely lost weight after body-contouring surgery.[18]

Such has certainly not proved to be the case with educated millennium patients. Most patients in private practice have already pursued exercise and diet regimens, only to become discouraged with the resistance of "alpha fat." Once this fat is removed by liposuction, exercise becomes easier. Can you imagine running a 100-yard dash with fat thighs rubbing against each other? Continued weight loss and improvement in general health are the norm rather than the exception.

In the same 1983 Technical Forum issue, Dr. Simeon Wall (plastic surgeon, Shreveport) warned neophyte liposuction artists to "get in shape because it's a lot of work!"[19] In an initial series he was bold enough to use liposuction on patients older than 40 years, but only those with good skin elasticity.

Today we know that less than ideal patients can achieve acceptable improvement in contour, as well as lifestyle, by reducing fatty bulk. These are the patients who must be told the following in advance: "You will look better in clothes, but there will be irregularities when you stand in front of a mirror without clothing." Nevertheless, these patients are the most appreciative of the reduction in bulk and are the most eager to enjoy their lives with full participation in outdoor activity.

Staying out of Trouble in Abdominoplasty

The following words of wisdom are courtesy of Dr. Alan Matarasso (New York):

1. Consider the vascular supply (and do not destroy vascular inflow).
2. Limit the number of liposuction sites beyond the inframammary crease.
3. Limit the extent of liposuction in this area to avoid damage to the axial blood supply.
4. Maintain flap thickness by not suctioning between the skin and Scarpa's fascia.
5. Limit suction lipectomy on skin that will be undermined.
6. Avoid a T-closure.
7. Do not crisscross liposuction sites (especially laterally).
8. Screen patients according to their risk factors.
9. Incorporate seroma precautions.

PREVENTABLE PROBLEMS—DR. MELVIN SCHIFFMAN (COSMETIC SURGEON, TUSTIN)

Scar Indentation

Indentation of the scar occurs as a result of removal of excessive fat around the incision area. This problem is best corrected by incising attachments below the scar and injecting autologous fat. The indentation can be prevented by turning off the vacuum when removing the cannula or using the cannula with a hole in the thumb depression, which allows quick and easy release of the vacuum.

Excessive Bleeding

Excessive bleeding after liposuction may have multiple etiologies, but it is usually preventable. Bleeding must first be diagnosed and may not appear in the wound drainage or be recognized at the time of surgery. A patient with syncope or feeling faint or dizzy after surgery should have blood drawn for determination of hemoglobin and/or hematocrit.* All dressings are removed and new dressings placed over all areas of liposuction with sufficient compression (usually requires tape [I use stretch tape] and/or elastic bandages). All dressings are changed daily until the bleeding has stopped.

Editor's Note: Dilutional factors that artificially lower the reported levels must be taken into account, especially in the case of arm or thigh liposuction and in the first 24 hours. Compression devices produce elbow and foot edema, which also further dilutes the blood sample and gives erroneous hemoglobin and hematocrit values.

Bleeding can be prevented by preoperative and postoperative avoidance of aspirin, herbs, and non-steroidal anti-inflammatory drugs. In addition, reducing the vacuum on the machine or venting the aspirating syringe by keeping 1 to 2 cc of air or saline solution in the syringe can help prevent bleeding. All patients with a history of bleeding or easy bruising or a family history of bleeding problems should be evaluated with appropriate laboratory studies. Sufficient epinephrine, 1 mg/1000 cc, should be used in the fluid to produce

> **CLINICAL PEARL**
> Looking back at his experiences with liposuction after retirement, Matt Gleason (plastic surgeon, San Diego) offers the following words of advice:
> Do not be afraid to take off less fat, especially in the thighs. Symmetry is what counts.
> For small areas of liposuction such as the neck and knees, use a small cannula hooked up in tandem with a specimen collection bottle. Not only can you get an accurate measurement of the fat removed, but it is also ready to use immediately as a fat graft.

> **CLINICAL PEARL**
> Visible "dents" are not always the result of untrained practitioners operating without surgical skill or knowledge. The standard procedure for correction of these preoperative or postoperative deficits is to lower the surrounding abnormal prominent fat by liposuction with small cannulas. The area of the "dents" is then elevated from the underlying fascia by blunt or sharp dissection, and fat grafts are placed in the subcutaneous zone in multiple overlapping crisscrossing tunnels. Deep grafting into the fascia or muscle beneath the deficit is performed as well. Overcorrection is advised, with the realization that if the overcorrection persists beyond 3 weeks, simple crushing massage can lower the profile of the area as much as desired.

> **CLINICAL PEARL**
> Be forewarned: In two cases in the medical literature, patients were given chilled infusates for liposuction, and disseminated intravascular coagulation developed from this iced fluid; the patients died.
> For liposuction in large people, consider warming the infusate to a temperature well above room temperature. The easiest way to do this is to place a temperature tape on the saline bag and place it in a microwave oven.

vascular contraction, and suctioning should not be continued in a tunnel that shows gross blood in the aspirate.

Liposuction without Skin Excision

The effect of liposuction is limited, even with the assistance of UAL and XUAL skin shrinkage. The decision to undergo this procedure, however, is reached with full understanding by patients.

Case in point
As is typical of patients older than 65 years, the patient shown in Figures 1-51 to 1-57 asked only for improvement and did not agree to any form of skin resection except a "limited abdominoplasty." The repair work was limited to the lower part of the abdomen, and XUAL was used over the abdomen, the anterior and interior aspects of the thighs, the knees, the arms, and the hips, with regrafting in the "X-ed" areas of the buttock. She was unable to participate in the postoperative ultrasound and massage regimen because of time and distance constraints. Nevertheless, at 6 weeks, the remarkably rapid shrinkage had occurred in the areas treated, with the usual residual edema just above the small abdominal incision (see Figs. 1-58 to 1-62). Operating within the limitations of liposuction without skin excision is an acceptable choice for patients in this category.

Liposuction Machines

Objections to the early-generation UAL machines included the prolonged operating time and its complications and side effects such as burns and seroma, rippling, and painful recovery, including dysesthesias. To eliminate or reduce these complications, a group of investigators led by Mark Jewell (plastic surgeon) discussed VASER-assisted lipoplasty with UAL. Operative time was reduced and blood loss appeared to be minimal. Pretreating the fat by pulsed continuous

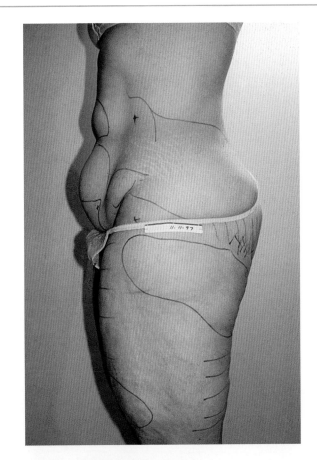

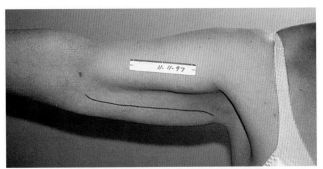

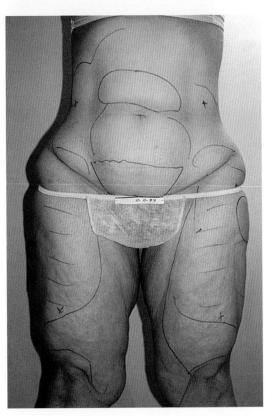

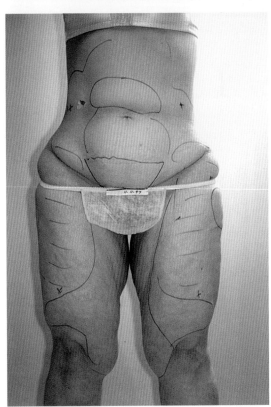

Figures 1-51 – 1-57 *Redefining goals according to the patient's wishes. In this woman older than 65 years, a less than ideal reduction allowed her to regain an active lifestyle. A "limited" abdominoplasty and single-stage partial-volume liposculpture with XUAL are planned.*

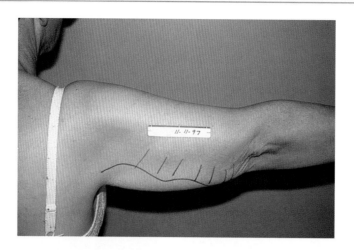

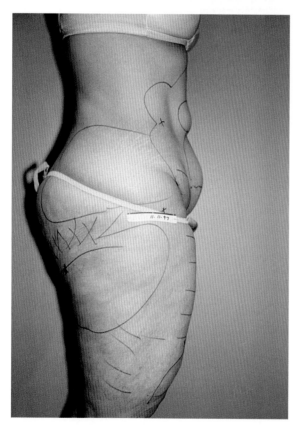

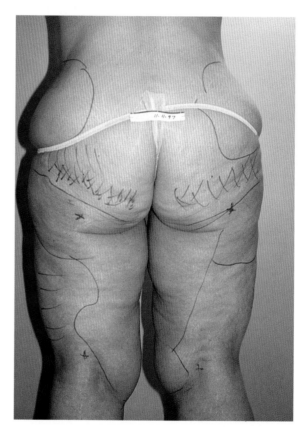

Figures 1-51 – 1-57 Continued

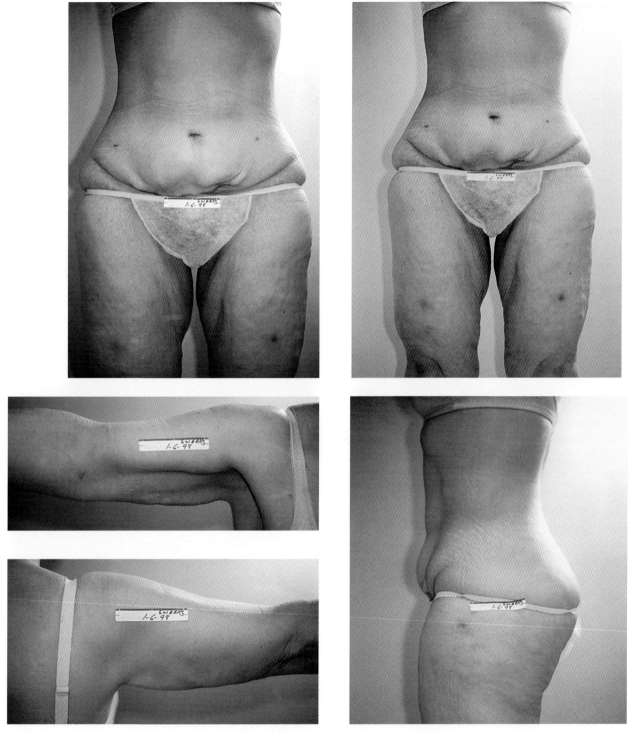

Figures 1-58 – 1-62 *Reducing the bulk of the arms and legs to this degree, plus the health benefits of the realigned abdomen, was a correct choice for quick recovery.*

ultrasound delivered through this new grooved small-diameter probe was both efficient and safe with greater efficiency of fragmentation and reduction of complications. An additional benefit is that the single probe should have a service life of approximately 100 cases according to the manufacturer. These investigators believe that it is worthwhile to consider abandoning suction combinations in hollow UAL designs because of the high power requirements of these devices and their limited aspiration capability. An interesting theory is that the suction attachment within a UAL probe may draw nerves, collagen, fibers, vessels, and lymphatics into the range of the destructive power of the ultrasound.

Reference had been made in the preceding discussion of machine versus syringe techniques of lipo-extraction. Although use of the syringe technique as advocated by Dr. Luiz Toledo has been designated as liposculpture and is described in the numerous teaching courses that I give with Dr. Toledo and Dr. Alan Matarasso, it has evolved into a useful technique for several reasons. The Gram machine, as well as those provided by Byron Medical, are still noisy and somewhat bulky. The power assist devices, which will be discussed, have advantages that outweigh this single disadvantage. With power assist, especially the air-driven devices, movement of the tip of cannula reduces the physical effort on the part of the surgeon. There is also a variable-movement tip, a device similar to power assists, but with more circumferential motion incorporated into the design. "Both are excellent in dense areas," such as the axillary tail of the breast, the upper part of the back, gynecomastia, and areas that have previously been liposuctioned. Combining the use of these devices with preliminary softening of tissues by external ultrasound is considered a safer alternative in many surgeons' view.

The machine liposuction technique often requires cannulas with "finger stops." In certain cases, if one wishes to immediately reduce the suction, the finger stop hole is released to decrease the suction. With the syringe technique, the degree of "pull back" of the syringe determines the degree of suction.

For a smaller degree of liposuction, particularly in office surgery, the syringe technique has the advantage of reduced staff involvement and a major advantage of allowing one to regraft all the aspirated fat. Various sterile traps have been used, but the fat that was removed by the machine technique was often badly damaged. With lesser degrees of suction, fat recovered with the syringe technique can be immediately regrafted (for filling dimples or hip depressions, or it can be concentrated and then regrafted with a pistol-type injection device for smaller contour irregularities such as the face or subcutaneous atrophy spots in which fat must be placed in small tunnels directly beneath the dermis).

The syringe technique requires only a "Toomey" open-ended syringe, which is readily available in most operating rooms, and a variety of metal devices to hold the plunger once the cannula has been inserted. These devices are available for 10-cc syringes as well as the larger Toomey syringes.

In many cases I will choose the machine technique because it is faster and offers continuous suctioning without the necessity of stopping and emptying syringes. We will use the syringe technique to harvest enough fat for regrafting into the face or lips and for direct regrafting underneath the deepest posterior buttock dimples and complete the procedure with the more efficient machine technique.

PROCEDURES

Combining Safe-Area Liposuction with Bichat Pad Removal and Fat Grafting

The patient in Figure 1-63 shows the typical jowl descent that can be treated with liposuction, provided that the skin retraction of youth can be counted on. No "bowing" or bending of her platysma is present. In addition, she requested lip enhancement and a change in her "moon face." Removal of the Bichat pad through an intraoral approach is no longer a difficult or rare procedure.

Under local anesthesia with intravenous sedation, the patient's face was infiltrated. Fat was suctioned with 3-mm cannulas from the jowl line and the submental triangle. Additional fat from the midportion of the abdomen was collected for grafts. This fat was placed in a multilevel fashion for enhancement of her lips, literally doubling their size. The Bichat pad was removed through a spreading maneuver with blunt-tipped scissors at the level of the second upper molar. With gentle compression, the Bichat pad was easily teased out and its base cauterized.

A photograph taken 2 years after these procedures shows the results of an aggressive skin care program with facial bleaching. Sun protection and topical lotions create the facial color that matches her new hair color. Hollowing of the cheek, absence of the jowl pads, the clean jowl line, and the fullness of the lip complete the transformation (see Fig. 1-64).

Obliteration of the Malar Pad with XUAL

The malar pad, the thickened area just lateral to the midline of the orbital rim, is problematic. Attempts to remove this sign of an aging face have included injection with steroids, direct excision, liposuction, and more recently, elevation and fixation. With large prominent pads, the latter procedure, which is usually helpful in face-lift procedures, may be contraindicated.

Before our experience with XUAL, the malar pads were always reduced with 2- and 3-mm cannulas by deep liposuctioning adjacent to the periosteum. This procedure was helpful and less problematic than others, but it often left a residual defect. With the popularity of elevation of the orbital and malar fat pads during blepharoplasty, including the "turned-down" orbital fat procedures (in which orbital fat is brought over the orbital rim or into the tear trough), surgeons have addressed the problem by wide undermining and fixation to the orbital rim or fixation laterally, with or without suspension sutures. Although this procedure is somewhat complex and damage to the infraorbital nerves is a possibility, it is valuable in many cases. Recently, we have used XU to reduce malar pads. The preliminary infusion in the nasolabial fold and on the malar fat pad allows ultrasound to produce excellent resolution of both areas and thereby avoid the extensive undermining that would be required.

The patient in Figures 1-65 to 1-67 is an excellent example of smoothing of the prominent pad without a direct approach. The area was infiltrated during the preliminaries of the face-lift procedure and after elevation and plication of the superficial muscular aponeurotic system (SMAS), internal repair of the anterior platysma was performed along with fat removal and posterior fixation, and tension-free closure was achieved with fixation of the posterior flap, temporal hair positioning, and the intratragal incision shown. The resultant face-lift is an improvement over results considered acceptable in the past. These minor points, possibly including fat grafting in the nasolabial groove, the lips, the subcommissural area, the wrinkling of the chin, and even the submalar area, are the small things that give face-lifting a more natural appearance without the "deer in the headlights" look of overcorrection.

In this patient's postoperative photograph (see Figs. 1-68 to 1-70), it is evident that the prominent fat pad has melted to an acceptable level. The fat pad was not undermined, elevated, or repositioned with sutures.

The addition of external ultrasound with fluid infusion (XU) to the face-lift procedure has improved recovery time. The comfort level, which is attributed to the ultrasonic influence of driving lidocaine and epinephrine into the soft tissues, is an additional benefit. Postoperative XU is used for its original purpose: to increase circulation and decrease tissue edema.

Our current practice is to use ultrasound in the operating room before making the first incision and apply XU from the malar and nasolabial area to the clavicle repeatedly in the postoperative recovery period. Ultrasound will also help individuals in whom localized edema develops, either from the natural gravitation of tissue fluid or from inadvertent tearing of the repair sutures in the platysma.

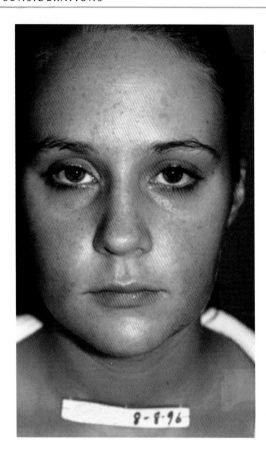
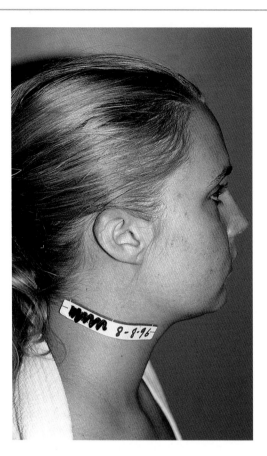

Figure 1-63   *The round cheek is a result of the internal Bichat fat pad. Bichat pads are removed in their entirety with an intraoral incision.*

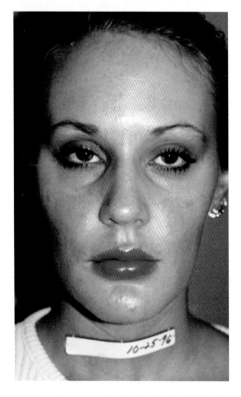
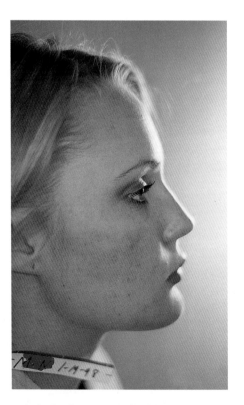

Figure 1-64   *This facial shaping accents the desired malar high points. Fat grafts for her lips were obtained from an abdomen donor site, not the potentially contaminated Bichat fat.*

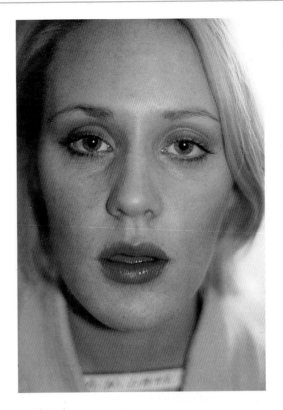

Figure 1-64   *Continued*

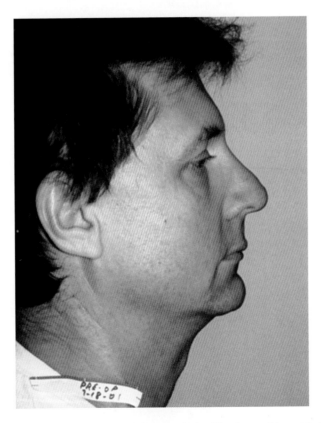

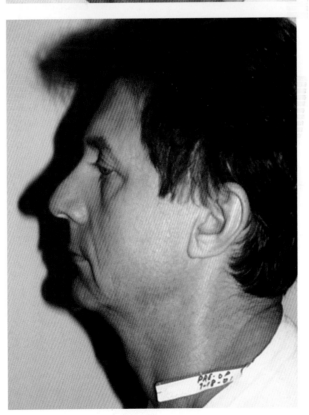

Figures 1-65 – 1-67   *The prominent malar pad has been addressed by liposuction deep under the surface, by steroid injection, and recently by repositioning via sutures during a face-lift. Each method has drawbacks. In male face-lifts, a "normal," not "operated on" result is essential. The face and malar pad were treated with ultrasound.*

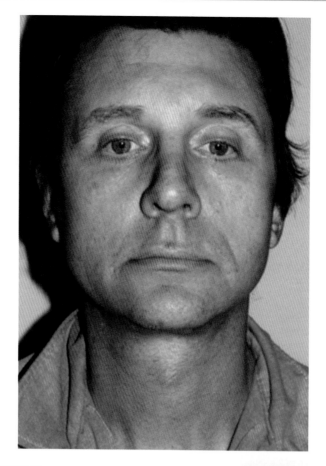

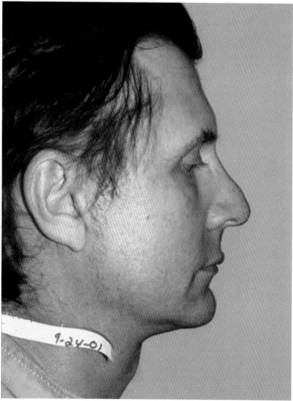

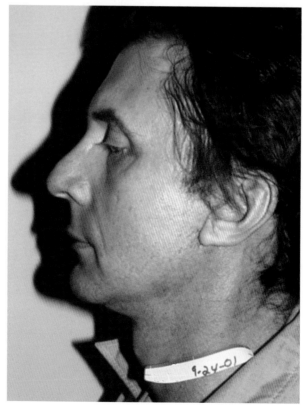

Figures 1-68 – 1-70 *At 2 months, the malar pads are flattened. At 1 year, a noticeable continuation of the ultrasound-induced skin contracture had removed the small skin folds of the cheek and neck.*

Small-Incision Abdominoplasty with Liposuction

Active young women frequently find that the general deposition of abdominal fat over the entire abdomen cannot be reduced without surgical help. The patient in Figure 1-71 is also scheduled to undergo a staged revision of a T-scar breast reduction in which the nipple-areolar complex will be moved to a normal position. Her complaint was that her nipples were above her bra, her T-scar was below her bra, and her abdomen was unattractive.

The corrective procedure involved revision of the breast scars and repositioning of the areolas. The addition of small-incision abdominoplasty with liposuction, a less invasive operation, made the combination of these two corrections safe and acceptable, with rapid recovery.

CLINICAL PEARL

When a simultaneous breast and abdominoplasty procedure is planned, dissection of the subglandular breast pocket can be accomplished through the umbilical liposuction entry point with a powered infusion pump and "super wet" solutions. The subglandular space may also be dissected in a periareolar entry to elevate the subcutaneous tissue from the breast mass in "internal" mastopexy or breast reduction. The use of XUAL and "super wet" infusion, which greatly reduces blood loss, has made simultaneous procedures commonplace and safe.

Postoperative recontouring photographs (see Figs. 1-72 and 1-73) show that the abdominal incision is covered by the equivalent of her thong bathing suit. Creation of the midline "champagne groove" with liposuction and recontouring of the lateral aspect of the abdomen produce desirable shadowing.

Correcting Arm Deformity

In women such as those older than 60 years (see Figs. 1-51 to 1-62), the arm deformity is primarily lax skin with a lesser element of fat deposits. XUAL with its concomitant skin shrinkage offers arm rejuvenation without surgical skin excision. Obviously, the degree of improvement varies from arm to arm in this category of patient. Shrinkage is virtually complete at 8 weeks. Skin excision with the often-unacceptable inner arm scar is no longer required for the overwhelming majority of women seeking arm improvement.

Case in point—A comparison of suction-assisted liposuction and XUAL

Only rarely is it possible to compare the results of two techniques in the same patient, but in this case, the abdominal repair prompted a second opinion and ultimately a secondary surgery. During a gynecologic procedure, abdominoplasty was performed through a "down-curving" unsatisfactory incision. Without regrafting, liposuction was performed on the hips and thighs. The results were less than expected (see Figs. 1-74 to 1-76).

After consultation our plan was three pronged:

1. Redo the incision line to place it in a more favorable spot by extending it upward from the edge of the hairline to repair the abdominal diastasis from the pubic area to just above the umbilicus via the "float" technique.
2. Save all available fat for regrafting into the dimples and depressions of the buttocks.
3. Redo the hip rolls, especially the folds beneath each buttock, with XUAL applied with a flat-bladed syringe cannula.

Little excess fat was available, not nearly enough to fill all the defects. Fat grafting had not been performed during her other surgery, so a significant amount was wasted.

The fat deposits in the upper part of her back were of a minor variety that could not be improved by liposuction. The postoperative contour is an example of the shrinking effect of XU with infiltration and compression, but without fat removal.

At 6 weeks, shrinkage was evident in all areas (see Fig. 1-77), and the abdominal incision showed no evidence of widening in its new position; grooving of the abdomen from aesthetic liposuction was not yet apparent.

At 5 months the results obtained are obvious (see Figs. 1-78 to 1-81): retraction of the buttock folds, a degree of correction of the dimpling and lateral buttock depressions with fat grafting, aesthetic contouring of the abdomen with the diastasis from the secondary repair flattened, and of special interest, complete smoothing of the upper part of the back. These results have persisted unchanged in the ensuing 5 years.

Because this patient is the ideal candidate for comparison, she was asked a series of questions about the two procedures. With XUAL and identical anesthesia she did not have the pain that she experienced with the

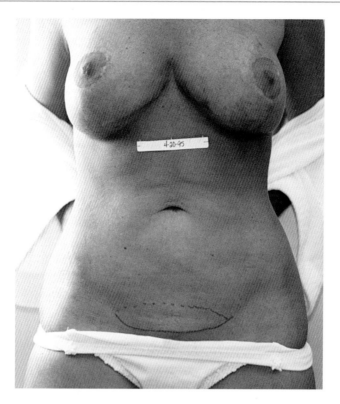

Figure 1-71 By limiting the extent of the skin resection in this abdominoplasty, liposculpture could be used with impunity to create the shadowing, and the operating time, including internal repair of her breast deformity, would not be excessively extended.

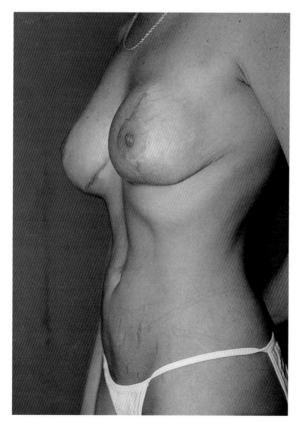 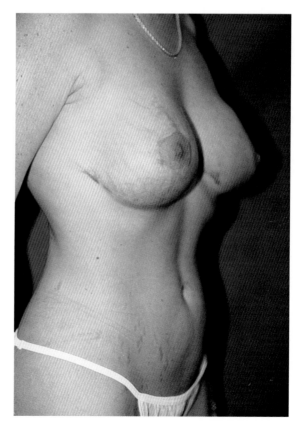

Figures 1-72 & 1-73 Adding this degree of liposculpture produces a favorable contour. Tension-free closure of the abdominoplasty "short-scar" procedure retains skin perfusion.

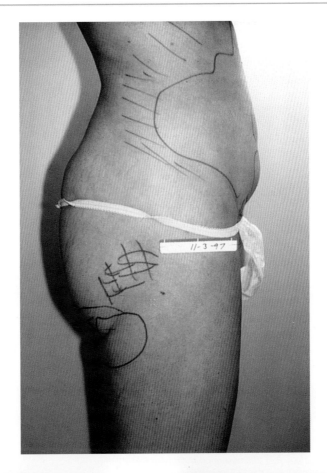

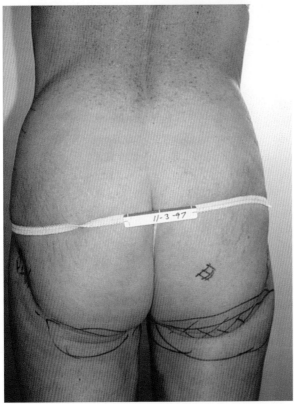

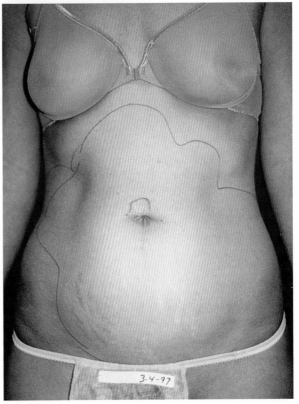

Figures 1-74 – 1-76 *The value of XUAL is illustrated by failure of standard liposuction in the abdomen and hips to achieve contouring. Markings show areas for XUAL regrafts, as well as revision of the abdominoplasty and repositioning of the hypertrophic down-curved mons.*

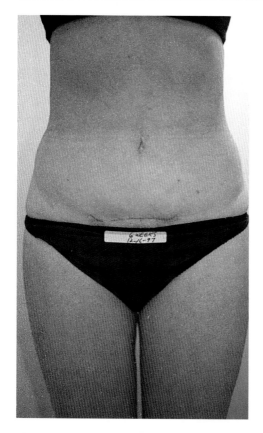

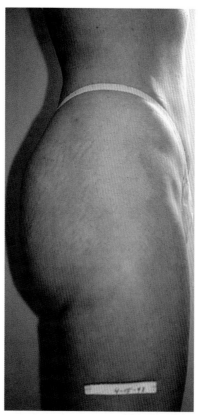

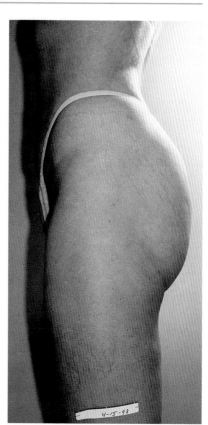

Figure 1-77 *At 1 month postoperatively, abdominal reshaping has progressed rapidly.*

Figures 1-78 & 1-79 *Continued shrinkage of the flanks occurred without fat removal by using infiltration and XUAL only.*

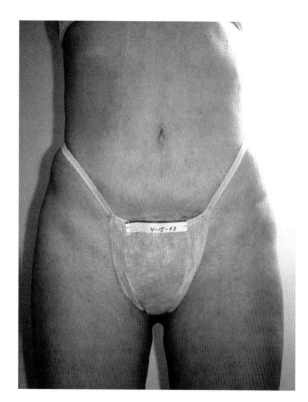

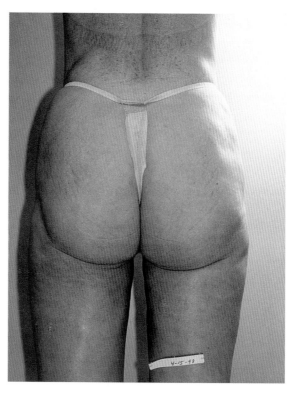

Figure 1-80 *Aesthetic contouring by XUAL was not apparent after standard abdominoplasty liposuction.*

Figure 1-81 *Rapid contouring of laxity in the buttock fold by XUAL, previously treated by suction-assisted liposuction.*

previous surgery. Our surgery includes the use of "super wet" pumps to place local anesthetics into the fascia of the rectus and oblique muscles. She did not have any recurrence of the previous muscle spasm and pain. Her recovery was more rapid also. This patient and others with similar comparisons indicate that the addition of XUAL and the newer techniques for complete abdominal repair make combined procedures more predictable and more natural in appearance.

Editor's Note: The patient's perspective: What our patients want to know. People seeking body sculpturing by liposuction and associated procedures come in all shapes and sizes, ages, races, and philosophies. To explore the variety and complexity and the vast differences between plastic surgery practices in other parts of the country outside Texas, I have asked knowledgeable writers to share with us their experiences in addressing the question of what people want to know and what they expect surgeons to deliver. Some aspects of the following information may be repetitive, but this information has been retained for consistency within each contributor's section. The following should be required reading by the office staff.

PATIENT EXPECTATIONS— SYDNEY BARROWS (NEW YORK)

Most patients find their way to a plastic surgeon's office to inquire about liposuction after years of dissatisfaction, unhappiness, or painful distress. Many have tried to solve the problems themselves, finally throwing in the towel after months, often years, of dieting and quality time at the gym. Others, especially those whose area of concern is noticeably out of proportion to the rest of their body, may have given up months or years before after having finally realized that no matter how many salads they ate or leg lifts they did, it really wasn't going to make that much of a difference. And, of course, there are those who really don't want to bother doing any work themselves when they can simply pay someone else to get rid of the fat for them. However, they all have one thing in common: they just cannot stand looking in the mirror and hating what they see for 1 more minute and they are determined to do something about it.

The Consultation

Many patients are painfully embarrassed by fat, especially when accompanied by a bad case of cellulite. Women especially have been conditioned for years that thin is good and fat is bad, thin people are good and fat people are bad, and thin people are desirable and fat people are disgusting. So it is with considerable trepidation that they approach the inevitable physical examination at their first consultation. Although many physicians have a nurse or other staff member in the room for legal reasons, to the patient this is just one more person, and a woman (presumed to be highly critical) at that, which just doubles the humiliation, especially if she is slender and attractive. And it is the rare female patient who will find the courage to take her clothes off in front of a handsome (read sexually attractive) doctor, which is why some prefer female physicians.

Of course with men, there is often an element of homophobia when nearly naked in the presence of another man, which is why they, too, sometimes seek a surgeon of the opposite sex. However, no matter how embarrassing the examination might be, having the fat is even worse, and their desire to hear you tell them that you can help temporarily overcomes their self-consciousness. Of course, what they really want to hear is that by the time you are done, they will have thighs that rival those of the latest supermodel, but most are realistic enough to know that such results are unlikely. What they need to hear is exactly what you can—and cannot—do for them in as much detail as possible. Using a closed pen or some other kind of pointer, indicate that you would take most off here, go lighter there, blend in this section, and so on. They want to see it, be able to imagine it, and get the sense that you see it too and have the solution. If you feel you need to address an area that they did not consider that much of an issue to get a more aesthetically pleasing result, explain why that area also needs to be done for their body to end up with a natural and pleasing appearance. Patients know doctors are in business to make money and are suspicious when the scope of the work expands because they know it is going to cost them more. If it is explained properly, they will appreciate that your motive is not financial, but a sincere desire to give them the best result possible.

And one last thing, if the area of concern is below the waist, do not require female patients to remove their brassiere. Yes, it happens, and the injury is compounded when the physician continues the consultation without indicating that the patient can put her dressing gown back on. Although it is probably true that the plastic surgeon has seen so many naked bodies that hers doesn't even register, she is so mortified that she will probably end up booking the procedure somewhere else and will warn everyone she can to steer clear of Dr. X.

Many prospective patients are so intimidated by the Great Doctor Himself that they save the "unimportant" questions for the staff person, usually the patient coordinator. After recent headlines in the genre of "Death by Liposuction," many patients are understandably concerned that the last face they see may very well be yours. Fear of anesthesia in general and general anesthesia in particular is extremely common, and if general anesthesia is to be used, the safety advantages need to be carefully explained so that the patient understands that general anesthesia is actually preferable and in this particular case safer. More than one patient has decided which doctor to go with based on anesthesia issues. It is during the initial consultation that hope temporarily triumphs over reality, so although it is important to go over the downsides and risks, most patients dismiss them because their desire to be transformed is so strong. The term, indeed the concept of "contour irregularities" is all but incomprehensible at this point, as is the understanding of skin elasticity and the fact that it may not be possible to remove as much fat as the patient might hope or expect because the skin will not retract enough to leave an aesthetically pleasing result. Those with the most unfortunate problems are usually the most forgiving in terms of these two issues; most of them are just so grateful to look more "normal" that a little ding here, a bit of loose skin there, or one thigh that is half an inch larger than the other is more than a fair tradeoff.

However, the ones with relatively minor imperfections who are accustomed to wearing skimpier, more form-fitting clothing will see every ding as a crater and one thigh that is half an inch larger than the other as "an elephantine leg." It is especially important that these more perfectionistic patients, whose expectations are more along the order of looking "fabulous" as opposed to "normal," be made very aware that surgery is not like sitting at a drawing board with a pencil, eraser, and a straightedge and that although in all likelihood you can give them an excellent result, they may not get a perfect result. At the same time, you or the patient coordinator should spell out just what other ancillary procedures such as endermologie, XUAL, and professional massage can or will be used to ensure the best possible outcome. A wise surgeon will draw on a series of choices to best meet the patient's needs.

The Preoperative Consultation

The decision process—whether to go through with it and which doctor to use—involves a combination of trust in the physician and staff, as well as the ability to finance the procedure. If these conditions have been met, the patient will be back in your office for the preoperative consultation. It is important for both of you to make sure that there is a thorough mutual understanding with respect to which areas will be addressed and how aggressively they can or will be treated. This is the time to make sure that patients understand the limitations of how much you can actually take out given the elasticity of their skin, to show them again where the entry point or scar will be, and to emphasize their part in the process, such as wearing the compression garment for the required amount of time; abstaining from smoking, drinking, and certain over-the-counter preparations; and performing postoperative self-massage, if that is a component of your protocol. If you include a series of endermologie, XU, or professional massage in your package—and this is highly recommended—remind them of the importance of adhering to the schedule that you have set up. It is important to make it clear that *both* of you are responsible for the most optimum outcome possible. Doing the Omnipotent God thing only sets you up to take all the blame if things do not turn out perfectly. Also, be clear that if they gain weight after surgery, those inches are going to pile on somewhere else. They may still have thin thighs, but thick ankles or sausage arms, too.

It is usually up to the patient coordinator or other staff member to go over the nitty-gritty details. At this point, most patients are very excited and much more focused on the results than the process, and they cannot and do not absorb much of what they are told during this meeting. This is why it is important to develop thorough and detailed written materials: consent forms, preoperative and postoperative instructions, your policy on touchups and revisions, and a schedule and checklist of preoperative tests with all the pertinent information included. Some practices require the patient to initial every item on the consent form, and they should be given the opportunity to discuss anything and everything that they do not understand. Make a photocopy of the initialed form for them to take home so that they can never rationalize to themselves that they were never warned in the hopefully unlikely event that they experience a problem. Have the staff member go over the preoperative and postoperative instruction as well. It is astonishing how many people "never get around" to reading them! In most cases, a second compression garment will be necessary (they can take up to 48 hours to dry). Many people, women especially, would prefer something a little more stylish than the standard-issue garment that most surgeons provide; a complimentary catalog from a company such as Veronique would be a very welcome addition to the information package. If the procedure is to involve removal of a sizable amount of fat, you may wish to note that they may need a garment in a smaller size once the initial swelling goes down. If you anticipate that more than a minor amount of tumescent fluid will be discharged during the first day or two, patients should be advised that they will probably need baby diapers or sanitary napkins to sop it up. Some patients may wish to have a rubber sheet on hand as well. Patients hate having to scramble at the last minute for something to soak up the fluid, and they appreciate the foresight of your staff to anticipate such a problem and offer a solution.

One last thing that many practices neglect to take into consideration is the availability and the caliber of help that the patient will have for the first day or so after going home. Obviously, someone who has had a relatively small amount of fat suctioned under local anesthesia is in an entirely different category from someone who has had a couple of liters or more taken under general anesthesia. The latter will not only be pretty much out of it for a few days because of the anesthesia but will also be very physically uncomfortable, and their ability to get in and out of bed without some assistance, for example, will be compromised. The presence of a responsible adult is imperative in these cases. A small-built 14-year-old, for example, with an uncertain maturity level is not going to cut it. Nor is a husband who works during the day and is not supportive of the surgery the appropriate person to be the designated caregiver. The staff must make sure that the patient has an adequate support system in place, commensurate with the level of care that the patient can be anticipated to require.

The Day of Surgery

Many surgeons have the anesthesiologist who will be assisting on the case telephone the patient the evening before. Often it is at that time that the patient is told what to expect on the big day. Most patients are somewhat apprehensive the night before, and contact with a member of the operating team, especially the one in charge of the element they fear the most, is extremely reassuring. If they have not spoken to the anesthesiologist on the evening before, that will need to be taken care of as soon as possible after the patient has arrived, and either the anesthesiologist or another staff member should walk them through what will be happening that day, including when they will be changing into a hospital gown, where they will be waiting, any preoperative medications, the marking procedure, the time they can expect to enter the operating room, approximately how long the procedure will take, what they will look like when they wake up (including dressings, compression garment, and most importantly, drains), where they will be recovering, and whether their designated driver can sit with them, as well as an approximate time that they can expect to be discharged. Postoperative instructions should be reviewed again, and this copy should be given to the driver, who is usually the caregiver as well. Ideally, caregivers should be given the opportunity to review the instructions and ask any questions that they may have.

If the compression garment will be covering the groin area or if sitting on a toilet will be problematic for at least 24 hours, or both, most patients appreciate any helpful tips that the staff may have concerning the logistics of answering nature's call. Most are much too embarrassed to ask or it never occurs to them until it becomes necessary, and if they are groggy and in physical discomfort, they might not have the wherewithal to figure out something on their own. Attention to minor details such as these is greatly appreciated. The marking experience can be terribly uncomfortable, both physically and emotionally. Patients tell of standing naked in a freezing cold room with two or more people present (most of whom are working and not paying any attention, but that is of scant comfort) and feeling chilled to the bone and terribly embarrassed. Conducting the marking in a warm and private room would be ideal. Tip: patients love those hot air blankets and report that they make them feel physically warm and comfortable, as well as emotionally soothed and safe.

Before patients are discharged, remind them again of the most important things that they can and cannot do for the next 24 hours, preferably in the presence of the driver/caregiver. Confirm that the caregiver understands the medication schedule and knows that some issues such as discomfort and oozing are normal and to be expected. Ideally, either the doctor or a staff member with whom the patient is familiar should speak to both the patient (if not asleep) and the caregiver. In addition, remind them of the date and time of their first postoperative appointment.

Postoperative Visits

Just about everyone hates to be patronized, so it is a far better policy to tell patients how terrific they are *going* to look rather than falsely gush about how much thinner they look already (unless they clearly do). You and your staff are the only ones whom the patient feels comfortable venting to (family and friends are less likely to be sympathetic and more likely to be anxious), so don't take the emotional unburdening too seriously. Genuine concerns will need to be dealt with, but more often than not the patient simply needs to share the experience and kvetch to someone. There are tricks to minimizing discomfort when getting in and out of compression garments that the staff should share with the patient, and if self-massage is part of the postoperative protocol, now is the time to begin demonstrating how to do it. In fact, the massage technique should be reviewed several times, not only to impress on the patient that it is important and necessary but also to give both of you the confidence and peace of mind that it is, indeed, being performed correctly. The staff should be warm, friendly, empathetic, and mature enough that patients have confidence in their experience. Having undergone liposuction themselves is a big plus and introduces a more intimate dynamic into the relationship, which patients find very gratifying.

Yes, some patients are very picky and can get extremely distressed over an imperfection so minor that you practically need a magnifying glass and a klieg light to see it. Others may get a result that is less than optimal but within the range of acceptability as far as the limitations of the procedure are concerned. Then there are those who fall on the downside of the bell curve in spite of your very best efforts. There is nothing more frustrating to a patient than to have a doctor claim they cannot see a noticeable contour irregularity or asymmetry. If the problem is minor and within the range of an acceptable result, explain again that surgery is not the equivalent of sitting at a drawing board with a pencil, eraser, and a straightedge and that minor irregularities are not uncommon, although they are certainly unwelcome. If you were clever and foresighted enough to include a series of endermologie, XU, or professional

massage in your surgery package, you might offer to extend the treatments half price for a certain number of sessions. In the hopefully unlikely event that the problem is not insignificant, you should offer to perform a revision as soon as medically advisable unless you do not feel that you have the skill to make the necessary improvements. Under no circumstances should you pretend that there is no problem, especially when there clearly is. The patient needs, wants, and deserves acknowledgement of the problem and to know that you have a game plan and are going to try to solve the problem. Patients are far more likely to accept the inevitable minor imperfections if they feel that you did everything in your power to correct them. More significant asymmetries and contour irregularities are very serious and need to be treated as such. Many surgeons, uncomfortable when confronted with their own fallibility in the form of a poor result that they themselves are clearly responsible for, lie, avoid, and in many cases, abandon patients in order to not face the fact that they screwed up. Unable to get the physician's attention (and sometimes that of the staff as well), these patients pursue the only avenue that they feel is left open to them. They sue and badmouth you all over town to anyone and everyone who will listen. If you are concerned that trying to improve their result is an admission that the result was less than perfect in the first place, consult with your attorney to determine ways that you can address the issue without coming right out and acknowledging culpability.

However, the one thing that you must never do is ignore patients with legitimate gripes. Instead, have a game plan, let them know that you will do everything in your power to improve their result, and be sure that you and your staff make them feel that you are genuinely committed to pursuing every avenue possible to help them achieve the best possible outcome. Experience has shown that patients who believe that their doctors have done everything possible to correct a less than perfect situation and have been there for them and held their hand every step of the way eventually accept that nothing more can be done and even praise the doctor for being so attentive and caring. Even patients who do not have a legitimate complaint can often be pacified by a series of ancillary treatments and attentive handholding. Surgery is not totally composed of the physical element, and some patients have an emotional element that needs to be addressed as well; a wise surgeon will remember this.

PHYSICIAN SELECTION— WENDY LEWIS (NEW YORK)

In a good surgeon, a hawk's eye; a lion's heart; and a lady's hand.

—Leonard Wright

Doctors fall into the vast category of professionals like lawyers, whose elevated stature is a matter of rank rather than explicit competence. It is ingrained in us to defer to doctors to some degree, and we are duly intimidated. The more specialized the doctor is (i.e., aesthetic plastic surgeons), the more reverence you engender. Patients are searching for special qualities, such as a sense of creativity, raw talent, innovation, and skills coupled with some ray of light that tells them you actually still care about your patients. Not all surgeons are warm and fuzzy; in fact, some are downright cool and arrogant. Although there is no substitute for skill and experience in a surgeon, we are more inclined to overlook a disinterested bedside manner in oncologic surgeons than in the realm of aesthetics. All things being equal—results, skills, and training—patients prefer plastic surgeons who are just plain nice.

Surgeons by their very nature are not always programmed to excel in handling the human side of patient care. For the patient, choosing a plastic surgeon to entrust one's face, nose, or breasts to is a very personal journey. Visiting a plastic surgeon can be a humbling experience. Take a moment to think about what brought the patient to your office. She feels vulnerable, as though her good looks are slipping away, and she feels old and less than her former self. She is also likely to be nervous and apprehensive. The first consultation is like a blind date and should never be rushed. No matter how busy a surgeon is, you can't really deal with an aesthetic surgery patient quickly. Patients have questions and they deserve answers from you or your staff (or both). One of the most important qualities a surgeon needs is the ability to listen and hear what patients are saying. The patient wants to feel special, like she is your most important patient. If you treat patients with dignity and respect, they are more likely to return the favor. Wash your hands before you touch a patient, and shake the patient's hand as a greeting. Sit down when you talk with patients, but stand up when the patient leaves your office. The worst offense is leaving a patient naked or exposed for longer than necessary. All exchanges between people leave things open to interpretation. It's not what you say; it's how they hear it. We are all looking for the kind of remark, warm smile, and reassuring gesture that makes us feel confident that you will do your best for us.

Although it may be true that a healthy dose of arrogance might not be a bad quality in a surgeon, too much of a good thing may just as easily get in the way of your patient relationships. At the end of the day, patients really aren't all that interested in the sum of your diplomas, accolades, and honors. Their main concern is "What are you going to do for my face?" Surgeons who favor flash over substance have missed a critical element that patients are looking for from their doctors—*trust*. We want to *trust* our surgeons. You're kidding yourself if you think that patients are impressed with doctors who are overly impressed with themselves. In the words of Patch Adams, "When you treat a disease, you win or lose. When you treat a person, you win every time."

Realities of Practicing Plastic Surgery in an Urban Setting

Ask any New York plastic surgeon what his patients are like, and you'll get a string of adjectives such as demanding, unreasonable, relentless, noncompliant, and downright tough. Look up the word "chutzpah" in a dictionary, and you'll find a picture of one of your patients. New Yorkers are natural-born shoppers. They want the best for the least, and they are rarely willing to wait for anything. They are programmed from an early age to hire a "specialist." Therefore, a guy who gets written up somewhere for breasts is not always considered "safe" for face-lifts. It is easy to get pigeonholed and known for doing only one operation. There is no guarantee that a patient who was happy with the eyelids you did will come back to you for her face-lift 5 years later. Cosmetic surgery is often a topic of interest at cocktail parties, and New Yorkers are as fickle about plastic surgeons as they are about restaurants and designers.

Running an efficient practice with you, the surgeon, in control quickly becomes something you only hear about at meetings. A patient who has a 2:00 afternoon appointment will often come at noon and at 12:15 complain that she hasn't been seen yet. The woman, who is scheduled for a face-lift with you, may also be booked with your colleague across town for the same day. If the forecast is rain, you can expect 25% of your patients to cancel or not show up at all. If it turns to snow, you can triple that number. They think nothing of bullying your receptionist to be "squeezed" in for an emergency collagen shot. The term "nonrefundable" preceding "deposit" loses all meaning when they cancel at the last minute and demand a full refund. You learn to not be outraged when you get paged on a Sunday morning by a patient you operated on last year who has a question about a scar, or when the pharmacist calls for a renewal on a prescription you wrote 2 years ago for Tylenol No. 3 for a patient you haven't seen since, or when an insurance company sends the check directly to your patient for the nasal fracture you set for her son and she spends it on a cruise to Bermuda.

The reason that New York patients treat surgeons no differently than they do their decorators and plumbers is simple: because they can. There are 153 American Society of Plastic Surgery members in the borough of Manhattan alone, about half of whom are in walking distance of my office and a dozen are within my zip code. This total does not include the hordes of dermatologists, oral/maxillofacial surgeons, and obstetricians/gynecologists practicing some form of cosmetic surgery. In addition, four other boroughs in New York City are within half an hour traveling time, plus the suburbs of Westchester, New Jersey, Long Island, and Connecticut, all of which are dotted with doctors performing cosmetic procedures.

Although there is surely more competition than ever before in all markets, New York is a unique place to practice. To undergo an extensive procedure such as a face-lift or large-volume liposuction in any of the major New York hospitals, your patient is expected to pay upward of $5000 in advance for use of the operating room, a semiprivate room, and anesthesia. At one time hospitals offered "cosmetic packages" for your patients at fairly reasonable fees, until they discovered that they lose money on these deals. Private nurses have priced themselves at more than $50 an hour, and some of them make more in one night putting ice packs on a lady's eyes than Oxford pays you for a TRAM (transverse rectus abdominis myocutaneous) flap. Office space is at a premium, and most plastic surgeons work and operate in 1500 square feet. Anything over 2500 is considered a palace and big enough to be shared. Getting your operating room accredited is also no small feat because most existing spaces have to be totally gutted to comply with any codes. For any construction or electrical work that you do to your office, you are required to get approval by that other great New York institution notorious for punishing doctors, the dreaded "co-op board." Another challenge for plastic surgeons is the New York labor pool, who take a crash course on employment law before you hire them. There is no such thing as "terminating at will" in New York. You need a reason, and it better be a good one. Stealing meperidine (Demerol) or being rude to patients does not qualify. Any possible violation that could remotely be construed as discrimination can result in you being named as a defendant in a lawsuit. Dealing with attorneys quickly becomes a way of life for us because New Yorkers are trained to sue at the slightest provocation in the blink of an eye.

In contrast, I have been told that patients in other regions are more likely to be loyal, generally follow your instructions, keep their scheduled appointments, and actually say "thank you" some of the time. "There are some days when I wish I were just a country doctor."

References

1. Franklyn R: Surgeon claims machine vacuums fat away in minutes. *Midnight Globe*, December 12, 1978, p 20.
2. Gorney M: Sucking fat: An 18-year statistical and personal retrospective. *Plastic and Reconstructive Surgery*, 2001; 107:608-613.
3. Hoefflin SM: *The Beautiful Face*, limited 1st ed. March 2002.
4. Coleman S: Indications and complications of autologous fat transplantation. Paper presented at the American Society for Aesthetic Plastic Surgery, Seattle, 1991.
5. de Jong RH: *Anesthesia Patient Safety Newsletter*, 1999; 14:25-26.
6. American Society for Aesthetic Plastic Surgery and the Lipoplasty Society. Press Release, New York, October 2000.
7. Rohrich RJ: Discussion. *Plastic and Reconstructive Surgery*, 1998; 101:1752.
8. Hoefflin SM, Bornstein JB, Gordon M, Waddle J, Coleman J: General anesthesia in an office-based surgical facility: Report on more than 23,000 consecutive office-based procedures under general anesthesia with no significant anesthetic complications. *Plastic and Reconstructive Surgery*, 2001; 107:256-257.
9. Rohrich RJ, Beran SJ: Is liposuction safe? *Plastic and Reconstructive Surgery*, 1999; 104:819-822.
10. Grazer FM, de Jong RH: Fatal outcomes from liposuction: Census survey of plastic surgeons. *Plastic and Reconstructive Surgery*, 2000; 105:436-446.
11. Rankin M, Borah GL, Perry AW, Wey PD: Quality of life outcomes after cosmetic surgery. *Plastic and Reconstructive Surgery*, 1998; 102:2139-2147.
12. Iverson R: Discussion. *Plastic and Reconstructive Surgery*, 2001; 107:254-255.
13. de Jong RH, Grazer FM: Perioperative management of cosmetic liposuction. *Plastic and Reconstructive Surgery*, 2001; 107:1039-1044.

14. Rohrich RJ, Beran SJ, Kenkel JM, Adams WP Jr, Dispaltro F: Extending the role of liposuction in body contouring with ultrasound-assisted liposuction. *Plastic and Reconstructive Surgery*, 1995; 101:1090-1102.

15. Fodor PB: Wetting solutions in aspirative lipoplasty: A plea for safety in liposuction [editorial]. *Aesthetic Plastic Surgery*, 1995; 19:379-380.

16. Grazer FM, de Jong RH: Fatal outcomes from liposuction: Census survey. *Plastic and Reconstructive Surgery*, 2000; 105:436-446.

17. Perry AW: Avoidance of disaster in liposuction. In: Habal MB, Himel HN, Lineaweaver WC, Colon GA, Parsons RW, Woods JE (eds): *Key Issues in Plastic and Cosmetic Surgery*, vol 16. Basel, S Karger, 1999, pp 100-121.

18. Hodgkinson D: Regarding suction lipectomy [opinions]. *Technical Forum*, 1983; 7:9.

19. Wall S: Regarding suction lipectomy [opinions]. *Technical Forum*, 1983; 7:9.

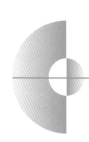

Superficial Liposculpture

Standard liposuction has a high patient satisfaction rate and an acceptable safety record. Originally, surgery was performed with large cannulas in the deep fat layers, thus protecting the blood supply and viability of superficial fat. Inevitably, surgeons would "extend the envelope" to seek further methods of improving appearance and to enhance skin retraction. Ultrasonic and power-assisted forms of liposuction were far in the future when American surgeons were introduced to the concept of superficial liposuction. Those in the audience who saw the first presentations by foreign surgeons were shocked and disturbed by illustrations of surgeons holding abdominal skin that was tissue paper thin. We knew then, as we know now, that there would be a flood of complications. The major complications of liposuction quadrupled when superficial liposuction was introduced; such complications included contracted and scarred skin, folds, skin sloughing, and other inoperable complications. I have personally seen cases in which superficial liposuction resulted in scarring and deformity of the inner thigh region and abdomen that were difficult to convert.

Dr. Simon Fredricks of Houston was the first to raise the warning during a national meeting when he accurately predicted the dangers that would occur from interruption of the blood supply and damage to the deep dermis. Careful surgeons such as Dr. Luiz S. Toledo of Brazil modified superficial liposuction in selected patients, and it has become a part of the armamentarium of trained and experienced plastic surgeons. I would only warn those with less experience to be extremely careful. It is far better to come back and treat small fatty deposits or areas that are not completely smooth with external ultrasound or secondary liposuction with 3-mm cannulas than to run the risk of major complications. As Dr. Toledo discusses in his books and presentations, superficial liposuction can be performed with care so that a layer of fatty tissue and superficial blood supply still remain, and the goal of enhanced contracture has been reached. The discussion in this chapter precedes other advances in plastic surgery to induce greater skin contracture.

SUPERFICIAL LIPOSUCTION

Superficial liposuction is an attempt to modify skin architecture and quality by liposuction in the immediate subdermal area. In the introduction to the 1993 textbook *Superficial Liposculpture: Manual of Technique,* Carson M. Lewis (plastic surgeon, La Jolla) teamed with Marco Gasparotti (Rome) and Luiz S. Toledo to present the relatively new concept of superficial liposculpture.[1] My first encounter with this concept was at the Review of Aesthetic Plastic Surgery (RAPS) meeting in São Paulo hosted by Dr. Toledo. One could not argue that the smoothness of contouring shown by Drs. Toledo and Gasparotti was not impressive. Only later, to our dismay, did we realize that there were far more disasters than successes with this concept. The initial successes

> **CLINICAL PEARL**
>
> Presentations by Drs. Gasperoni and Gasparotti of Italy in the summer of 1990 convinced North American surgeons that superficial liposculpture was a safe and desirable procedure and that if one did not use it, the surgeon would be remiss. Convinced that the subdermal layer of fat must be treated to avoid waviness and that small cannulas (1.3- to 2-mm "Mercedes" type) were needed to break the "arch phenomenon" peel for further shrinkage, many surgeons abandoned their conservatism and obtained often disastrous results: rippling, scarring, and untreatable deformity. As a corollary, in 1979 American surgeons learned to their dismay that European colleagues had abandoned direct curettage of subcutaneous fat because of its extremely high complication rate. This led to questioning of suction-assisted lipoplasty in an editorial in *Technical Forum* in which my readers were warned that removal of fat under direct vision, especially in the submental triangle or in the midline of the abdominoplasty, was a proven and safe technique that should be considered before embracing the "new" liposuction touted by French and Italian colleagues.[2]

were attributed as much to the syringe technique as to the skill of the surgeons who advocated syringe liposculpture as being "more precise and accurate" with shorter convalescence and less blood loss. We know that was certainly wishful thinking and not reality.

The concept of superficial liposculpture was to reduce skin flaccidity, thus leading many practitioners to attempt this procedure on less than ideal patients. Flaccid skin has minimal blood supply and is more easily damaged. No subcutaneous tissue and fat protect the skin and ensure contouring. Consequently, superficial liposculpture on such skin produces irregularities, scarring, lumpiness, and contractures, which are now well-known complications.

American surgeons were inundated with unsatisfactory liposuction patients who had dents and irregularities. Thus, Dr. Toledo, de Souza-Pinto, and others formalized repair surgery that included the release of scar tissue and autologous fat regrafting. Fat regrafting therefore moved from the accepted filling of "dimples and dents" and mid-gluteal flat areas to become an important component of reparative liposuction.

PATIENT SELECTION

The concept of superficial liposculpture in the "ideal candidate" is valid.[3] In 1989, large cannulas were used exclusively in the deepest layers. Many surgeons were beginning to work closer to the surface, but not directly beneath the skin. In reviewing *Superficial Liposculpture: Manual of Technique*,[1] which is now over 10 years old, one must not be too critical. Nonetheless, it was naïve to believe that thin skin draped over cannulas with no subcutaneous tissue would result in a smooth contour with normal healing. In patients with larger fat deposits and in healthy young adults, "superficial" liposuction added another dimension and was indeed helpful.

> **CLINICAL PEARL**
>
> There must be a category of patient in whom simple skin excision can complement liposuction of the abdomen. Dr. Ed Dalton (plastic surgeon, Oklahoma City) removes a propeller-shaped ellipse with wider excisions laterally rather than medially. If there is some laxity of the abdominal wall, he will repair it. If there is laxity of the entire abdomen, he frees the umbilicus as in the "float procedure," with or without plication of the rectus fascia. In "large liposuctions," which make up a goodly portion of his practice, there is so much laxity that excision is required, but often the musculature is still intact and taut, thus indicating that there is no reason for abdominal repair of the internal structures.

Today, all the surgeries that we do are "liposculpture." We are no longer content to simply remove large deposits in "ideal candidate" patients, but offer this procedure with its many variations to different age groups and those with differing needs, anatomy, and less than ideal skin qualities.

At Least We Know This

Fat distribution differs in men and women, in different races, in different subgroups within those races, and at different ages. Some men and women begin with the hip and thigh fat distribution that requires correction by liposuction in their early teens. In others, the mid-abdomen and "love handle" deposits develop in their early thirties. Fat deposits appear in the jowl and submental triangle, fat disappears in the perioral area, and the lips also shrink with age.

The actual number of fat cells is stable during adult life. Fat cells become larger with weight gain and shrink with weight loss. I recommend that patients make no effort to lose weight before liposuction so that these cells are "fat and happy." Weight loss after liposuction is inevitable during the recovery period, and it improves our results. On the other hand, weight gain after liposuction means that fat will be deposited somewhere, and that is often in "embarrassing" places. Better safe (re-do it) than sorry (over-did it).

> **CLINICAL PEARL**
>
> **To Gain or Lose Weight**
> Initially, in the rush to establish that liposuction should not be used in obese patients, mandates from university surgeons declared that all patients should undergo a trial of weight loss and not be considered for liposuction unless this trial was successful. This is ridiculous. As we know now, 99.9% of patients have already tried exercise and weight loss without success. The bulk of the fatty deposits, either from an inability to exercise or because of heredity, do not respond to dieting. Many summaries of laboratory cell studies conducted 20 or more years ago concluded that "those fat cells are the last ones to shrink, the first ones to come back."[4] A more practical approach is to insist that the patient maintain a steady weight or even gain weight before surgery. The reason? If a patient has been dieting, the fat cells in question will have a degree of shrinkage. We judge the liposuction according to the amount of fat that is left behind, not the amount that is removed. If the patient is a successful dieter, these compressed fat cells will certainly rebound in a few months after surgery. It is wiser to have the fat cells "fully loaded" so that the amount that is left in each area may decrease with natural variations in weight rather than rebound. In other words, tell patients to not "crash diet" before undergoing liposuction.

In general, women have a proportionally higher percentage of body fat than men do, especially in the hips, upper part of the thighs, and buttocks. Intra-abdominal fat often accumulates with age, especially in men. Generally speaking, men and women can lose intra-abdominal fat with diet and exercise but cannot lose the fat deposited in outer areas such as the hips, thighs, flanks, and abdomen.

INSTRUMENTS

The first successful liposuctions were performed in Europe with suction machines designed to perform abortions. The cannulas used would be considered unacceptable by today's standards. Use of the dry technique with various suction machines produced results that intrigued surgeons in many countries. "Superficial" cannulas differ only in diameter, whether for "pump" suction or "syringe" suction.

CLINICAL PEARL

In the interesting "political" revision of the history of wet solutions for liposuction, it is not mentioned that Dr. Illouz, considered the founder of modern liposuction, visited Dr. McCarthy at New York University in 1982 to discuss Dr. McCarthy's use of hypotonic fluid to lyse fat cells. Initially, liposuction was performed with hypotonic solutions. However, experience revealed that balanced salt solutions were not only safer but also equally effective.

Dramatic changes have occurred in instrumentation. Cannulas were designed with various suction tips and included single-holed cannulas, multiple-holed cannulas for deeper areas, flat-bladed cannulas for freeing the skin, and various pickle-fork combination cannulas for use in contiguous suctioning and release of adhesions in dimpling and even re-injection. In addition, many manufacturers developed liposuction machines that varied in design but produced the same degree of efficiency.

With the advent of syringe liposculpture, instrument redesign included standard tips for the cannulas and various shapes, diameters, lengths, and disposable products. Many surgeons objected to the awkward loss of suction with the syringe technique, but improved designs have eliminated this problem to a large degree. The choice of machine rather than syringe liposuction is not only a personal one but also depends on whether one intends to use the fat for regrafting. For larger cases, many surgeons prefer to harvest fat with a syringe technique and then proceed with machine liposuctioning for greater efficiency and conservation of operating room time.

In summary, the choice of cannulas ranges from the larger diameters originally used for all levels of liposuction to the present concept of restricting large cannulas to the deeper, heavier fat deposits in larger individuals. Most liposuction is performed with 3- and 4-mm cannulas of various design. For superficial and subcutaneous liposuction, the choice of cannulas depends primarily on the physician's experience and the designs with which the surgeon is most comfortable. The instruments designed for gynecomastia, which were originally rather large and bulky, have been refined. Individual surgeons often promote instrument designs that are essentially minor modifications of the standard ones. Surgeons who are learning to perform liposuction should try a variety, but the "open-ended" tiger tip, Mercedes tip, and single-lumen types that protect the subcutaneous fat are good choices. Multiple-holed cannulas allow greater efficiency in harvesting and produce acceptable results, but careful monitoring is required. In cases in which "bulges" are primarily due to deep dermal thickening/scarring, small cannulas with serrated flat tips are useful. Any fluid, tissue, debris, or blood is aspirated as the "crosshatching" of the pre-marked thick area proceeds. As often stated, the success of liposuction is not based on the equipment, but on the skill and dedication of the surgeon.

THE PROCEDURE

Deciding to Perform Superficial Liposuction

The primary advantage of superficial liposuction is that it induces a greater degree of skin contracture than standard liposuction does, but there is more bruising and a greater risk factor. In the typical patient, the mid-abdomen has an excessive amount of wrinkling, greater than what would be expected to conform if ultrasound-assisted liposuction (UAL) or external ultrasound-assisted liposuction (XUAL) were used. The markings are made such that the deeper fat deposits are circled, as well as those in which there is little fat, usually lateral to the midline or into the flank areas.

A minimal infusion is a better choice than the "full tumescent" technique, with approximately 600 cc of the standard formula used for the typical abdomen; superficial liposuction is also performed in saggy arms because contracture in these areas is a greater goal than smoothness. Patients who are chosen for superficial liposuction have healthy skin with wrinkling. They are in good health and less likely to refuse exercise or massage or to follow other instructions postoperatively that are essential for obtaining a smooth contour.

After the infusion has been allowed to penetrate the tissues, small separate stab wounds are made at intervals. It is most important in superficial liposculpture to use the nonoperating hand to judge the degree of thickness and to pause frequently to measure the remaining thickness of soft tissue by the "pinch test." First, liposuction is performed in the deeper areas of the pre-marked bulges with 4- and 6-mm cannulas. Whether one uses the syringe or the machine technique is immaterial. The syringe technique is chosen if regrafting is planned. Many women in this category who have only small amounts of fat and greater degrees of laxity will also have dimples and depressions in the hips and buttocks. The syringe technique allows one to harvest all the remaining fat for regrafting in multilevel techniques underneath these depressed spots.

After a crisscross fanning application of liposuction in the deeper tissues, a change is made to a 3- or even a 4-mm cannula, usually with a single hole placed so that suction can be directed away from the subdermis. Superficial liposuction is then approached in all these areas, and a small amount of blood will be noted as the upper areas are breached. Care must be taken that the dermis is not damaged. For this reason, only extremely experienced surgeons should use UAL for superficial liposculpture. The risk of damage is also greater from UAL than from standard cannulas. It can be helpful to reduce the degree of suctioning with the syringe technique by filling the syringe only partially. This reduces the actual suction applied to these areas and gives a small additional safety margin.

Crisscrossing is done in the usual manner, but an attempt is made to crisscross in the opposite directions of the deeper liposuction. Frequent evaluation of the remaining dermis and retention of small amounts of subcutaneous fat are essential. One should never attempt to remove all the subcutaneous fat because the risk factors are greatly magnified. After completion of the superficial liposculpture, the superficial fat and skin will still give a positive pinch test result and will not be "transparent." At this point a compression dressing may be required to aid in smoothing. A number of foam devices are used. The danger, of course, is that excess pressure can destroy the skin. If one chooses to use a compression device of any type, it is essential that the pressure be released every 3 to 4 hours for at least 30 minutes. This can be accomplished by the patient at home.

For experienced surgeons, the change from soft, yellow fat extraction to a slightly more difficult passage with blood-tinged fat indicates that superficial liposculpture is being accomplished. Many surgeons believe that the small entry points for superficial liposculpture should be left open because there is a greater degree of bruising. If the blood remains in the deeper tissues, it can induce fibrosis.

One technical point that is helpful is to reinsert the infusion cannula that was used to place the "super wet" solution and use the remaining fluid to flush out the entire area. Several hundred cubic centimeters is passed through the tunnels and then allowed to drain into soft compressive dressings.

As noted in this chapter, the main complications of superficial liposculpture were scarring and banding of the dermis, dermal destruction with tissue loss, and even larger areas of tissue necrosis from disruption of the blood supply. Because the only advantage of superficial liposculpture is the greater degree of contracture that can be achieved, this procedure is not recommended in many areas of the body. If fatty arms are being reduced without skin excision and if laxity is judged to be typical of an older patient, primary and secondary use of superficial liposculpture has merits. The same applied to the upper part of the abdomen, but rarely to the thighs, flanks, breasts, or other areas that are treated. One should never perform superficial liposculpture on the face and neck! The deformities resulting from over-resection are almost impossible to repair.

Measurement

Weight and tape measures are objective, whereas photographs are frequently too subjective, according to Dr. John Kelleher (plastic surgeon, Amarillo). Preoperative documentation is the single most important aspect of liposuction in his practice. Each patient is weighed and measured. A certain number of patients complain that they do not see a change, but a 3- to 4-inch change in measurements is often eye opening.

CLINICAL PEARL

CLINICAL PEARL

"Touchups" Are Going to Be Required; You Can't Prevent Them

Although compression after surgery helps distribute damaged fat cells that are still in the resolution phase and the use of super wet techniques plus careful attention to detail should eliminate the need for secondary procedures, they do not. A patient can gain 3 ounces and put it just where it shouldn't be. Facing this situation, only two choices are possible, and each involves a form of intervention. The simplest choice is to infiltrate the area, with a very small amount of corticosteroid added, and then apply ultrasound for 2 days directly over the area to break up the remaining fat. Skin contracture may be responsible for a problem because the underlying fat that was thought to be of adequate thickness now occupies a small space and will inevitably bulge upward. The second approach is one that was used in a very athletic male just recently. He had excellent resolution of his "love handles," but by 3 months a small midline fatty deposit had developed. He also asked whether further resolution of the love handles could be accomplished. Physical examination showed little if any fat in the area, yet there is an approach that will improve the result. Local anesthetics were used to infiltrate both areas, small pinpoint openings were then made, and 3-mm cannulas were passed into each zone. Surprisingly, about 40 cc of fat was removed. Ultrasound was then applied over the reduced area to enhance the degree of skin retraction. Subcutaneous "breakup" of tissues may also be required. These minor procedures can be performed in an office facility under local anesthesia at the cost of a "reduced facility fee." Such practice is good public relations and good patient care.

CLINICAL PEARL

Why Does Superficial Liposuction Improve with UAL?

Before we discuss all the warnings about skin burns, sloughing, and irregularities, experienced surgeons such as Jim Grotting believe that a thin layer of residual emulsion from UAL will thicken and make the superficial plane more even, thus making superficial liposuction more effective and aesthetically pleasing.

After hearing a presentation of XUAL for skin retraction after arm liposuction, Dr. Grotting agrees that there is not enough skin retraction with UAL to avoid skin excision in similar patients.

Superficial Liposuction of the Posterior Leg and High Hip Areas

Case in point

As shown in Figure 2-1, the patient is slightly turned away from the operator, who places a hand beneath the roll to suction. This is especially useful in gauging the depth and amount of fatty tissue to be left in place. Palpation with the fingertips and the "pinch test" after a

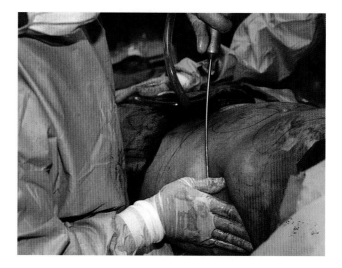

Figure 2-1 *Superficial liposuction is used in "safe" areas such as this lateral abdominal deposit. After deeper suctioning, the hand is used to judge the position of the cannula to ensure that sufficient subcutaneous fat is left undisturbed.*

first run should prevent over-suctioning with its unfortunate sequelae. The fat removed by superficial liposculpture is blood stained, in contrast to the clear yellow of the fat removed from the deeper tissues, which is a clear warning to proceed slowly and with caution. The blood loss is not a significant amount to warrant concern.

Case in point

Preoperative markings indicate the thicker areas for liposuction, and superficial and deep suctioning will be used in the abdomen (see Figs. 2-2 and 2-3). Placing the nonoperative hand over these areas allows one to gauge the amount of fat that remains. Entry points are at the mid-pubis and umbilicus, as well as at a lateral position (see Figs. 2-4 and 2-5), to allow liposculpturing centrally and laterally. The supine position is maintained throughout the procedure, and curved cannulas are passed from the anterior to the mid-back area. A second entry point allows cross-suctioning in a horizontal manner in the flank position. See Figure 2-6.

COMPLICATIONS

The two layers of subcutaneous fat are the deep and superficial layers. Liposuction usually focuses on the deeper layer where contouring is more predictable. Suctioning in the superficial layer must be done with caution because of the added risk of injury to the skin's

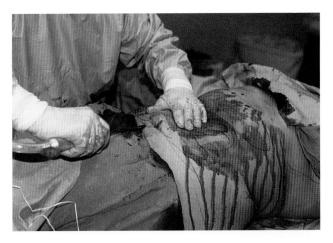
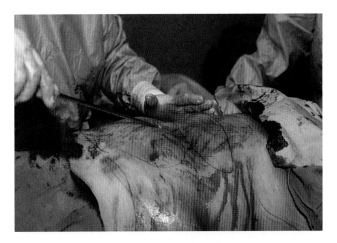

Figures 2-2 & 2-3   *An advantage of standard liposuction of the machine type during superficial liposculpture is the ability to continue "fanning" without interruption. It is essential that one gauge the depth of removal so that the most superficial fat layer is left undisturbed; placing a hand as shown allows one to intermittently assess the contour, as well as direct the tip of the cannula. By wetting the skin with providone-iodine, the surgeon can slide the guide hand.*

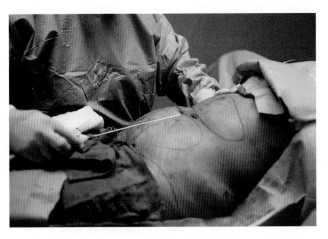

Figure 2-4   *Superficial liposculpture in the midline before abdominoplasty is permissible if the closures are performed without tension. An entry point at the umbilicus also allows one to create the grooving for contour aesthetics.*

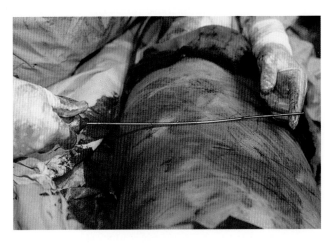

Figure 2-5   *The use of smaller cannulas with adjustment of the curve is important for reaching difficult areas. At this point, the patient may be elevated and turned on the side, but we rarely find it necessary to turn the patient prone.*

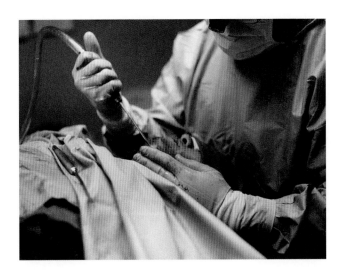

Figure 2-6   *It is particularly important to leave subcutaneous fat when sculpting the occasional patient who does not require muscle surgery in the submental triangle. Placing a protective finger at the junction of the jaw line and the neck also prevents damage to nerves by inadvertent puncture of the muscle layer.*

blood supply, as well as contour irregularities from scar formation.

The complications that have been seen personally and that have been reported through *Technical Forum* correspondence are frightening and inevitably related to superficial liposculpture, even in trained hands. The first complication is mottling and fibrous pebbling of the surface and is due to an interrupted blood supply, scar tissue, effects of postoperative bleeding, or direct injury to the dermis itself. Removing the superficial layer of fat, which adds contouring to the skin surface, induces irregular skin contraction to fill the void, thereby leading to these deformities.

The major complication is loss of skin and subcutaneous tissue. Such loss has been reported more often after superficial liposculpture of the abdomen than other areas, but case reports of large skin sloughs in the inner aspect of the thighs after liposculpture are well known. In discussions of these problems in our teaching seminars, it is stressed that the once-proposed ideal of tissue paper–thin skin that can be elevated like a fine silk handkerchief is a dangerous goal. Even in experienced hands, the lack of blood supply to these tissues and the variability in patient response not only to surgery but also to changes in blood pressure, ambulation, overly tight garments, and other unknown factors can produce a disaster. Once the soft tissues have sloughed, there is little to do except skin grafting, which is a most unsatisfactory compromise for returning the patient to society. These deformities were once considered common complications of liposuction in the earliest applications, and they occurred during the curettage phase as well as the early dry phase in the evolution of the current technique. The fact that these complications are now occurring with efforts to produce greater skin retraction with superficial liposuction indicates the need for a text such as this and the attendance of all surgeons in competent teaching courses and refresher seminars.

CONCLUSION

Extending the range of liposuction to more superficial levels was a result of surgeons' interest in further cosmetic improvement in a very safe and dependable procedure. The first improvements came with changes in cannula diameter, the use of "super wet" rather than tumescent infusions, and postoperative care regimens that included skin preparations, massage, compression, XUAL, early ambulation, and so on. Although the goal of skin retraction was a worthy one, achieving it by an extremely risky degree of superficial liposuction is certainly unacceptable. It only takes one disaster. The same corollary should be made for the initial phases of UAL, for example, in which perforation of the skin, fascia, and even internal organs occurred in the learning phases. Again, it only takes one disaster, and that is true whether it is one life in a large metropolitan area or in a small community.

"It's a Notta' My Fault" was the title of an editorial in *Technical Forum* that addressed the audience's quiet acceptance of a presentation by an Italian surgeon whose name is linked to the development of superficial liposculpture.[6] In his opinion, anyone who has complications with the procedure that he promoted (extreme thinning of the surface of the abdomen down to bare dermis) would have them only because they could not match his skill, and moreover, it was not his fault that they could not produce the same results. One wonders when such a pronouncement is heard whether the audience stays quiet because of embarrassment, because they have had these complications, or because it is impolite to laugh out loud? One unfortunate problem in national presentations is the tendency of the presenters to show only excellent results, gloss over mediocre results, and absolutely refuse to discuss complications.

CLINICAL PEARL

Superficial Liposuction

Those of you who have followed the exchange of letters in the white journal from a California plastic surgeon who advocates facial *superficial liposculpture* (scraping the undersurface of the dermis) are reminded of the many warnings against this practice. Disaster lurks.

After running a brief note in *Technical Forum* regarding his original presentation, I received mail from unhappy, litigious California patients regarding the surgeon "who destroyed my face."[5] According to these letters, there were many lawsuits related to superficial liposculpture, and the California State Board was involved.

As with laser rejuvenation, one must ask, "Is it the procedure, the instrumentation, or the surgeon who is responsible for this complication rate?"

On a well-deserved vacation I ran into a very nice lady from our state who had undergone superficial liposculpture of her abdomen and face. After the fourth repair surgery, which included facial fat grafting at a major university, she is almost presentable. The surgeons who took over her care were not as successful with her abdomen; they eventually had to resect a large portion of abdominal skin above the midline. The lady was not happy.

On a similar note, during the presentations of our Innovative Procedures Committee, a report was given on the severe complications from a procedure inaccurately described as a "weekend face-lift." The complications seen by surgeons in the La Jolla area reflected the ill-advised method of excessive liposuctioning of the neck followed by laser burning of the dermis, presumably to induce contracture. The resultant scars and deformity that were described were labeled as unrepairable. Just because a procedure is widely advertised, as these two were, and is touted by the media is not an indication that a wise surgeon should embrace them wholeheartedly and abandon surgical training and, indeed, common sense.

References

1. Lewis CM, Gasparotti M, Toledo LS: *Superficial Liposculpture: Manual of Technique.* New York, Springer-Verlag, 1993.
2. Follow up: Section removal of fat. *Technical Forum,* 1979; 3:6.
3. Matarasso A: A superficial suction lipectomy: Something old, something new, something borrowed. *Annals of Plastic Surgery,* 1995; 34:268-272.
4. More than you really wanted to know about fat metabolism. *Technical Forum,* 1986; 9:10-11.
5. No good. Big mistake. *Technical Forum,* 1993; 16:9-10.
6. "It's a notta my fault." *Technical Forum,* 2003; 28:1-2.

CHAPTER THREE

Ultrasound-Assisted Liposuction, External Ultrasound-Assisted Liposuction, and Power-Assisted Liposuction

In this chapter we will explore the modalities that have enhanced our results with liposuction in contouring difficult areas. Surgeons were certainly wary of internal ultrasound-assisted liposuction (UAL) after anecdotal reports of cannulas burning through the skin and fascia and even injuring intra-abdominal organs without any warning to the operating surgeon. Each of these modalities, UAL, external ultrasound-assisted liposuction (XUAL), and power-assisted liposuction (PAL), has one major advantage, a reduction in surgeon fatigue and operating time. Surgeons may prefer one or a combination of these modalities and, with care and experience, use them to their advantage in inducing skin contracture and contouring superior to what we had achieved with our standard techniques.

The change in technology, which included hollow and solid UAL cannulas and teaching courses that emphasized safety and limitations on the use of this modality, has been offset by the cost of the equipment and the added personnel necessary. For some surgeons, the cost is not worth the advantage, except in very large patients, in whom the reduced blood loss from UAL and ease of deep fat dissolution are certainly advantageous. XUAL was introduced as an alternative. Even with its limitations, it has induced a safer degree of skin contracture but has not reached full acceptance. Perhaps this is due to the technology and perhaps it is due to the means of application. As is often discussed, XUAL must be allowed to penetrate into tissues infused with "super wet" solutions. "Tumescent fluid" makes the tissues rigid and will not allow penetration. In addition, the slow careful application that is advised by those who successfully use this technique is essential. Although this concept is not difficult, failure to follow these simple guidelines makes XUAL ineffective. One major advantage—and the technique that illustrates the efficacy of the various XUAL technologies—is facial contouring without surgical intervention. It is now apparent that small amounts of superficial fat are dispersed or destroyed by XUAL, and the degree of skin contracture, which we did not expect, can range from "improved" to "spectacular."

PAL was abandoned in France where an oscillating tip was introduced, but a new version is being marketed. In its semiannual conferences, the Emerging Trends Committee of the American Society for Aesthetic Plastic Surgery is advised on liposuction improvements such as "VASER" and the newer air-driven and gas-driven power techniques. One weighs the advantages of the ease of the liposuction, particularly in difficult areas such as the breast or a previously operated area, against the weight of the handle, any awkward handling problems, and the expense of the machines. The change from nitrogen tank technology to air-driven devices seems to be a major advantage. PAL has proved to be an exceptionally effective technique in larger cases by reducing operating time and surgeon fatigue.

ULTRASOUND-ASSISTED LIPOSUCTION

Ultrasound has been used for selective tissue destruction in neurosurgery, ophthalmology, urology, and liposuction. Adipose tissue is changed through microfibrous disruption and cavitation, which is the more important mechanism. Vapor bubbles are created by sound wave energy that fragments the fat cells and diffuses the lipid materials into the intracellular space. The physics of ultrasound makes it tissue selective, with tissues that contain more collagen and/or elastin and tissues that are denser fragmenting poorly. Ultrasound can disrupt blood vessels, ligaments, and nerves, but the sound energy is more easily transmitted through soft tissues such as fat. Its clinical effectiveness is achieved by additional fluid infusate, which decreases the structure and organization of the fat and concentrates the sound energy more effectively. Theoretically, the thermal energy from ultrasound should be inconsequential, but in clinical practice, this has proved to be a major concern.

Patient Selection

Because ultrasound has a thermal component, a number of devices have been improved to extend the scope of patient selection. The newest external device, "Smart Sound," incorporates a change in engineering to ensure that a steady level of ultrasound is delivered percutaneously. External ultrasound and electrical stimulation have been evaluated separately, but not as a combination for our purposes. The application of XUAL to promote the use of external cosmetics or skin care products and facial rejuvenation with electrical stimulation is often reported in the lay press. These cosmetic applications therefore give credence to the more powerful system that will deliver the wattage desired for softening of fat and skin contracture by XUAL. Our preliminary trials show that this system is effective for both body and facial liposculpturing. Patient selection for facial reshaping with XUAL includes individuals with localized fatty deposits and relatively normal-appearing skin. Although we do not exclude the proto-typical "thin-skinned redhead," one must take care to avoid thermal damage. In body liposculpture, the use of XUAL is not limited except by the expectations. It will definitely *improve* the results of standard liposuction and facilitate PAL. The use of UAL should be confined to more obese individuals, and at this point it is not recommend for use with abdominoplasty. XUAL and PAL may be used with relative impunity in abdominoplasty.

For very fibrotic areas such as the male breast, flanks, and areas that have previously undergone liposuction, each modality is advantageous when there is a degree of skin damage present from over-resection. These patients should be treated only with gentler procedures of standard liposuction and, perhaps in certain cases, the use of XUAL to relieve some of the fibrosis. For physicians who are accomplished users of UAL, it may be considered as an adjunct to all these procedures, except in the aforementioned instances. Thinner individuals are more likely to suffer "end hits" and have a painful recovery than are those in whom larger volumes of fat are to be removed. In essence then, UAL is considered safe and effective in removing thicker fatty deposits by primarily concentrating on the deepest fat layers. PAL and UAL give a degree of control and ease of application of liposuction in more superficial fat, but XUAL is unlikely to add any benefit in the deeper layers because of the limitation of penetration of the sound waves.

> **CLINICAL PEARL**
> Although surgeons have been cautioned that liposuction should not be used for obesity, the pendulum of opinion is beginning to swing toward liposuction as an adjunct to encourage patients to continue with weight loss. By removing the bulk of abdominal fat, patients are able to exercise and are often motivated to continue their improvement. Although one would argue that gastric stapling or other procedures are indicated for massive obesity, the role of liposuction is being re-evaluated. At the Lipoplasty University Conference in 2003 hosted by Dr. Robert Ersek (plastic surgeon, Austin), discussion of reduced insulin requirements, decreased blood pressure, and other beneficial effects of large-volume liposuction indicated the need to apply this modality to a larger number of patients previously excluded. There is no doubt that UAL is valuable in overweight patients of this category because there is less effort and the cannula is in the deeper fat layers. Over-resection is still a problem today, and distortion of the skin and subcutaneous tissue can be accentuated by the use of an ultrasonic device versus a liposuction cannula. As discussed in the chapter on superficial liposuction, the use of any potentially hazardous procedure close to the surface that may result in dissolution of the essential final layer of subcutaneous fat must be viewed with caution.

Patients who benefit most from the addition of XUAL are those who have "transition zones," or areas commonly seen in the flank and anterior of the leg with little subcutaneous fat but visible irregularities. Because XUAL is responsible for freeing the adhesions of frozen joints in orthopedics and physical medicine, it stands to reason that the beneficial effects on "cellulite" have to do with dissolving a portion of the fibrous band in the subcutaneous tissue that is responsible for this doughy, irregular pitted appearance. Patients with larger body fat deposits are best served by UAL because the softening effect of XUAL is not as great an advantage. Another group of individuals who benefit from XUAL are those who have relatively taut abdominal musculature but a small excess of skin that results in visible folds in addition to body fat deposits. Our series included these individuals, who would have undergone skin resection if it were not for the constricting effect of XUAL, which resolved the rippling or hanging pannus that was otherwise expected to require resection.

Other patients who benefit from XUAL are those who do not have the severe "bat wing" deformity of the arms but, instead, have hanging fatty deposits that would normally be addressed by skin excision.

Therefore, practically any patient who is considered a good candidate for liposuction may be included in the selection of patients for one of these adjunctive modalities, with the exception of abdominoplasty and the scarred and distorted skin associated with over-resection. Treatment of scarring in deeper tissues is certainly facilitated by UAL, but because of the energy component, superficial scarring must be addressed with standard techniques such as the "pickle fork," release of scar tissue, fat resection and regrafting, and external skin care.

Advantages and Disadvantages of UAL

Experience with UAL: Lessons from the University of Texas Southwestern Medical Center—Rod J. Rohrich, M.D., and Evan S. Sorokin, M.D. (plastic surgeons, Dallas)

Liposuction quickly became the most frequently performed plastic surgery procedure after the introduction of SAL to the United States in the 1980s. Foremost among the new developments and refinements was the introduction of UAL, which was initially developed by Zocchi and introduced to the United States in the 1990s. It has quickly become an essential part of the plastic surgeon's armamentarium and enables surgeons to safely sculpt the human body with accuracy and consistency. Initially, UAL was met with uncritical enthusiasm spurred by media and consumer demand. Only after time, experience, and a critical assessment of indications, results, and complications have appropriate applications been defined. UAL is an excellent adjunct to SAL. Proper patient education is vital to successful body contouring. Informed consent is more than a signed document—it's part of the education process. Weight loss is known to preferentially occur from visceral fat stores rather than subcutaneous stores. Circumferential body contouring is ideally suited to addressing these subcutaneous adipose stores. Adherence to the tips that follow, awareness of the aesthetic human form, a clear understanding of anatomy, and attention to detail will allow the surgeon to truly become a sculptor of the living body.

The following is the currently accepted consensus on techniques in performing UAL:

- The primary UAL end point in aspiration is loss of tissue resistance.
- Short periods of initial UAL decrease total the surgery time by 40% to 50%.
- UAL is best performed with bullet-tipped cannulas for soft tissue sculpting.
- The "super wet" technique, in which the ratio of room-temperature infiltrate to aspirate is 1:1, is used.
- Large-volume liposuction (>5 L) requires resuscitation with crystalloid, "super wet" infiltration, and intravenous replacement of aspirate at a ratio of 0.25 cc of crystalloid to 1 cc of aspirate. Communication between the surgeon and anesthesiologist is crucial.
- Use a skin protector or an external sheath and do not torque or bend the cannula.
- UAL progresses from superficial to deep areas, whereas evacuation and final contouring with SAL progresses from deep to superficial areas.
- Avoidance of zones of adherence is mandatory. These areas include the gluteal crease, the lateral gluteal depression, the posterior inferior and distal lateral aspects of the thigh, and the middle of the inner portion of the thigh. The gluteal crease is inviolate to both UAL and SAL.
- UAL is used in fibrous areas and SAL in nonfibrous areas.
- UAL is ideal for areas of scarring from previous SAL.
- Concave areas should not be treated from convex areas to avoid inadvertent fascial penetration and visceral injury.
- Asymmetrically placed incisions give a less "surgical" appearance.
- UAL is a dynamic, bimanual technique in which the nondominant hand tracks and guides the position of the cannula.
- The long-term success of large-volume liposuction depends on changes in lifestyle patterns, with an emphasis on the importance of diet and exercise.

CLINICAL PEARL

Dr. Grady Core (Birmingham) has excellent low-complication outcomes with ultrasound liposuction. The simple guidelines that are taught in UAL courses should have alerted surgeons that UAL cannot be used as cavalierly as SAL. Naomi Lawrence and William Coleman III (dermatologic surgeons) also agree that ultrasound provides greater ease of fat removal in fibrous areas.

CLINICAL PEARL

Reviewing comments made by Michele Zocchi in 1992, one is struck by the overly optimistic view of UAL that unleashed a Pandora's box of complications on the surgical world. Zocchi stated, "In this new method all vascular structures—arterial or lymphatic—as well as nervous structures remain undamaged, thus allowing a quicker and favorable postoperative course."[1] However, many of us know that this is untrue; the structures may not remain undamaged.

CLINICAL PEARL

The use of microwave energy for liposuction was evaluated extensively, and the decision was made to not pursue this modality. The bulky equipment and clumsy technique were less acceptable than UAL and more expensive.

CLINICAL PEARL

Despite changes in technique and instrumentation, the introduction of hollow as well as solid cannulas, and growing conservatism among surgeons, UAL has become a valuable adjunct to liposuction in carefully selected cases. In the hands of a skilled practitioner, UAL has a role in the initial breakup of scar, fibrosis, and fatty tissues and in subsequent removal of the residue by liposuction. Other experienced surgeons have discontinued the use of UAL altogether because of cost, the time involved, the extra personnel required, and the risk of injury to nerves, blood vessels, and skin, even in the hands of the most experienced surgeons. Patients risked skin deformities, soft tissue deficits, and internal "hits" (burns). The realization that the results were identical to those of standard liposuction, although less effort may have been required, led some to revert back to PAL, SAL, and a search for new toys.

Apparent disadvantages of UAL

If you don't want to have any complications at all with UAL, turn off the volume. Don't use it.

—Richard Mladick (Virginia Beach)

It seemed likely that UAL would be an important part of every aesthetic surgeon's life, especially after seminars devoted solely to UAL were conducted. It is hard to be objective about anything involving liposculpture, however. The procedure has come a long way—from dry techniques to overfilling tumescent techniques to the compromise "super wet" technique. The original ultrasound machines were removed from the market because of the high complication rate. The 1996 American Society of Plastic Surgeon's Task Force and reports from enthusiastic surgeons discussed over 800 procedures performed over a period of 3 years with four different machines. Only 10 patients suffered permanent sensory loss, it was a breakthrough. Many surgeons believe that blood loss is reduced and, with experience, "no more skin burns" will be produced. Those who witnessed presentations noted that the fat-to-blood ratio in the aspirate, when compared with the results of standard suction, seemed the same, which meant that the blood loss with UAL was the same as with conventional liposuction performed with the wet technique. Blood loss should not even be an issue with the "super wet" technique. In fact, blood loss in all studies was less than 1 cc per 100 cc of fat aspirate.

CLINICAL PEARL

It is impossible to actually quantify the amount of blood loss and fluid changes in any liposuction procedure. Nevertheless, enthusiastic surgeons continue to voice their opinion that UAL reduces blood loss and that with experience, one should not encounter skin burns or the permanent sensory losses that plague this procedure. Therefore, when Dr. Luiz Toledo rose to address his experience with UAL, the audience was not prepared for his conclusions. First, he stated that the ultrasonic technique is not easy to perform simply because the instrument weighs so much. Syringe liposculpture equipment is lightweight by comparison. Patients had itchy paresthesias and more edema with the ultrasonic technique. Two major hematomas were noted. In addition, it took longer to perform the ultrasonic technique. Entry skin incisions had to be wide and thus required extra sutures to close. Luiz reported never before having a hemorrhage in his extensive syringe liposuction series, and his XUAL patients bruised more. True hemorrhages are being reported by other practitioners.

Another disadvantage of UAL is that one cannot reinject the fat. In most American women, the liposuction fat is immediately placed in the buttock flat zones and dimples in multiple subcutaneous and deep deposits by using a tunneling "skin tether release" technique.

Finally, the ultrasonic technique is much more demanding in terms of time, personnel, and equipment. The conclusion: Don't change over! UAL offers some advantages but carries a great deal more risk, and it requires much more of your time and the patient's time to achieve a result that is certainly not superior to and in some ways less attractive than the result with other techniques. In short, except for large people, the advantages of UAL may not outweigh these concerns.

Anesthesia

With any of the adjunctive devices, anesthetics are a requirement. The danger of local anesthesia is primarily that of pain rather than overdosage. With the popular intravenous sedation techniques, such as propofol, or diazepam (Valium)/ketamine, or other short-acting intravenous anesthetics, such as methohexital (Brevital), one may safely infiltrate the entire area with the super wet concentration. The other alternative, preferred by many experienced surgeons, is general anesthesia supplemented by lesser degrees of infusion into the area to be addressed. It is the wet environment that enhances the effect of UAL and XUAL, and it is the ballooning of the soft tissues that allows a greater degree of aggressive removal of fat with power liposuction and, indeed, in all aspect of liposculpture in which one gauges the procedure by the amount of soft tissue (fat) left beneath the dermis.

Except for extremely small areas of liposuction, use of the adjuncts with monitoring is considered the standard of care.

Instruments

UAL instrumentation is divided into solid and hollow probes. With increasing regularity, surgeons conducting teaching courses now seem to favor use of the solid probe for most procedures as noted in the experience in this chapter. A number of manufacturers have entered the field, and their equipment is comparable. The VASER has a new vented design that allows a small amount of air to pass through, and it releases ultrasonic energy throughout the entire length and circumference of the cannula rather than simply at the tip.[2]

Richard Ellenbogen (plastic surgeon, Los Angeles) is convinced that the VASER-assisted cannula has changed his perception of liposuction. With the standard PAL devices, he noted fatigue secondary to the vibration, although the units were faster than those used for standard liposuction: "In both cases these advantages were not worth the financial expense. The actual shortening of time or effort in my hands did not warrant their purchase."[3] The VASER-assisted machine,

with its new vented design, allows a small amount of air to pass through, which keeps the fat moving freely without the occasional clogging of the cannula that occurs with standard liposuction. Because the VASER releases ultrasound energy throughout the length and circumference of the cannula, more volume of fat is treated and fragmented at a quicker rate and the device is less cumbersome. The pulsed ultrasound option in which ultrasound energy is released with less heat production allows safer use with less risk of skin burning.

The Silberg instrumentation is a variation on the previously available external ultrasonic devices widely used in physical medicine and rehabilitation. The change in instrumentation increased the power and wattage to the degree that was effective in the initial evaluations discussed by Silberg and associates.[4] When XUAL articles began to appear in the medical literature, a number of manufacturers prepared machines for clinical use in sterile environments. The original Silberg design, initially manufactured by the Wells Johnson Company, was promoted as a more efficient method of energy delivery. Because of the configuration of ceramic heads, steel head delivery systems that did not require a sterile cover were introduced by Byron Medical and the Snowden Pencer Company. The advantages of each machine lie in the design of the handle; the on and off switches, which are located either on the machine, on a foot pedal, or on the handle itself; and most importantly, a cable and delivery head that can be detached and sterilized by gas before surgery. As noted earlier, the new ultrasound system that combines XUAL with electrical stimulation is commercially available.

The original PAL devices with propulsion systems are still preferred by many surgeons, but newer devices with air-driven power or lighter, less-fatiguing instrumentation weight are safe and in use. A vibrating head liposuction device has been reintroduced in the American market, but we were unable to obtain the "Lipomatic" device for trials before the publication date.

CLINICAL PEARL

The vibrating head liposuction device has been reintroduced as "lipomatic." We were unable to obtain this unit before the publication date, but the current literature shows practically identical preservation of internal structures (endoscopy) after the liposuction procedure. In contrast to the PAL devices with which surgeons are becoming increasingly familiar, this device has a "whipping" effect with a rotation of the tip that is claimed to enhance results by greater contact with larger amounts of subcutaneous fat. This remains to be seen.

Procedure: How I Do It—Ron Finger (Plastic Surgeon, Savannah)

I use the UAL unit for the following cases:

1. Malar pads. A solid cannula is used for malar pads. A stab wound with a No. 11 blade is made lateral to the pad. The setting on the Contour Genesis unit is at 40% to 45%. Very few passes are done, perhaps 10 or so. The fat is rolled or milked toward the incision site. Occasionally, a second procedure is needed a few months later if the correction is insufficient.

2. Neck and lower part of the face. Open-type cannulas are used at a setting of 50% to 60% for the neck and lower portion of the face, followed by a few passes with the traditional SAL cannula. The cannula is generally two holed and 2 to 2.4 mm in size. After elevating the cervical flap during a face-lift, the UAL open cannula is also used very effectively to melt and vacuum any remaining undesirable fat in the cervical and jowl regions under direct vision. This has replaced excision with scissors in my practice, and bleeding with this UAL technique is nonexistent.

> **CLINICAL PEARL**
>
> Don't do this unless you're extremely experienced. Only a few surgeons promote the use of a small UAL cannula in the face. They believe that the contour is smoother with melting of fat. Other surgeons report disastrous facial burns and irregularities.

Remember that the safe zones are the thicker jowls and the upper part of the neck, not the cheeks and certainly not the lateral portion of the neck. Liposuction of any form in these areas has caused more grief for plastic surgeons than any procedure in recent memory.

(**Editor's Note:** An advantage of XUAL is that these peripheral areas, the so-called transition zones, will show a degree of fat dissolution without the risk of furrowing.)

3. Abdomen and extremities. I use UAL followed by traditional SAL. Traditional SAL works, but UAL makes the procedure much easier because of lack of resistance to the cannula. Bleeding is virtually absent during UAL. I did not use infiltration through the cannula during the UAL procedure because it makes a mess, adds time to the procedure, and in my opinion, adds to postoperative swelling. One must,

of course, be aware of the location of the tip of the cannula to prevent burns from the end of the cannula pressing against dermis. I have not seen this complication, however. For the head and neck region a shorter cannula is used, which can become fairly warm and require the placement of a wet sponge on or around the incision site. Before the use of a wet sponge, I did see first-degree burns at the incision site when using short cannulas. Whenever I perform UAL, it is standard procedure to follow with traditional SAL. The end point for using UAL that I prefer is the presence of blood in the fat removed or when resistance of the cannula is reduced to nil.

Another difference between UAL and SAL is that in the former, the cannula moves more slowly, for example, once per second, as opposed to SAL motion, which is about twice per second. The patient tends to be less "beat up" with UAL.

Cannulas for SAL are 3 mm and 4 mm with holes on one side. The former is used to smooth and contour the final result and to obtain more skin retraction by suctioning close to the skin. When done close to skin, the holes are directed away from the skin. I use about 1 cc of infiltrate for every cc removed, and my solution contains 1 g of cefazolin (Ancef) per 1000 cc.

Regarding skin retraction, there may be a little more skin retraction with UAL than with SAL, but this is difficult to quantify. I originally began ultrasound liposuction with XUAL and thought it very useful, but I noticed that its effects seem to be limited to fat within the first 0.5 to 1 cm below the skin. My own rotator cuff injury made me seek further physical ease with UAL, and I have been very pleased with its use and results.

My use of XUAL is not limited to postoperative recovery. It softens suctioned areas, and patients believe that such softening reduces the swelling. In addition, I use it postoperatively in patients who have undergone a face-lift and believe that it similarly speeds recovery and softens the tissue. Generally, the patient will undergo XUAL once a week postoperatively for 3 to 4 weeks. One must be careful to keep the hand piece moving with the external ultrasonic unit, however, because the patient may have decreased sensitivity and burns are possible. I do use the maximum setting of 3 with the Silberg ultrasonic unit. After the first week, XUAL may be followed by massage. It is difficult to quantify here, but it does appear to be helpful for the patient both physically and emotionally, and it is my impression that the postoperative course is shortened.

All my efforts in plastic surgery have been directed toward results looking natural, postoperative recovery being shorter, and achieving these objectives in the simplest, most predictable manner. The transmalar subperiosteal mid-face–lift was designed with these goals in mind. In these cases, UAL has helped during surgery and XUAL for postoperative care and reduction of the malar pads, as mentioned already.

In addition, for my face-lift patients, I have used nandrolone (Deca-Durabolin), 100 mg, on the day of surgery and again in 1 week. I am convinced that this anabolic steroid in low dose increases the healing rate and speed. I first learned of this with a few of my own broken bones that occurred during my automobile racing career.

Other tricks to consider in an effort to reduce postoperative care are to eliminate the intake of aspirin, nonsteroidal anti-inflammatory drugs, vitamin E, *Ginkgo biloba*, tuna or salmon, fish oil, and even garlic, all of which reduce clotting ability. The life of a platelet is supposedly 3 weeks, so my patients are asked to follow this regimen for 3 weeks before surgery.

Another Viewpoint

According to Dr. Edward Lack (cosmetic surgeon, Chicago), "One cannot mitigate the long learning curve and the expense of the UAL equipment, and for this reasons it has become a tool used by only a subset of cosmetic surgeons in the United States and Europe." Dr. Lack advises that it is prudent to "retumesce" the tissues after 1 minute of exposure before resuming UAL for another 2 to 3 minutes. In his opinion, a continuously moving cannula can be safely used in the superficial portion of the subcutaneous tissue and will result in better surface reduction. Keeping a low vacuum pressure of SAL to finish the procedure will also avoid increasing tissue trauma. Dr. Lack advises that a SAL pressure of 10 mm Hg be used during the UAL portion and 15 to 20 mm during the SAL portion of the procedure.

Skin retraction is elusive in the medial aspect of the thighs, pendulous aprons, and the female bra lines. The advantage of UAL is consistent skin retraction. The disadvantage, in addition to burns, persistent edema, and longer healing time, may be avoided by combining power assist with UAL. Keeping the setting for UAL at about 50% of the maximum allowable excursion reduces the heat production. Ideally, the lowest possible excursion should be chosen, but for practical purposes, 2% or less is advised.

Technical guidelines include avoiding moving the cannula in a new direction during partial withdrawal, which should prevent tissue damage and heat necrosis. Dr. Lack advises withdrawing the cannula to the opening in the skin with each stroke before passing forward in any direction. Other surgeons disagree and argue that damage at the entry point is more likely with this technique.

> **CLINICAL PEARL**
> In the early experience with UAL, seromas occurred in over 50% of abdominal liposuction procedures. With experience and planning, however, seromas are less frequent, and the additional time requirement can be shortened even though areas must be liposuctioned first with UAL and then again with traditional liposuction.[5]

Before embarking on a UAL program, surgeons must be aware that costly probes need to be replaced, maintenance and repair costs are increased, and there is, in addition, a costly extended warranty.

In contrast, the 3-year experience of plastic surgeons George Commons and Bruce Halperin indicated fewer problems with liposuction of back rolls, the lumbar area, the male chest, and especially "bodybuilders and athletes with fibrous fat." Skin contraction was not consistently seen, nor was it "reliable or predictable." Although the surgeon's work effort was reduced in all areas, "no contour or skin contraction benefits were seen in the thighs, buttocks, lower extremities, arms, and in many abdomens."

Dr. Jorge Perez presents the examples that follow to illustrate the points made regarding safe and effective use of UAL. First, markings are placed to guide radial removal from fewer entry points, with a second color marker used for cross-suction (see Figs. 3-1 to 3-4).

Case in point

This 27-year-old underwent UAL liposuction of the flanks and the hip and thigh area and is pictured at 1 month. Resolution is continuing at this point. See Figures 3-5 and 3-6.

Case in point

This 33-year-old underwent liposuction of the saddlebag areas, the inner portion of the thighs, and the upper part of the back. At 6 months, resolution is complete, with good skin retraction. Skin retraction has always been a problem for patients with this degree of lipodystrophy and poor quality of trunk and extremity skin. See Figures 3-7 and 3-8.

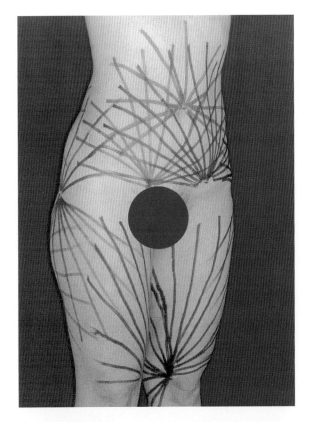

Figure 3-1 *Preoperative markings for UAL to indicate areas for crisscross and overlap.*

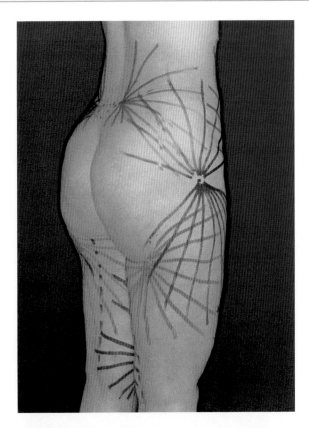

Figure 3-2 *Limiting entry points for circumferential UAL to as few as needed.*

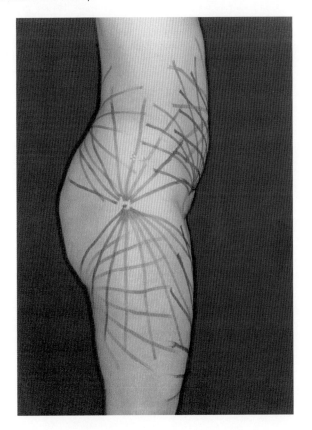

Figure 3-3 *Crossing fan pattens for outer thigh and flank.*

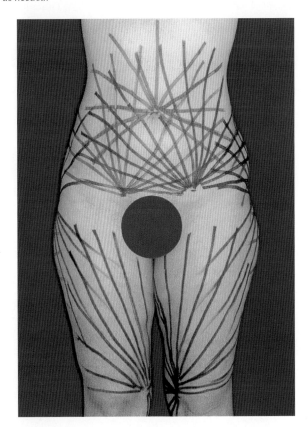

Figure 3-4 *The umbilical entry allows "etching" of a midline groove.*

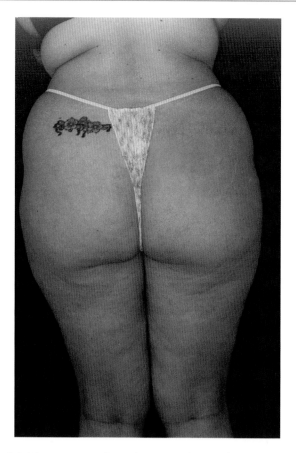
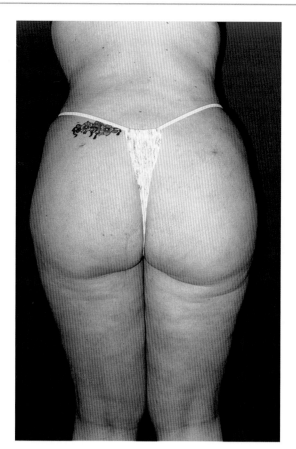

Figures 3-5 & 3-6   *Preoperative and postoperative UAL liposuction.*

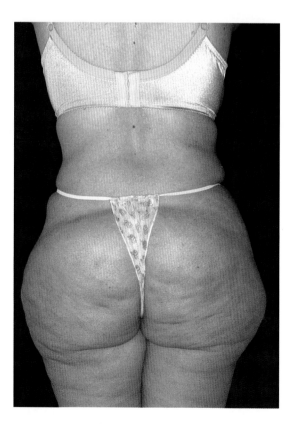
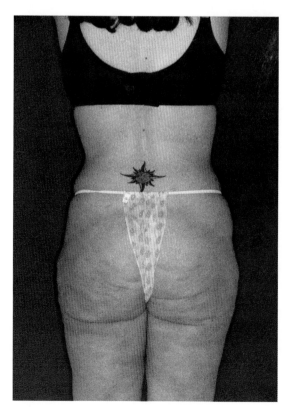

Figures 3-7 & 3-8   *Even patients with less than ideal cases benefit from the additional skin shrinkage offered by ultrasound.*

Case in point

The patient is a 41-year-old man who had undergone UAL liposuction of the "love handle" area. Note that upper buttock hip roll has been included. This degree of skin retraction rarely occurred with standard liposuction. See Figures 3-9 and 3-10.

Case in point

This 47-year-old has undergone UAL liposuctioning of the lower part of the body, including the inner portion of the thighs, the saddlebag and outer thigh regions, the anterior of the thighs, and the abdomen. At 6 months, Dr. Perez advises his patients to discontinue compressive garments. See Figures 3-11 and 3-12.

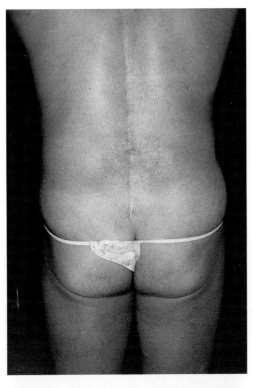
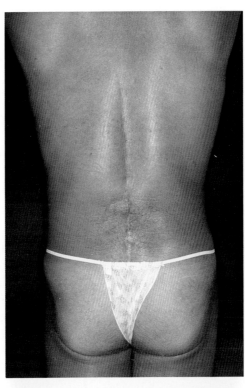

Figures 3-9 & 3-10 *Male patients often do not shrink as well because of thicker subdermal tissue. Shrinkage is enchanced with UAL.*

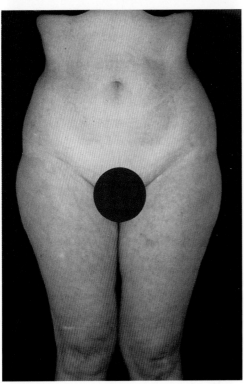
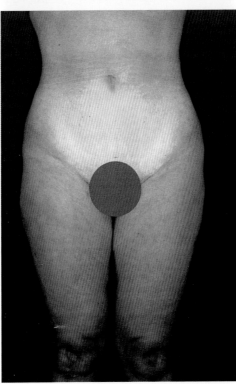

Figures 3-11 & 3-12 *Inner thigh shrinkage was less successful with SAL than, as shown, with UAL.*

Technical Concerns

Dr. Joe Hunstad (plastic surgeon, Charlotte) likes UAL, but doesn't "really love it." Even though he's using less energy, inadvertent skin burns and 3- to 5-month-long dysesthesias still occur in a significant number of patients. One suggested reason is that the ultrasonic energy changes a wet environment to a dry environment, thus leaving the tissues more vulnerable.

On the other hand, Dr. James Grotting (plastic surgeon, Birmingham) uses UAL in his cervicofacial surgery. He believes that it is more of a sculpting procedure than the ablation of standard liposuction and considers the results smoother and more even. One uses ultrasound melting. That said, it is good to remember his advice, which we believe so strongly: "Facial fat is a precious commodity."

It is important to pre-tunnel before you introduce a small UAL probe. Dr. Grotting prefers the Mentor Contour Genesis. He no longer uses a skin protector or sheath. About 2 minutes of work is enough. Stop using the device when it begins to slide easily through the tissues, and most importantly, he advises surgeons to always *undertreat!* In addition, when you aspirate, take out the oil at low suction pressure to avoid any grooving from the aspirating cannula.

> **CLINICAL PEARL**
> Remember that the marginal mandibular nerve is vulnerable to UAL at the point where it crosses the mandible. It is a good idea to palpate the notch and mark it.

> **CLINICAL PEARL**
> With current wet techniques, the common approach is to infuse 2 L for every liter of fat that is to be removed. One can achieve a similar result with lesser degrees of infusate. This alternative becomes particularly important if XUAL is used. The overinflated and stiffened tissues will not allow adequate transmission of the external ultrasound energy to break fat bonds apart and lyse fat cells. The drawback in the "super wet" technique is the temporary hemodilution that renders blood counts wildly inaccurate for up to 48 hours. This is more of a problem with XUAL because infusion fluid is not extracted from "transition" areas.

> **CLINICAL PEARL**
> Safety parameters publicized by the American Society of Plastic Surgeons indicate that 5-L removal is the limit of safety. That's 5 L of aspirate, not 5 L of fat. Even if one might be tempted to go beyond the guidelines, don't do it! Observe the guidelines for reasons that are medicolegal, as well as for patient safety.

Complications and How to Avoid Them

Experienced surgeons such as Dr. Ralph Kloehn (Milwaukee) have reduced major complication rates after UAL to less than 5%, but "slight irregularities" do occur, especially in obese patients. By adding XUAL to "soften the fat" for UAL breakup, he related easier sculpting and cannula penetration, with "somewhat less" bleeding than without preliminary XUAL.[6]

Dr. Kloehn's advice can be summarized as follows:

1. Keep the amplitude of UAL at a "reasonable level."
2. Never stay within one channel for more than two to three passes.
3. Avoid subdermal channeling. Leave "corn rows" of untouched dermal fat intact between the channels to avoid making a "free flap of the skin."

Indeed, Dr. Kloehn believes that "UAL in any of its forms should take a bad rap because it is done technically inadequately. If one follows simple tenets, the average surgeon can achieve excellent results if he has basic knowledge in how to perform ordinary liposuction. Before combining the two modalities of external and internal ultrasonic liposuction, however, I believe that a teaching course should be taken so that the surgeon has the confidence and at least some hands-on experience."[6]

Dr. Kloehn was an early pioneer with UAL and published a landmark article in 1996 in which he described his 6-year experience in over 600 patients. It is his contention that the skin burns, necrosis, and complications result from using solid cannula devices, which deliver a higher amplitude of ultrasonic vibration. His success is credited to use of the "super wet" technique and less surgeon fatigue, plus the learning curve.[5]

> **CLINICAL PEARL**
> A possible explanation for the complications of UAL with the hollow-cannula suction device is that the suction creates a dry environment leading to greater tissue damage from the ultrasonic energy at the tip.

> **CLINICAL PEARL**
> Reports from Europe confirm that there is actually more blood loss than we thought with internal ultrasound in liposuction. Apparently, blood is continuously oozing after the surgical procedure, which was documented by serial hematocrit determinations after 48 hours.

In 1997 in my editorial in *Technical Forum* I discussed problems with UAL that were largely ignored in national publications and presentations.[7] More and more reports of painful dysesthesias, skin discoloration, and internal burns from experienced surgeons were discouraging. Little mention was made of the additional cost of the extra nurses and increased operating time. Hospitals passed on the cost of new equipment to patients, often adding enormous surcharges. It is interesting that in the early experiences of XUAL, Michele Zocchi, the originator of UAL and its most ardent advocate, stated publicly that "disadhesion" could not possibly occur with XUAL. Whatever "disadhesion" means, subcutaneous tissue destruction and over-resection were common occurrences, even in skilled hands.

So many people repeated the belief that UAL produced less bruising and quicker recovery that comparative studies were ignored. Reports of extensive bleeding, such as the presentation by Luiz Toledo, became more frequent but were dismissed as aberrations. Wrong again. These complications are less frequent today, but they are the reason that many surgeons have abandoned UAL.

CLINICAL PEARL

In addressing the question of blood loss in UAL, Dr. Jeffrey Kenkel (plastic surgeon, Dallas) noted in a review that if a surgeon waits a period of 10 to 20 minutes between injection of the solution and commencement of UAL, a dry environment is created, which will result in a very high degree of blood loss. He believes that surgeons reporting their experience must be more specific. End points such as loss of tissue resistance or blood-tinged aspirate are more important than an arbitrary length of time for use of the cannula. In their group's experience with "super wet" UAL beginning in 1995, advantages of UAL included improved contouring, decreased revision rate, less surgeon fatigue, easier treatment of fibrous and scarred areas with less bruising, and "possible skin retraction" from removal of fat in the middle layer. In addition, if extensive body sculpture was required, a better overall contour was achieved when UAL was used circumferentially.

Decreasing the incidence of seromas and other UAL-related complications such as burns and tissue damage, as well as overcorrection, is certainly facilitated by reducing the application time and the time of contact with any tissues. It is far safer to perform a secondary procedure than to over-resect and face the consequences of inadequate techniques for restoration. Experienced surgeons indicate that they are able to determine the loss of resistance to movement of the cannula as an "end point," as well as a change in the aspirate from

pale yellow to pink or tan. In addition, because UAL cannulas cannot be bent, burns on the undersurface of the skin are a risk. Manipulating the tissue to the cannula is suggested. Furthermore, "feathering," which is quite important to avoid irregularity, may be done with the UAL cannula or with standard liposuction cannulas.

Summary

The adjunctive use of ultrasonic cannulas to facilitate liposuction has been a mixed blessing.[8] Advantages include the use of ultrasonic energy to selectively break down fat cells, release liquid fat for later removal by suction, break down fibrotic tissue in gynecomastia and previously liposuctioned or damaged tissues, and ease the physical effort. Disadvantages include the cost of the equipment, the extra personnel, and the likelihood of complications during the "learning curve."[8] A major drawback for a solo practitioner is the cost of equipment, as well as maintenance and replacement of the liposuction probes after a period of use.

EXTERNAL ULTRASOUND-ASSISTED LIPOSUCTION

Ultrasound energy has been evaluated in the laboratory and in clinical settings to facilitate liposuction and body contouring. Drawbacks of UAL include engineering and developmental problems associated with a new technology, equipment, design and expense, increase in operating room time, and the discovery that sound waves have a deleterious effect not only on fatty tissue but also on dermal and neural components. Patients' complaints included protracted dysesthesia, prolonged discoloration, and irregularities from "end hits" in which ultrasonic energy produces an internal thermal burn. When external ultrasonic delivery systems were introduced, they were naturally greeted with skepticism. Dr. Barry Silberg (plastic surgeon, Santa Rosa) developed the first practical external ultrasonic device, which was then evaluated by a number of plastic surgeons. Early reports were encouraging and indicated that the physical aspect of liposuction was easier for the surgeon. However, I was not convinced until I conducted a study for the American Society of Aesthetic Plastic Surgeons in which I compared treated and untreated areas in the same patient with measurement and photography.[9] When evaluating the initial cases, a degree of skin shrinkage in the second or third week after surgery was observed by patients and independent observers that had not been seen with standard liposuction.

> **CLINICAL PEARL**
>
> Dr. Greg Rouscher (Hackensack) agrees that the physical therapy units that are readily available do not generate the amount of ultrasonic energy needed to replicate Dr. Silberg's experience. Agreeing that XUAL is a "tremendous asset," he has evaluated other units providing collimated sources of ultrasonic energy rather than convergent energy that he believes are at least as good as the Silberg unit if not superior. "I believe Barry has come across a great idea which in my hands has given in more than seventy-five patients unparalleled results. I completely agree that there is no seroma development with XUAL. Patients generally have less pain."

Advantages of XUAL

XUAL improved the results of liposculpture without causing perforations, burning at insertion sites, seromas, or irregularities. It has a long history of reducing swelling and discomfort in physical medicine and rehabilitation. Before the study, I reviewed much of the published literature. Both UAL and XUAL devices use injected fluids to increase transmission of the ultrasonic waves, similar to edema in trauma rehabilitation. It soon became apparent that overinfusion (3:1 "tumescent") prevented penetration of the sound waves, thus limiting the effectiveness of XUAL.

> **CLINICAL PEARL**
>
> In the first group of published reports on the benefits of XUAL, Dr. William R. Cook, Jr. (dermatologic surgeon, Coronado), and his observers concluded that pretreatment of the infiltrated area with XUAL was "easier for the surgeon, required less physical effort with less operating time and less bruising, swelling and discomfort for the patient."
>
> Subsequent formal and informal left-side, right-side comparative studies have convinced operating surgeons that less effort is required and that patients are more comfortable postoperatively. All these patients had no trouble identifying the liposuction areas that were not pretreated with XUAL because they experienced prolonged discomfort, tenderness, and usually an increase in bruising in these areas.

The advantage of XUAL is that there is no direct contact with the deep-lying tissues. One can shrink and contour the flank in abdominoplasty without traumatizing the incoming blood vessel area. A word of warning: Until we're absolutely sure about this, do not use XUAL

in the triangle between the mons and the umbilicus. With 7 years of experience using XUAL in "limited" or "complete" abdominoplasty procedures, no deleterious effect has been observed. XUAL fat was used successfully in grafting for lip enhancement and filling of the nasolabial line and to aid the small-incision technique of weakening frown muscles. My first description of this minimally invasive means of reducing glabellar folds, weakening the ability to frown, and eliminating reflexive frowning was described in 1989.[9] In this technique, a small dissector is introduced through a stab wound in the scalp (the Wilkinson rhytid dissector, Byron Medical) and used horizontally to elevated the frown wrinkle lines from the deep dermal attachments. The instrument is then withdrawn and turned vertically to shred the corrugator, procerus, and depressor muscles. The void created subdermally and intramuscularly is now filled with autologous fat. XUAL fat was as effective as liposuction fat in reducing frown excursion, eliminating habit-type frowning, and elevating the depression of the frown lines.[10]

In theory, XUAL energy fractures the collagen septa and intercellular bonds, which allows fat cells to become separated into smaller groups for easier removal and transplantation. In the initial unpublished investigational work by Silberg and the subsequent manufacturer's summaries, the process was described as follows: A transducer produces the ultrasonic field by way of a device transmitting energy through hundreds of piezoelectric crystals. A minute variation in the orientation of the crystals results in rapid diffusion of the energy as soon as it begins to pass into the tissues, thereby resulting in areas of increased power produced by harmonics within the fields. These "harmonics" act on fluid absorbed by the deep dermis and on the intercellular bonds between saturated fat cells. Thus, liposuction would be less traumatic. The diminished bruising and discomfort that we observed seem to result from increased blood flow dispersing epinephrine into the subcutaneous tissues. What works, works.

> **CLINICAL PEARL**
>
> Because of the absence of significant aesthetic differences between SAL and UAL in comparative evaluations and because of reports of delayed healing, itching, and pain with no decrease in bruising with UAL, standard liposuction still has a place in the armamentarium of plastic surgeons who are pleased with the results of careful liposuctioning by syringe or machine techniques.

Patient Selection—Robert A. Ersek, M.D. (Plastic Surgeon, Austin)

When blunt lipoplasty was first described at the meeting in Hawaii in 1983, Yves-Gerard Illouz, Greg Hetter, and other leaders in the field were very concerned about creating unrealistic expectations, and it was therefore decided that liposuction would not be advertised or promoted as a means of obesity treatment or weight control, but would be advocated only for figure faults. In fact, the safe amount of tissue to be removed in those early days was thought to be between 2 and 3 L. As the procedure has developed and has currently become the most frequently requested cosmetic surgery procedure in the world, our knowledge has expanded and it is now reasonable to recommend liposuction as a means of treating endogenous obesity. Recent metabolic studies have clearly demonstrated that liposuction can and does alter metabolism favorably, and it may be a means of preventing or delaying the onset of adult type 2 diabetes.

Materials and methods

With the development of the "super wet" technique whereby large amounts of lactated Ringer's solution containing lidocaine (Xylocaine) and epinephrine are infiltrated into the subcutaneous tissue before liposuction, it is now possible to remove 10 or 20 lb of tissue at one time safely. Infiltration of this fluid mechanically squeezes blood out of the fat and subcutaneous tissue so that there is less blood present, and the adrenaline, of course, causes the precapillary arterioles to shrink down, thus further minimizing the amount of blood in the tissue to be removed so that far greater amounts can be removed safely without significant blood loss.

The development of diazepam and ketamine sedation has enabled liposuction to be performed on an outpatient basis under local anesthesia so that patients go home the same day without the occurrence of deep vein thrombosis or pulmonary embolism, thus substantially increasing the safety of outpatient liposuction. The development of serial procedures in which one area may be treated at one time and, after a wait of 6 weeks, another area may be treated has enabled us to remove any amount of subcutaneous fat over a prolonged period. There is no limit.

Our methods

When patients first enter our facility, they are given 20 mg of Valium by mouth. Because of its amnesic properties, it leaves many people with no memory of the event or even entering the operating room. After an intravenous line is started, patients are given droperidol (Inapsine), 0.125 mg, and atropine, 0.3 mg subcutaneously, and are taken to the operating room where the area is prepared and draped. They are then given Valium intravenously until their speech is slurred. For some patients, as little as 5 mg will be sufficient; for others, as much as 150 mg is required. Once the speech is slurred, we can be certain that the limbic system has been tranquilized. This is then followed immediately by 75 mg of ketamine intravenously. This amount will render most patients insensitive, and within a few minutes they are completely relaxed and it is possible to infiltrate the area to be treated. We then infiltrate a solution of lactated Ringer's solution containing one vial of Xylocaine with epinephrine, red label, per liter. This comes out to about 0.25% Xylocaine. The 1:100,000 epinephrine, diluted with 50 cc of saline, results in a 1:2,000,000 ratio of epinephrine. If the entire body is to be treated, the patient is first laid prone so that the entire back from head to toe is infiltrated with the solution. In a large patient, we may inject as much as 6 L into the posterior aspect of the body. Then, with the use of long cannulas 5 or 6 mm in diameter inserted through a single 3-mm incision at the top of each buttock crease, we are able to reach all the way from the neck to the knees to remove large amounts of fat by careful liposuction.

After completion of the procedure, the single incision is closed with a 4-0 Vicryl subcuticular stitch, the patient is repositioned on the back, and essentially the same procedure continues for the front. After surgery, patients are placed in a compression garment that may go from their wrists to their ankles, depending on the areas treated. These garments remain in place for 1 week religiously. For the next 2 weeks, they can be removed for an hour or so at a time. Then, for the following 3 weeks, the garments are to be worn most of the time.

Metabolic modulation

Through the years we have treated several diabetic patients who reported that their insulin needs decreased and/or their oral glycemic drugs were either decreased or eliminated. However, because these patients had previously been taking a variety of medications before they had lost weight during and after the procedure, we were unable to verify that our liposuction had a direct effect on improving their carbohydrate metabolism and thus lowering their blood sugar. Recently, we had a patient who is a nurse. She had gestational diabetes and measured her fasting blood sugar every Monday morning for several years. It has always been between 150 and 200. Subsequently, after we removed 10.5 L of fat by liposuction and a few weeks later performed a mini–tummy tuck in which another 2 L of tissue was removed, her blood sugar dropped below 100 and has remained there now for over 2 years. Just as important, she has lost an additional 60 lb in that 2 years.

The history

Dr. Sharon Giese presented a significant study wherein she monitored 14 patients over a 2-year period. All these patients were young women who were substantially overweight (body mass index greater than 27). As a result of what she considered large liposuction (more than 4 L at one time), all these patients had a substantial reduction in their serum insulin levels and substantial weight loss that continued even during the 2-year follow-up. All of them also experienced a reduction in systolic blood pressure.

The theory

Clearly, subcutaneous fat is the target organ for insulin. Insulin, of course, is produced by the pancreas and responds to an elevated blood sugar level, and circulating insulin then allows that blood sugar to be transported across the cell membrane into fat cells, where it is stored as fat or oil. Thus, the more fat that is present, the more insulin may be required to maintain hemostasis, and conversely, the less fat that is present, the less insulin may be needed, and therefore a borderline functioning pancreas may be able to produce enough insulin to provide for a greatly reduced fat storage capacity. Every endocrinologist and diabetologist agrees that reducing body weight will reduce insulin needs and is one of the prescribed treatments for all diabetics. Of course, attempts are made to control body weight by diet and exercise. By reducing the fat surgically, it is accomplished in 1 day and it is a certain accomplishment. That is, the fat that is removed from that body and ends up in the bottle is gone forever.

We have noticed through the years that many of our liposuction patients continued to lose weight over the next few years. However, it was thought to probably be a psychological benefit whereby when they found themselves down a few sizes in their clothes, it was motivational for them to not ask for that second dessert. Furthermore, anyone who has ever attempted to exercise realizes that exercise is a lot more fun, a lot more comfortable, and more possible if one is not carrying an

extra 10 or 50 lb around. So, the rapid reduction in body weight accomplished by liposuction was thought to encourage people to exercise more and eat less. However, it is only after Sharon Giese's published studies that it became clear that this is the most effective means known to control body weight. There is no other program that is so successful that 100% of the patients lose weight and stay lean for a 2-year follow-up. Even gastric bypass, as dramatic as it is in controlling body weight, has the occasional failures and is also associated with substantial mortality.

Hemoglobin A_{1c}

Hemoglobin A_{1c} is a new test that is an average of the blood sugar for the preceding 3 months.

As hemoglobin is made within the hematopoietic system, hemoglobin A_{1c} is formed stoichiometrically with circulating blood sugar at the time of formation of that hemoglobin molecule. Red cells have a life span of about 120 days, and therefore a measure of the amount of hemoglobin A_{1c} present is a measure of the average blood sugar over the preceding 3 months. It has recently become a routine screening test for diabetes and a means of testing the effectiveness of glycemic agents. In fact, we have begun routinely measuring hemoglobin A_{1c} levels at the time of surgery, which of course is an average of the blood glucose for the preceding 3 months, and then at 3 months, 6 months, and a year. We are correlating this change in hemoglobin A_{1c} and therefore average blood glucose concentration with the amount of fat removed, body weight, blood pressure, and other measures. The Lipoplasty University has established a website at ersek@ersek.com where practitioners throughout the world can log on with their patients and enter their data into our secured website so that a large amount of clinical experience can be rapidly assimilated, evaluated, and published. From these preliminary studies, it is clear that liposuction can modulate metabolism to the benefit of patients who are prediabetic and frankly diabetic. These findings mean that liposuction will become a treatment of obesity, and therefore, because it is effective therapy for a chronic illness, insurance programs may cover it.

Instruments

The most difficult areas to avoid rippling with liposuction are the face, the inner aspect of the thigh, the anterior of the thigh, and the flanks. These difficult areas are often best left alone or treated exclusively with XUAL and no invasion.

The discussion of ceramic heads versus metal heads for XUAL will never end. Each delivers 30 W of power. Each can have surges. With ceramic heads (Wells Johnson), XUAL seems to be faster than with the metal head devices of other manufacturers. On the other hand, the metal heads are warmer, which is both a plus and a minus. The new "Smart Sound" XUAL/ETS system (Smart Sound, 429 S. Main St., Oswego, IL 60543) is said to be designed to deliver a steady unvarying 3 W of energy.

XUAL: A Clinical Trial

After the pioneering work of Dr. Steven Hoefflin (plastic surgeon, Santa Monica), who in applying XU to anesthetized areas of the face for redistribution of fatty tissues noted facial skin shrinkage, each patient in our initial 1997-1998 evaluation group was offered XU to anesthetized facial tissues without invasion at no additional cost. Jowl, submental, and even subplatysmal fat pads slowly dissipated with a concomitant shrinkage of cheek and neck skin.

On completion of the first 3 months of the initial study, each patient was interviewed. Each could easily identify body areas that were not pretreated with XUAL as being more tender, "not as comfortable," and often more bruised. Even patients who "bruised easily" could identify the nontreated areas as being less comfortable. Equalization did not occur until 3 to 6 months after surgery.[11]

Part of our evaluation was in "transition zone" areas such as the upper part of the flank or the anterior of the thigh where there was only a small amount of fatty tissue, not sufficiently thick to warrant removal by liposuction. Experience has shown that areas with little fat have a high risk of skin disfigurement and wrinkling. These "transition" areas were infiltrated with the same "super wet" anesthetic solution used in all other areas (a total of 3000 to 4000 cc of normal saline with 0.125% lidocaine and 1:800,000 epinephrine delivered with a pump system). Transition areas also showed remarkable redistribution of fatty tissue and skin shrinkage.

The upper arm and inner thigh areas, where skin shrinkage rarely occurred to a satisfactory degree in our previous experience with standard liposuction, also showed a significant degree of skin shrinkage and smoothness with XUAL that was not anticipated. Several patients who had been advised to undergo skin removal with "limited abdominoplasty" and refused this procedure were treated with XUAL alone. To our surprise, there was little, if any, rippled skin in these individuals. The study group also included individuals who had the "Victoria's Secret" short-incision abdominoplasty of the complete or limited abdominal repair types.[12] Skin shrinkage occurred in these individuals as well. At the conclusion of 1 year, follow-up examinations indicated that several of the individuals had gained weight. In those who gained weight, return of fat occurred in the breast area and lower part of the abdomen, but not in the face where no fat had been removed.

Patient categories

All patients evaluated between September 1997 and December 1998 were divided into three facial categories. Category I included individuals who chose to have rhytidectomy with submental repair of muscles, removal of the deep fat pads as well as liposuction in the "safe areas" of the jowl and lower part of the neck, and fat grafting. Category II individuals chose to have only submental repair with liposuction of the "safe area" of the jowl and upper part of the neck and fat grafting. A number of these individuals had fatty cheeks as well as fat rolls low in the neck that were not liposuctioned. The most interesting group was Category III, in which the individuals had only a small amount of cheek, jowl, and submental fat, visible nasolabial folding, and excess superficial and deep fat in the upper and lower parts of the neck. These patients refused the suggested surgical removal of skin and/or fat.

In four individuals, the Bichat deep cheek pads were removed during the primary procedure.[13] In each case, the Bichat fat did not seem to be affected by previously applied XU, nor was the deep fat pad beneath the platysma muscle in individuals in whom reparative surgery in this area included surgical removal of the fat pad.

Evaluation of improvement in facial contour in group I patients is purely subjective in that internal and external tissue recontouring was performed. Nevertheless, it was my impression that a lesser degree of postoperative edema, more rapid resolution, and additional skin shrinkage occurred in the weeks after rhytidectomy.

These nuances can be demonstrated photographically but vary because of individual differences in swelling, skin type, and extent of the procedure. Category II patients all demonstrated a greater degree of skin shrinkage than did patients undergoing identical procedures before the addition of XUAL. Fatty low neck rolls, thicker cheek fat, and other "transition zone" deposits beyond the "safe zone" of submental and jowl liposuction that were not liposuctioned uniformly regressed.

Of special interest was a similar degree of smoothness and shrinkage observed in XUAL-treated arms and inner thighs and adjacent "transition zones" in patients who refused recommendations for inner thigh–lift or upper arm skin resection. "Transition zones" such as the anterior of the arm and thigh, as well as the upper part of the back, are areas without significant fatty deposits to warrant fat removal by liposculpture. As in the face, these areas were infiltrated with the anesthetic solution and treated with XU.

Whereas the application of XU to an anesthetized face without physical removal of fat is not the best choice for a patient who would benefit most from superficial musculoaponeurotic system (SMAS) plication/resection rhytidectomy, skin shrinkage, and fat remodeling, these "transition zones" plus the skin shrinkage areas have made the less invasive approach an acceptable alternative. For patients who were originally considered suitable candidates for arm or inner thigh surgical excision, XUAL and "transition" ultrasound proved to be a better choice.

Category III patients agreeing to facial ultrasound without skin or fat removal were evaluated by surgeon and office personnel and were photographed at weekly and monthly intervals. Patients were asked to compare their facial appearance with preoperative photographs and note the change in jowl, cheek, and submental fat and the laxity of the face and neck skin as (1) very good, (2) good, or (3) no change. Photographs were compared for evaluation at 60 and 90 days and after 6 and 12 months. All parties concluded that each patient had visible improvement in facial appearance. Over 90% rated their facial recontouring as "very good," an opinion shared by independent observers who judged from photographs and direct observation. Long-term 5-year follow-up examinations confirm the published photographic 4-year results.[6]

The use of XU to "fractionate" and redistribute facial fat is a valuable adjunct in facial plastic surgery. In addition to body liposculpture, the patients enrolled in my preliminary evaluation of XUAL under the auspices of the American Society of Aesthetic Plastic Surgery Innovative Procedures Committee were treated by XU applied to "super wet" anesthetized face and neck regions, with or without physical removal of fat or skin. When no excision or liposuctioning was performed, there was visible and photographic improvement in facial contouring. Interview comments ranged from "I can see my cheek bones now" to questions regarding whether a face-lift had indeed been performed. Individuals who underwent submental resculpturing ("submental tuck") or simple "safe zone" liposuction in the submental area, jowl, and nasolabial zones also showed a remarkable degree of skin tightening and contouring beyond the area of actual fat removal. The individuals who have been closely observed for over 5 years still have the improvement. The redistribution of fat and skin tightening initially noted between the second week and months thereafter have persisted unchanged, often in spite of fat accumulation elsewhere from weight gain.

Case in point—Rapid recovery and improved skin shrinkage in body sculpture

The 1997-1998 and subsequent volunteer patients were questioned regarding bruises, discomfort, and time of recovery. Instead of the usual prolonged period in which moving about was difficult, they reported driving to a nearby mall, resuming aerobics classes, or even golfing 24 hours after liposuction! At this point we realized that external ultrasound added one more valuable part to the solution of body resculpturing: early mobilization without pain, as well as early shrinkage of the external ultrasound-treated areas. The early pain-free activity certainly contributed to the overall surgical results.

The patients shown in Figures 3-13 to 3-16 were the first volunteers for the XUAL trial. To our surprise, the hip- and flank-recontouring edema disappeared in the XUAL-treated areas rapidly, and fat grafts obtained by XUAL gave the same correction as fat grafts obtained by SAL before the 1997 trial.

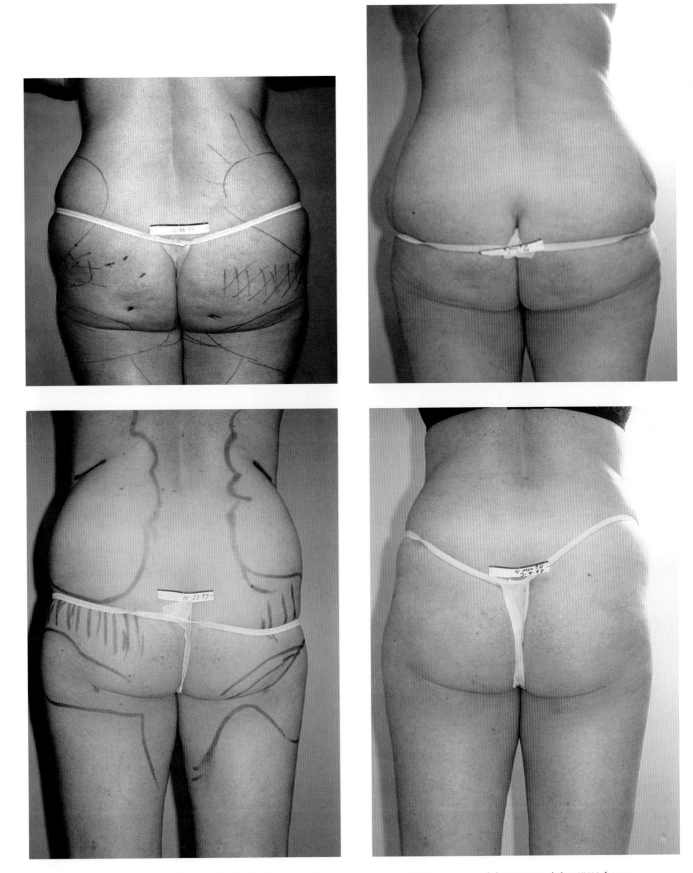

Figures 3-13 — 3-16   *The first volunteers for XUAL showed rapid, unexpected, less painful recovery and demonstrated that XUAL fat was successful as a regraft to the mid-buttock.*

Procedure

As shown in Figures 3-17 and 3-18, a contact lubricant must be used to ensure transmission of ultrasonic energy into the infiltrated subcutaneous fat. A slow, steady "ironing" motion is used, with return to the thicker areas outlined in the upper part and midportion of the abdomen. The crease between the lateral flank rolls is avoided. In our initial trials, we found that fat softening in a larger abdomen and flank was complete in 12 to 15 minutes (see Fig. 3-18). Longer application times did not affect the consistency of the fat or the ease of removal. Lesser time periods produced the effect in only the upper fat, as judged by the ease of removal. In this patient, shrinkage of the flank and abdomen was complete at 14 days, with additional favorable recontouring occurring for months afterward. Liposuction of the traditionally "tough" flank rolls was accomplished with less effort.

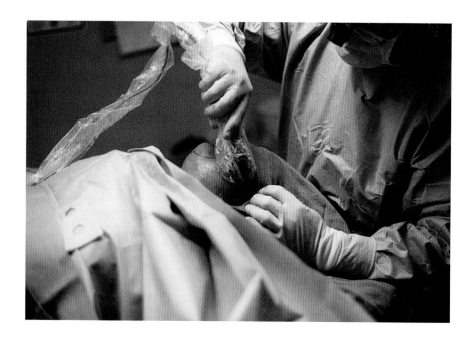

Figure 3-17 *XUAL is applied in a firm "ironing" manner with constant motion. We stop at 1-minute intervals to assess skin temperature with the fingertips. In the face, we move from side to side with extra attention to the jowl, subjowl, submental pads, malar pads, and prominent nasolabial folds.*

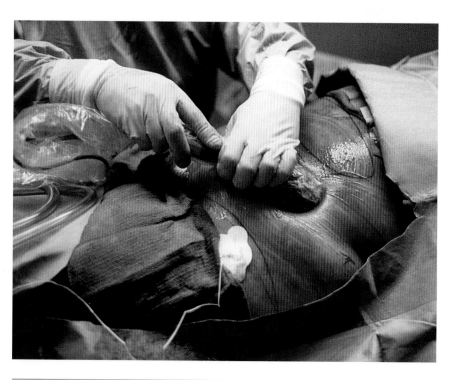

Figure 3-18 *The danger of skin burns is less in the abdomen, but more passes are required over the thickest fat rolls.*

The temperature probe shown in the left lower quadrant of the abdomen is no longer commonly used because the data available from this superficial probe are not clinically useful see (Figure 3-27). The Wells-Johnson XUAL machine used in our initial trials was designed for operating room procedures and had the infiltration pump incorporated into the body of the machine. This pump mechanism with adjustable pressure allowed full infiltration in a minimum of time. It also taught the lesson that overinfiltration, that is, "tumescent" infiltration in a 3:1 ratio, voided the advantage of external ultrasound by preventing penetration into the mid and deep layers of fat.

Case in point—Contouring of the flank with ultrasound but without liposuction

The patient shown in Figures 3-19 and 3-20 is undergoing breast repair surgery, small-incision abdominoplasty, XUAL of the hip roll and saddlebags, and regrafting in the buttocks area. The flank areas will be treated with ultrasound alone. At 3 months there is good contouring of the buttock fold, filling of the mid-buttock depression, smoothing of the upper hip roll, and ongoing shrinkage of the nonsurgical flank (see Figs. 3-21 and 3-22). This progress of ultrasound without surgery is a continuous one, as illustrated by continued improvement in the contour of the flank at 6 months (see Figs. 3-23 and 3-24). These nonsurgical changes induced by XUAL appear to be permanent. Patients who participated in my 1997-1998 trials have not had any recurrence of the fat deposits and folding.

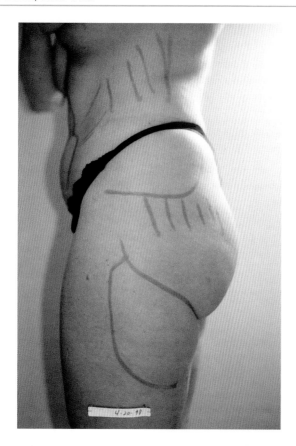
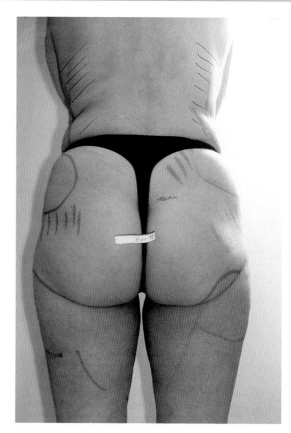
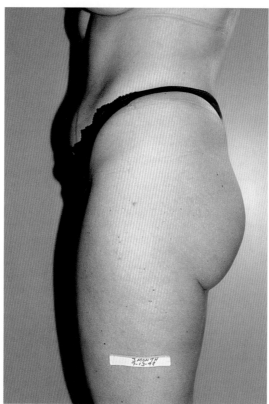

Figures 3-19 – 3-24 Limited abdominoplasty with XUAL, XUAL-obtained fat grafts for the mid-buttock dimples and depressions, and XUAL of the hips and thighs resulted in too rapid recovery. Returning pain free to work in 48 hours, she tore the lower abdominal fascial sutures! Secondary repair was required. Note the ongoing contouring of the anterior of the thighs and flanks. No fat suctioning was performed, only ultrasound.

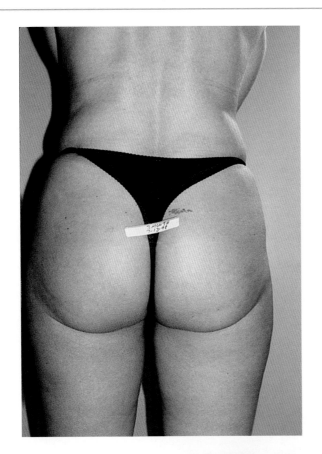

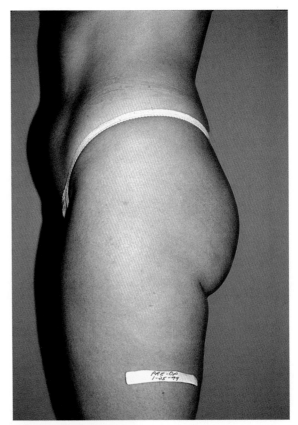

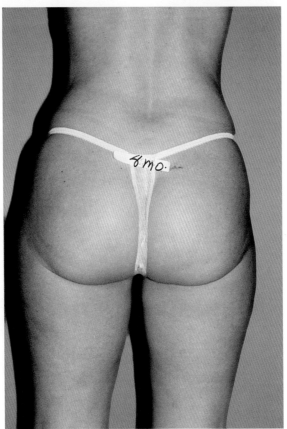

Figures 3-19 – 3-24 *Continued*

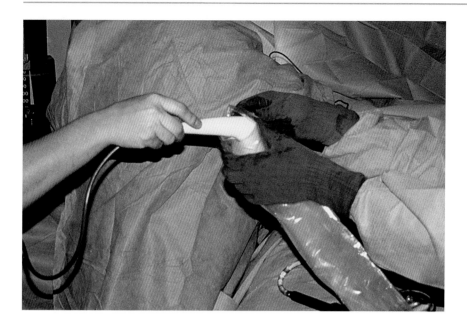

Figure 3-25 *Gas sterilized, or with a sheath as shown, the Mettler and the Byron Medical ultrasound, which are less expensive and ideal for postsurgical treatment to reduce edema and enhance buttock contouring as seen in Figures 3-21 through 3-24.*

More on Instruments

Case in point—Sleeves

Coverage of the XUAL delivery heads for sterility is required because entry points have already been made into the skin for the super wet infusions (see Fig. 3-25). Our preference is to clean the heads thoroughly before inserting them into a cover sleeve. One advantage of the metal head Snowden-Pencer and Byron Medical XUAL devices shown is that they can easily be sterilized with gas or just cleaned with glutaral (Cidex), Betadine, or alcohol. No sleeve is required for sterility. Recommendations for the Wells-Johnson ceramic head delivery system are to place the unsterile device in a closed-end sleeve filled with ultrasound gel. One may choose to have the cleaned head protrude through the sleeve at the end for more certain contact. However, this unnecessarily complicates the duties of operating room nurses.

The advantages of ultrasound are dissolution of fatty tissue and skin contracture. In contrast to UAL cannulas, XUAL cannulas can be bent and curved to reach areas such as the lateral aspect of the flank as shown in this patient (see Fig. 3-26), thus limiting the number of entry points needed.

> **CLINICAL PEARL**
>
> Dr. Luiz Toledo prefers titanium-coated cannulas for SAL with XUAL but no longer uses internal ultrasound. The syringe technique allows him to accurately judge the amount of fat removed. "You avoid the problem of dimples because suctioning stops when the syringe is full."

All the steel cannulas that were evaluated can have their shape altered as required by the individual case.

Although it is recommended that surgeons supply their own cannulas, which are purchased according to their individual preferences, UAL patients must be

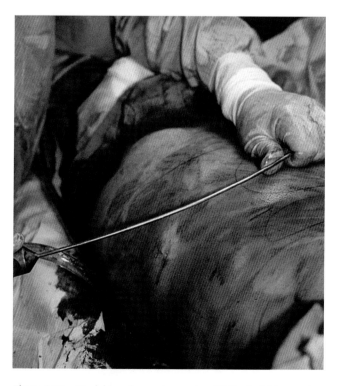

Figure 3-26 *Straight and curved cannulas: XUAL; straight cannulas only: UAL. An advantage of XUAL is that standard in-house cannulas are used with bending to meet surgical requirements. Curved cannulas that follow the body contour make it easier to judge the amount of fat that is not removed and to access distant spots.*

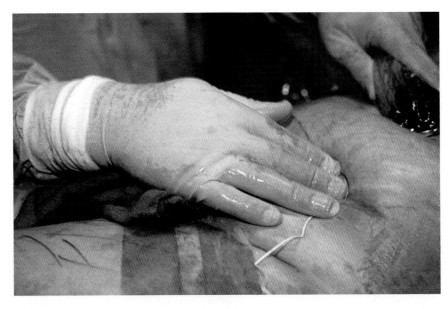

Figure 3-27 *Irregular fat distribution in the abdomen. A useful maneuver with the XUAL head is to manually create folds that can be treated from the top and sides for the full XUAL effect.*

treated with straight cannulas, usually supplied by the facility. These cannulas have a limited life and are expensive to replace. XUAL patients can be treated with standard cannulas that each surgeon and facility have in stock; they can be modified by hand pressure for the degree of curvature as shown if one has a problem reaching a particular area from an entry point selected before surgery (see Fig. 3-26).

CLINICAL PEARL

Dr. Victorio Belo (Philippines) commented in a news report on his XUAL experience. He observed improved intraoperative surgeon comfort through increased ease of cannula movement. As originally reported in his 1997 trials, more fibrous areas such as the back and flanks in males and secondary liposuction areas were also easier to correct with XUAL: "I was experiencing numbness and tingling in my hands with my technique of tumescent liposuction. I was becoming increasingly concerned about my ability to continue this caseload. With the use of external ultrasound my symptoms have mitigated and my patients benefit as well with a better recovery."[16]

Food for Thought

Case in point—Irregular fat distribution in the abdomen

A useful technique is to manually elevate the mid-abdominal rolls while applying external ultrasound energy. This technique protects the thinner areas from the effect of ultrasound and the potential for over-resection and concentrates the delivery system into areas that will be removed (see Fig. 3-27).

Case in point—Skin retraction

Traditional liposuction has always been limited by patient expectations of a smooth result with no excess skin. In the patient pictured, conventional wisdom would be to advise limited abdominoplasty and excision of excess arm skin from the elbow to the axilla. The goal of skin retraction has been reached by several means, including superficial liposuction, UAL, and XUAL. In the patient in Figures 3-28 to 3-30, after discussion it was believed that she could restore her abdominal musculature with an exercise program, and she agreed to not have an abdominoplasty so that we could evaluate the effects of XUAL. Typically, this patient totally rejected arm reduction by excisional surgery. In the postoperative photographs (see Figs. 3-31 to 3-33), skin retraction proceeded very rapidly in the abdomen, hips, and arms. These changes have been maintained. At the end of a year, her exercise has not produced complete flattening of the abdomen (see Figs. 3-31 and 3-32), and this patient is now contemplating abdominal repair.

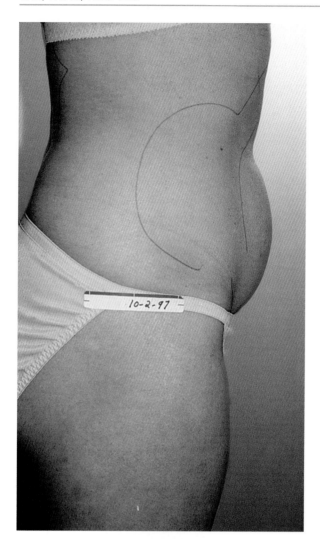

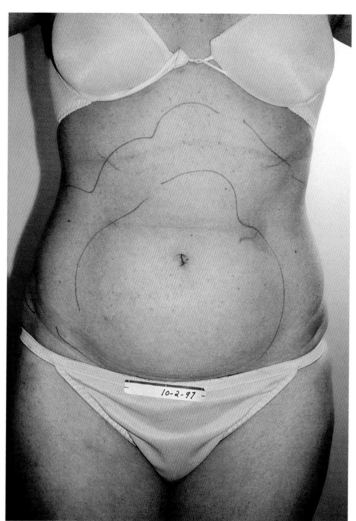

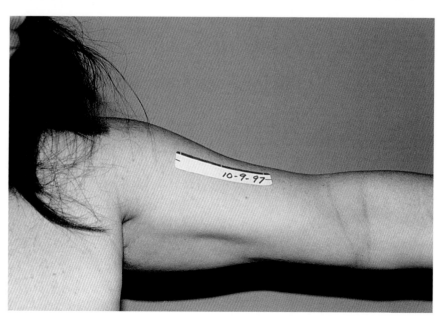

Figures 3-28 – 3-33   *Offered a choice between skin excision arm sculpture with limited abdominoplasty and the new technique of XUAL, the lady chose "no incision" XUAL with the degree of shrinkage shown at 1 year. She was quite satisfied with this improvement, which would not have been possible with SAL.*

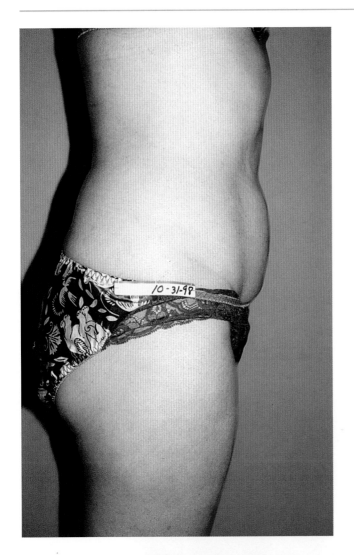

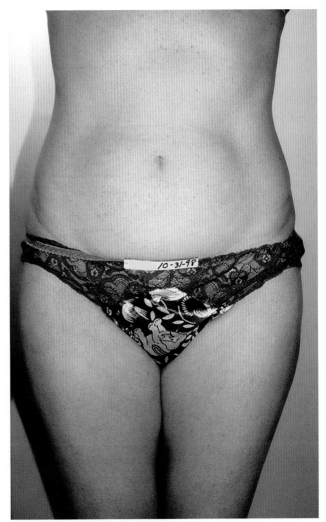

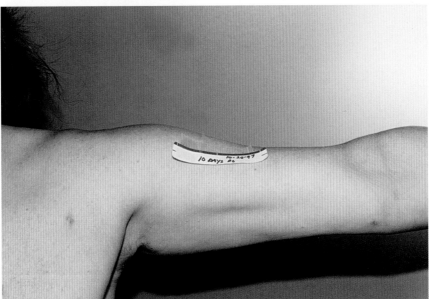

Figures 3-28 – 3-33 *Continued*

Does XUAL reduce bruising?

The general consensus today is "yes." This patient illustrates the visible difference in bruising in patients treated with external ultrasound during our initial study. She had the typical feminine distribution of fat below the waist in the outer thigh, upper hip, and inner thigh areas (see Figs. 3-34 and 3-35). These photographs, taken 1 week after an XUAL procedure in which only the right hip was treated with standard liposuction, illustrate the difference in the degree of bruising (see Figs. 3-36 and 3-37). Decreased bruising was evident in most patients, but not all. We observed that in all instances the bruising in the ultrasound-pretreated area regressed more rapidly.

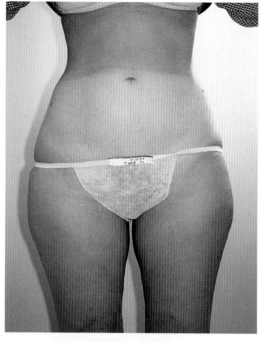
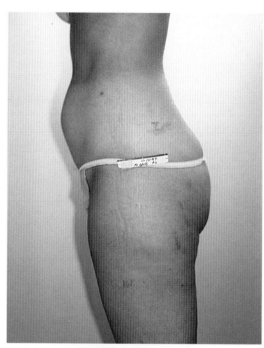
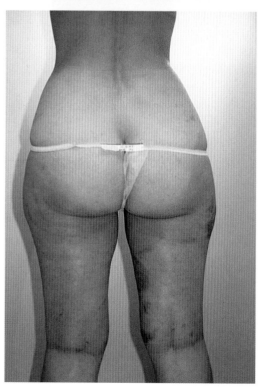
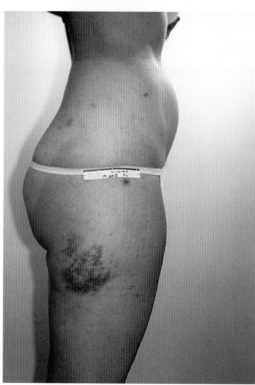

Figures 3-34 – 3-37 *The "left side, right side" evaluation of XUAL was a double-blinded critique. The upper portion of the right thigh was the only SAL area, and bruising and discomfort exceeded that in the XUAL-treated opposite side. Final resolution is shown in Figures 3-75 to 3-79.*

Initial evaluation of XUAL

In assessing the effectiveness of XUAL in skin shrinkage and reduction of bruising, one area was treated by standard liposuction and comparison photographs were taken in the immediate recovery period. The patient in Figures 3-38 to 3-41 was assured that liposuction alone would leave a hanging panniculus and have little effect on fatty descent of the platysma fat and jowl fat. There was no doubt in his mind that the right flank had been treated with standard liposuction and the left flank and entire abdomen with XUAL. Not only was the bruising more prominent, but the right "love handle" area also remained tender and swollen for 3 months after the procedure while the other areas regressed rapidly (see Figs. 3-42 to 3-44). Even at 3 months, there was almost total retraction of the abdominal skin aided

by an exercise program to tighten the abdominal musculature (see Figs. 3-45 and 3-46). Total regression of the "love handle" area was slower on the left side than on the right (see Figs. 3-47 to 3-50). There was even disappearance of the submental fat pad (see Fig. 3-51) along with contracture of the skin of the cheek as well as the neck.

This patient certainly would have benefited from a mid-face–lift and complete repair of the platysma. The remaining platysmal bands as illustrated and the remaining excess skin in the submental triangle indicate that XUAL alone is not a substitute for internal surgery and skin removal, but the contouring of the cheek and jowl and the reduction of the neck protrusion allowed him to defer this procedure to a future date.

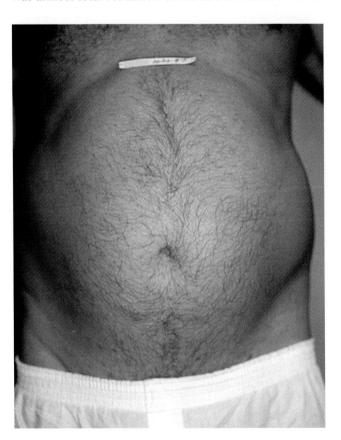 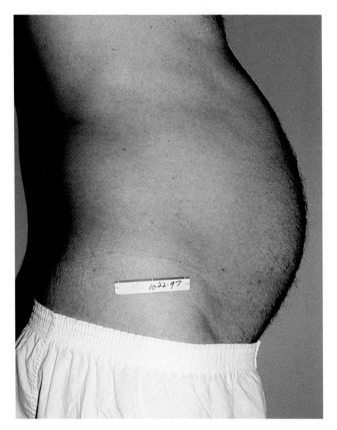

Figures 3-38 – 3-42   *Unable to exercise properly or do "crawl space" work, this gentleman was cautioned that even the new XUAL procedure would leave an unsightly apron of loose skin. He agreed to a trial of ultrasound without fat removal in his jowl area (see Fig. 3-42). The SAL-treated right flank shows a greater degree of bruising than the XUAL-treated left flank does.*

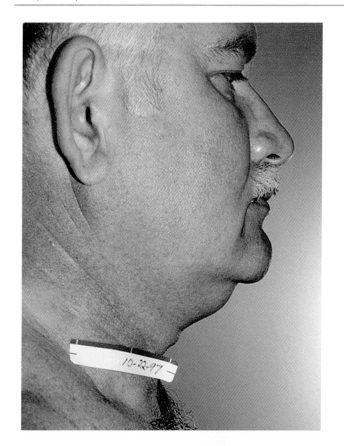

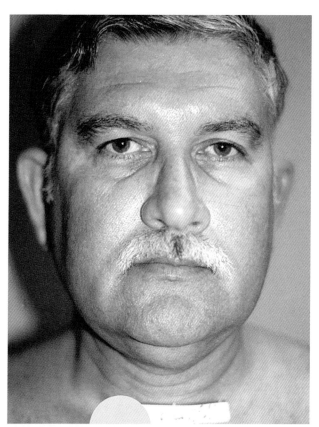

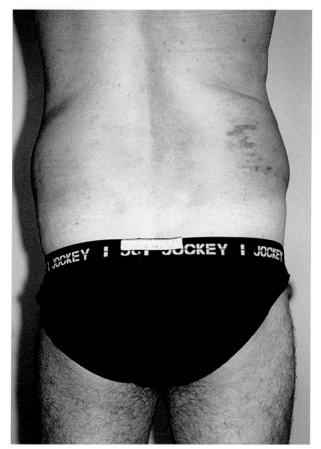

Figures 3-38 – 3-42 Continued

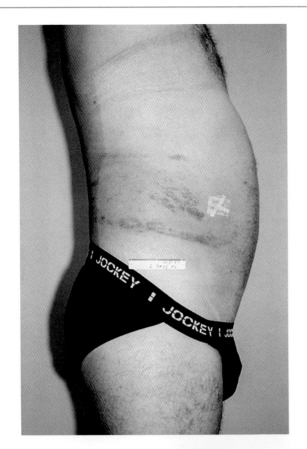 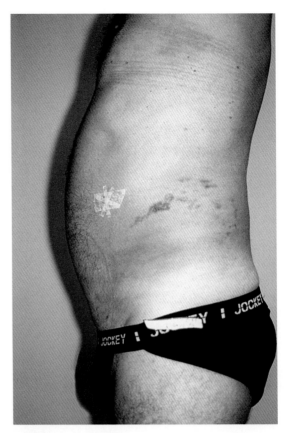

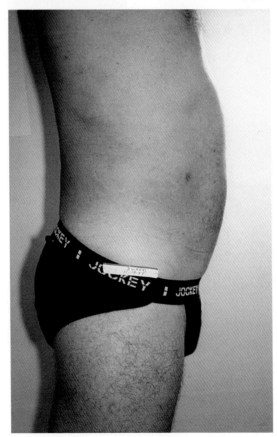

Figures 3-43 – 3-45   *Rapid shrinkage and resolution of edema 3 weeks after XUAL.*

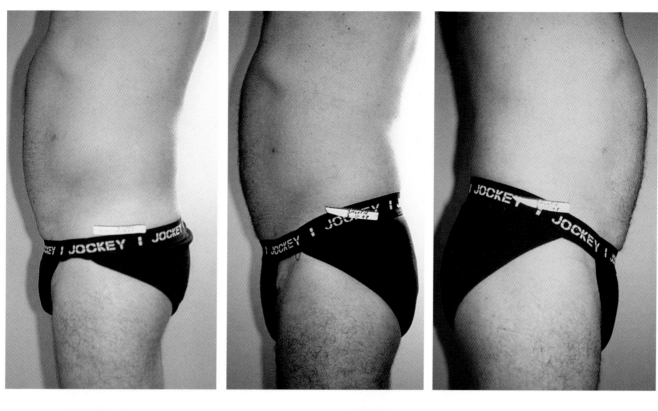

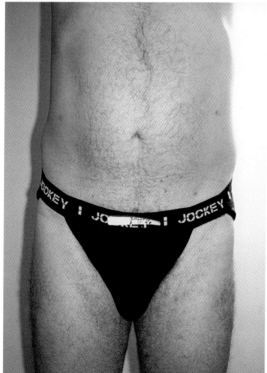
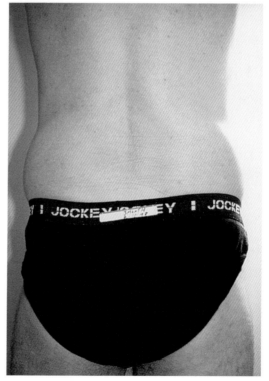

Figures 3-46 — 3-50 *Continued shrinkage with no "apron" 3 months after XUAL.*

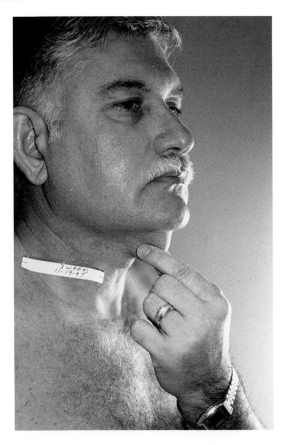

Figure 3-51 *A fat-free submental zone accompanied jowl regression.*

The Facial- and Body-Contouring Effects

When evaluating patients 5 years after the initial application of XUAL for facial contouring, several facts became apparent. All patients showed "improvement" in facial contouring ranging from subtle to dramatic. In certain patients, absence of the jowl pads and flattening of the nasolabial line were sufficient to create a more youthful appearance. With added experience and further application to the nasolabial line and the submental triangle, we were able to reduce not only the superficial fat pads but also the deep fat underneath the platysma to such a degree that a certain amount of retraction was apparent in the submental triangle. An ideal combination then developed. The classic "submental tuck" approach with direct resection of the deep fat pad, division of the platysma, and anterior plication is accompanied by infiltration from the malar area to the clavicle and the application of XUAL for 5 to 6 minutes or until redness appears. XUAL is reapplied on the second, third, and fourth days. It appears to be effective as long as tissue edema is present. These patients wear compression dressings for 5 days.

> **CLINICAL PEARL**
> Dr. Gary Rosenberg (Delray Beach) noted that the fat is emulsified and an oil level develops after XUAL treatment, and he presented microendoscopic demonstrations as well as a clinical series demonstrating the value of XUAL.

To our surprise, flattening of the nasolabial fold and retraction of the cheek were apparent at 2 weeks and increasingly smoother at 4 weeks, and at 60 days some patients demonstrated continuation of the contraction process. Individuals who did not undergo platysmal plication demonstrated bare platysma bands. Those who had the combination procedure showed sufficient improvement that they were often described by their friends as "having had a face-lift."

Surgeons with experience know that a face-lift primarily consists of internal repositioning of soft tissue, as well as external contouring. In our face-lift series, we noted that facial surgery patients did not show progressive stretching in the first 6 months. To our surprise, face-lift patients reported improvement in facial contouring beyond 6 months.

Clinical assessment of XUAL demonstrated that the theory of "breakup" of fat into individual cell clumps was correct. The "proof of the pudding" was that this fat could be regrafted into lips, lines, and buttock folds as successfully as standard liposuction fat. Dr. Nicanor Isse (plastic surgeon, Burbank) added to the confirmation in presentations that included videotaped demonstrations of ultrasound disruption of the fibrous tissue binding the fat cells. XUAL destroys some cells but also frees normal-appearing fat cells, which "float in the fluid." Melvin Schiffman (cosmetic surgeon, Tustin) reported pathologic evaluation of fat after XUAL and standard liposuction and stated in a letter to me that "There appears to be a 24% loss of fat cells by disruption, which is the same as liposuction alone."

CLINICAL PEARL

Lipodissolution Fluid

Building on his early success with XUAL to dissolve small facial fatty deposits that had been infiltrated, Steven Hoefflin (Santa Monica) deduced that a collection of fat cells could be isolated vascularly with vasoconstrictive solutions. If the area were injected with a microdose solution of "scientifically sound" medications to desensitize and lyse the fat cells, dissolution would be more effective with XUAL. Up to 250 cc of fatty deposits could be redistributed and/or lysed without invasive liposuctioning.

The Hoefflin "barrier vasoconstrictive" fluid is 1000 cc of lactated Ringer's solution with 1 cc of epinephrine 1:1000, 30 cc of 1% lidocaine with epinephrine, 30 cc of 0.25% bupivacaine (Marcaine), 10 cc of 8.4% bicarbonate, and 2 cc of hyaluronidase (Wydase, which is no longer available). After 10 minutes, a "lipotryptic" formula of 400 cc of normal saline, 600 cc of distilled water, and 0.25 cc of norepinephrine 1:1000 is injected. Norepinephrine was added to stimulate catecholamine-induced intracellular lipolysis and attract intravascular fluid into the cells. Another compound, verapamil, 2.5 mg, was included to inhibit the cell wall calcium-dependent transport mechanisms. Potassium chloride, 4 mg, was administered to assist in elevating the potassium-sodium gradient and also aid in attracting intracellular fluid. The final ingredient, 2 cc of absolute alcohol, was included to inhibit the cellular-lipid interface and lipid clumping and to assist in dispersion of the fluids. Last, triamcinolone (20 mg) was added to assist in "secondary resolution of edema." "One delightful outcome is the unexpected early shrinkage" of facial skin and subcutaneous fat.[17,18]

Case in point—Ultrasound-induced skin contracture for post–face-lift skin stretching

Experienced plastic surgeons know that a certain percentage of face-lift patients will require a skin "touchup" resection within 1 year of the procedure despite adequate internal repair and resection of the skin. The patient in Figures 3-52 to 3-54 is typical of those who will be expected to need a touchup. Three months after surgery, the jaw lines were clean, and a good contour of the face, eyebrows, and nasolabial areas was obtained with face-lifting and fat grafting. At 4 months, however, the patient reported a hanging band of skin in the submental area with bagging of skin in the nasolabial area and jowl (see Figs. 3-55 and 3-56). She agreed to undergo a series of external ultrasound infiltration procedures rather than skin resection to aid us in evaluating the process. Local anesthetics were infiltrated in February, and a series of external ultrasound applications lasting 5 minutes each were applied for 3 concurrent days. In May, retraction was evident (see Fig. 3-57). Another ultrasound series was applied and gave further improvement (see Figs. 3-58 and 3-59). The position of the tight skin in the lower part of the face has been maintained (see Fig. 3-60).

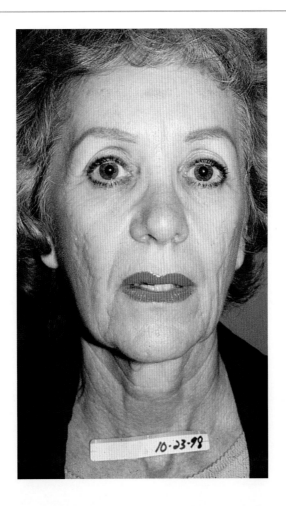

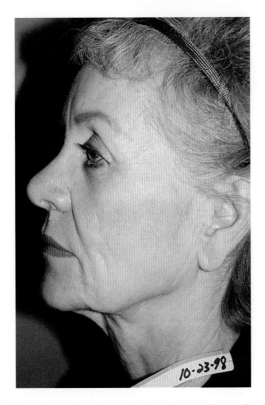 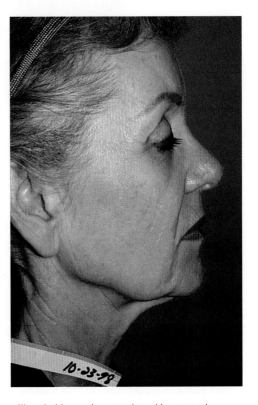

Figures 3-52 – 3-54   Typical face-lift candidate with poor skin quality that will probably require secondary skin removal.

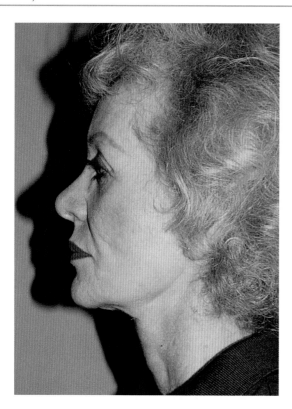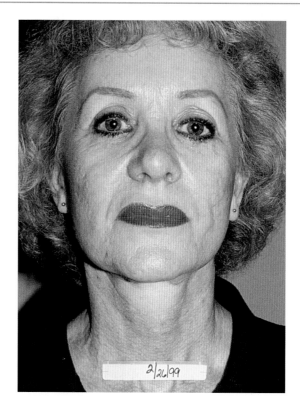

Figures 3-55 & 3-56   *Good contours after face-lift, 4 months postoperatively.*

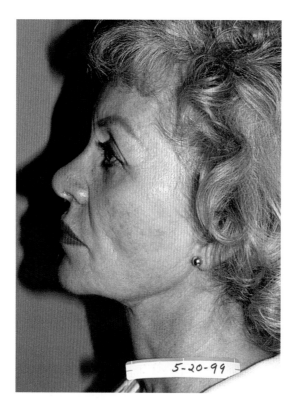

Figure 3-57   *Skin descent of the lower part of the face and neck 7 months postoperative. Normally, a secondary "skin tuck" would be recommended.*

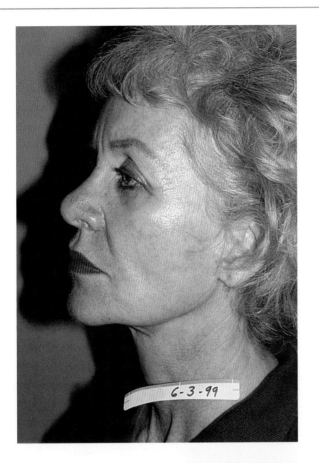
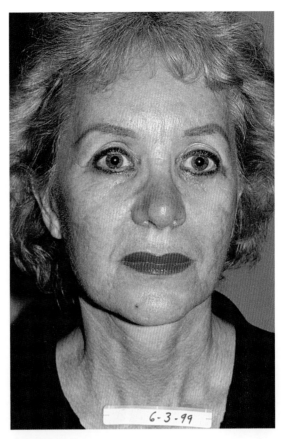
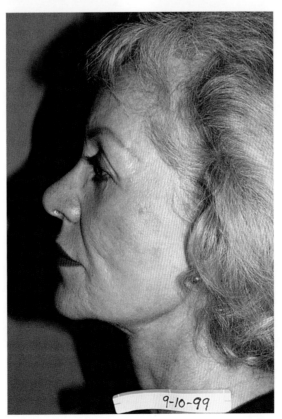

Figures 3-58 – 3-60   *Restoration of contour by the application of ultrasound without skin removal surgery. The reversal was noted by the patient and physician within 1 month of therapy, and the skin continued to regress to the original postoperative contour with ultrasound treatments.*

Case in point—Full-thickness burns from XUAL

Fortunately, only one patient in our experience suffered a significant burn from external ultrasound. When beginning her procedure it was noted that the thin areas of her arms were becoming warm, so the ultrasound time was cut in half. Liposuction of her arms, abdomen, and flanks proceeded without difficulty. In the left flank, a 4 × 8-cm full-thickness burn occurred and required excision and advancement enclosure (see Figs. 3-61 and 3-62). This case illustrates that XUAL is not without risk. An extensive review of this case failed to completely explain this complication. The reduced time of application was obviously insufficient to prevent damage. The operating room technician who applied the ultrasound was experienced. The only explanation was that this individual, who unknown to us was "on medication," was distracted at several points during the application of ultrasound on this side and may have inadvertently applied the energy in a single zone rather than the entire marked area. The lesson learned is that constant attention to the application of ultrasound by trained personnel is the responsibility of the surgeon and that as with all technology, there is no risk-free procedure. Since this single incident in November 1998, there has been no recurrence of second- or third-degree burns.

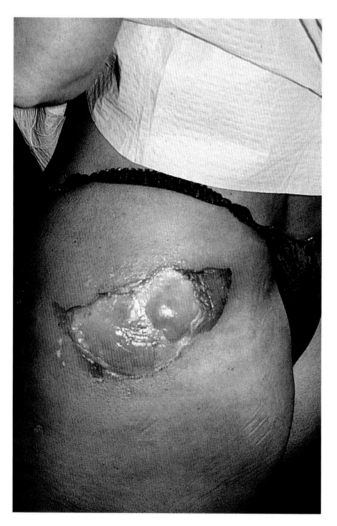

Figure 3-61 *Third-degree burn from ultrasound (see text).*

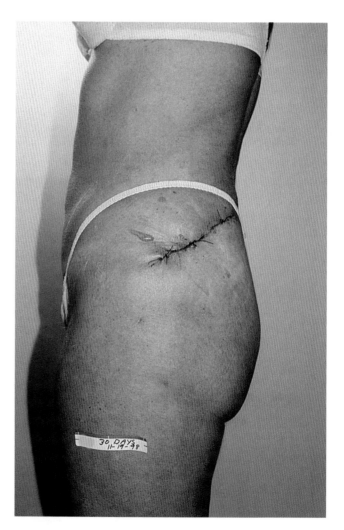

Figure 3-62 *Immediate excision and closure to lessen the impact of this situation.*

Case in point—Patients who bruise still achieve superior body recontouring

This mid-40s white female has fat deposits that are a challenge to the aesthetic surgeon. The flank rolls extend partially toward the midline, and transition areas between the rolls and the midline measured more than 2 cm in thickness (see Figs. 3-63 and 3-64). In addition, the entire buttock area is atrophic with dimpling and generalized concavity. The buttock fold and lateral hip area, though not as overdeveloped in fatty deposits, still require a considerable degree of skin retraction to achieve an acceptable contour. The abdomen exhibits the typical variation in thick zones, but her arms are the greatest challenge (see Figs. 3-65 and 3-66). Adamantly refusing surgical arm reduction, this patient agreed to join one of the first trials of XUAL for the "bat wing deformity."

In her preoperative evaluation she mentioned that she "always bruised." Such was certainly the case as noted from the immediate postoperative photographs (see Figs. 3-67 to 3-69).

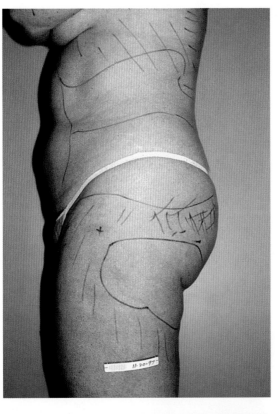
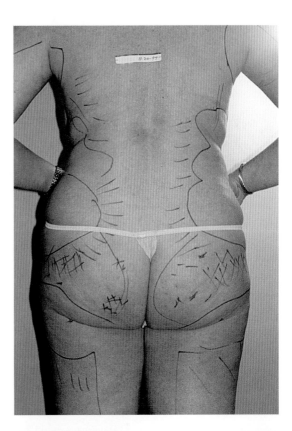
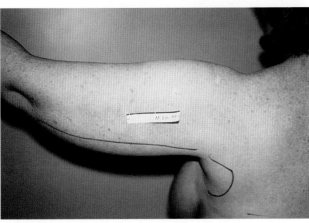
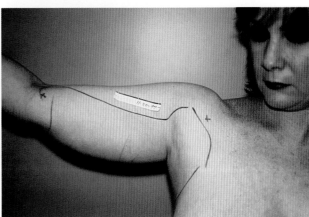

Figures 3-63 – 3-66 *The minimal blood loss associated with XUAL allows comprehensive rejuvenation. These figures show markings for XUAL and regrafts for the entire buttock.*

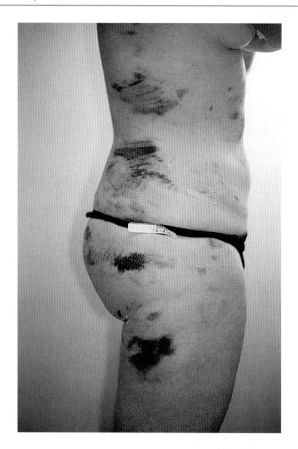
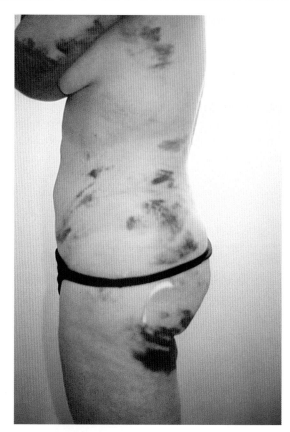
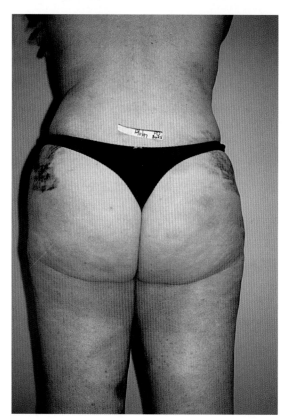

Figures 3-67 — 3-69   *Overall bruising may be genetic or related to medications. The SAL area (left hip) regressed less rapidly.*

As one of the initial volunteers for the evaluation of external ultrasound in body sculpturing, she agreed that one area would be treated solely by standard liposuction. We chose the left buttock area. This area continued to be more tender to the touch, although unbiased observers saw little difference in the degree of bruising. As is often the case, bruising occurs where more superficial liposuction is used, as in her arms versus the buttock or high hip roll areas.

In addition, this patient agreed to volunteer for nonsurgical sculpturing of her face and jowls with a 6-minute application of external ultrasound after infiltration (see Fig. 3-70).

Despite the degree of bruising noted in all areas except the face in the early postoperative photographs, hydrotherapy, massage, early ambulation, and resumption of exercise resulted in rapid clearing in the following 3 weeks (see Figs. 3-71 to 3-74).

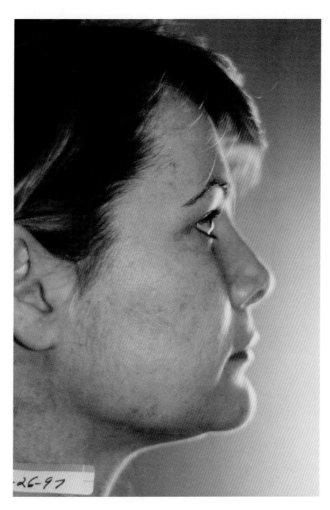

Figure 3-70   *Facial jowls to be treated with ultrasound alone.*

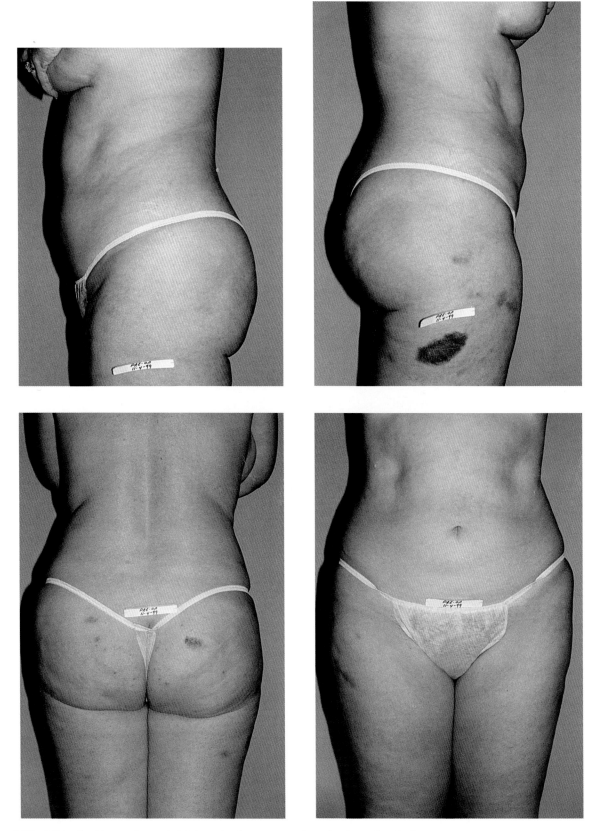

Figures 3-71 – 3-74 *Rapid regression and shrinkage despite an unprecedented ecchymotic episode.*

The 3-month photograph shows remarkable improvement in the upper part of the arms from XUAL and the 6-week period of compression and massage. The thick fatty rolls of the back (which were removed fairly easily after XUAL) also showed regression more rapidly than had been expected based on previous experience. The transition zones in the back regressed as well (see Figs. 3-75 to 3-80).

Comparable patients also had a minimal degree of residual thickening postoperatively, as noted in the out-lines of the inner thigh and the areas below the buttock fold. Note the retraction of the buttock fold, the contouring of the buttock area as a result of multilevel fat grafting, and the shaping of the face despite modest weight gain after surgery. This patient also illustrates that contouring of the face is a progressive ongoing process that can continue, as in this individual, for over 3 months after the initial facial ultrasound application. Contour has been maintained in the face as well as the body.

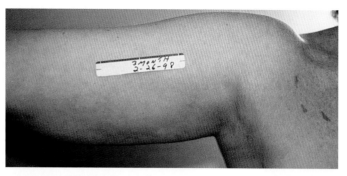

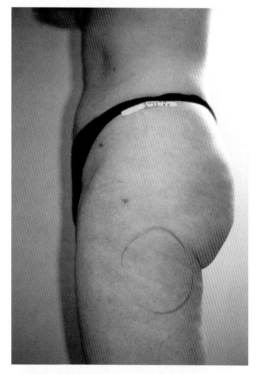

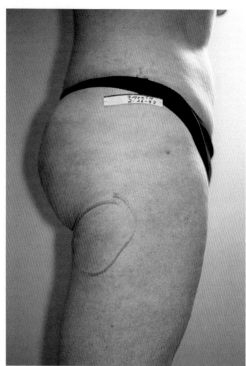

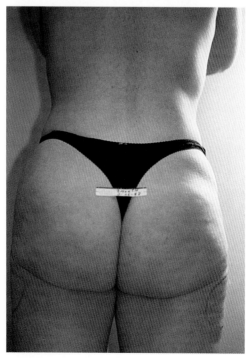

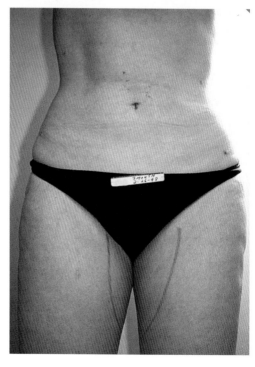

Figures 3-75 – 3-79
Continued shrinkage and remodeling. Marked areas show the only residual edema at 3 months postoperatively. (Refer to Figures 3-34 to 3-37)

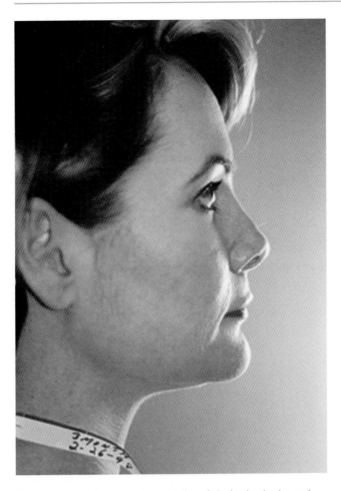

Figure 3-80 *Shrinkage and remodeling of the jowls, cheeks, and neck after a single ultrasound treatment.*

Case in point—Body and facial contouring enhanced by XUAL

One of the initial volunteers in the evaluation of XUAL led an active life. Without pregnancy damage, she could maintain her abdominal muscle contour easily. However, dieting and exercise alone did not reduce the fatty deposits in the inner portion of the thighs, mid-abdomen, and back. Simultaneous XUAL and breast enhancement were planned. In addition, she volunteered to have a single application of XUAL to her face after infiltration of the "super wet" solution.

Preoperative photographs (see Figs. 3-81 and 3-82) show the typical upper thigh deposits that do not respond to exercise and the high center zone of the abdomen fading into lesser fatty area zones in the flanks. The transition areas in the lateral aspect of the flank and back were outlined for treatment with ultrasound alone. The depressed central buttock area is typical of an active female even in this younger age group. This region was enhanced by fat grafting.

Expecting that there would be little improvement over standard liposuction, patients were initially photographed in our study while wearing standard underwear. We were not fully aware that external ultrasound–treated fat is more vulnerable to pressure. We discovered indentations from panty line pressure! Subsequently, all patients undergoing multilevel fat grafting in the high buttock area were instructed to wear thong underwear and bathing attire for a minimum of 4 weeks.

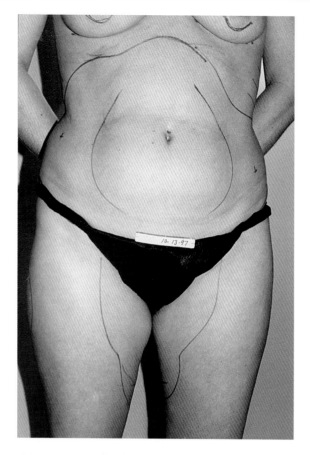
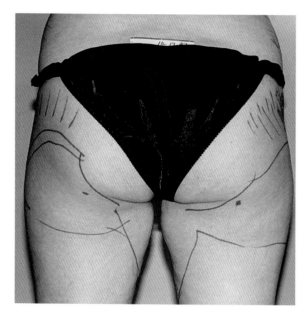

Figures 3-81 & 3-82   *Typical fat distribution that is resistant to diet and exercise in the abdomen and low flank and lower buttock area, with flat mid-buttock fat regression zones.*

This patient was featured in our initial report in the first publication of our trial of XUAL in 1999.[11] The article detailed her rapid recovery, melting of transition-zone fat, and shrinkage of the inner aspect of the thighs, which had not been expected (see Figs. 3-83 to 3-86). As was our custom, our patients in this age group were always advised that standard liposuction of the inner thigh region would leave irregularities. This has not occurred with external ultrasound. Shrinkage in these areas was improved. The appearance as the second month passed is shown in Figures 3-87 to 3-89.

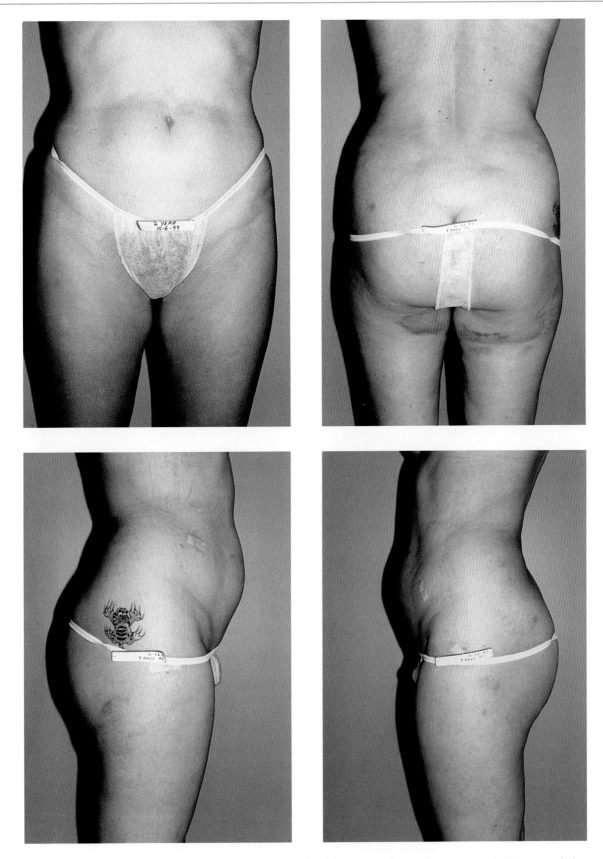

Figures 3-83 – 3-86 *Early regression at 7 days, with SAL performed on the right; XUAL on the left hip, buttock, and abdomen; and ultrasound only on the rippled skin and fat of the flanks.*

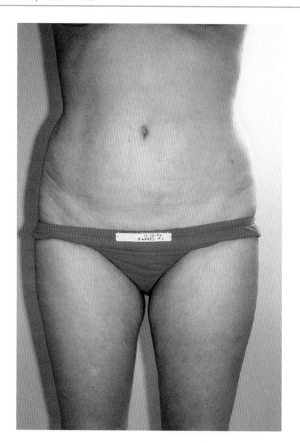
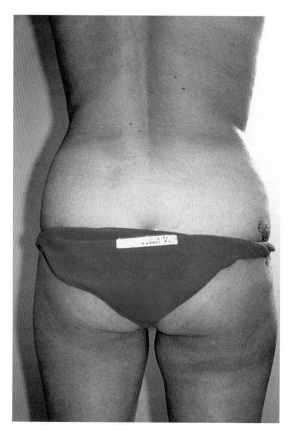
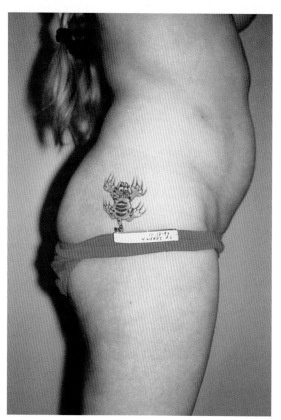

Figures 3-87 – 3-89 *One of the first volunteers for our evaluation of XUAL versus standard SAL agreed to a single ultrasound facial treatment and XUAL of the abdomen, hips, and thighs with buttock regrafting. Further improvement is noted 4 weeks after treatment, more rapidly on the left hip and buttock (XUAL) than the right (SAL).*

After her surgical experience, she returned to her home city where she subsequently married and gained 10 lb. Her fiancé had questioned her about whether she had a face-lift! This patient was presented to visiting plastic surgeons who viewed the preoperative facial photographs (see Figs. 3-90 to 3-92). They also raised the same question. The facial contouring is entirely the result of infiltration and 6 minutes of ultrasound at 30 W applied from the malar prominence to the clavicle. She reported that resolution of the jowl fat and submental fat, as well as the laxity in the skin, was progressive, as noted in the 2-year (see Fig. 3-93) and 3-year (see Figs. 3-94 to 3-96) postoperative photo-graphs. In addition, we noted an unfolding of the nasolabial fold. It was not aided by fat grafting or undermining.

Although the 2- and 3-year photographs indicated that she did indeed gain weight in the mid-abdomen, the overall result was better than we expected judging by the preoperative evaluation of her skin tone, transitional fat, and other factors (see Figs. 3-97 to 3-99). This patient was one of the first to demonstrate that nonsurgical resolution of fatty tissues in the flank could be achieved with external ultrasound and infil-tration alone.

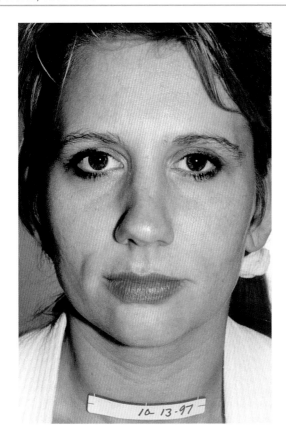
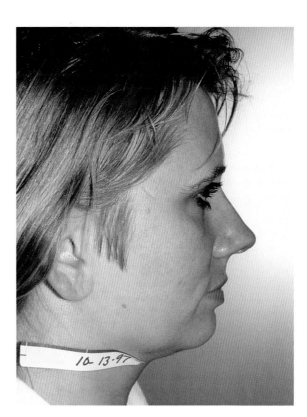

Figures 3-90 & 3-91   *At this point, we needed better photography because XUAL was obviously effective.*

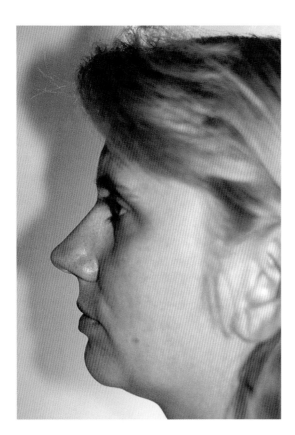
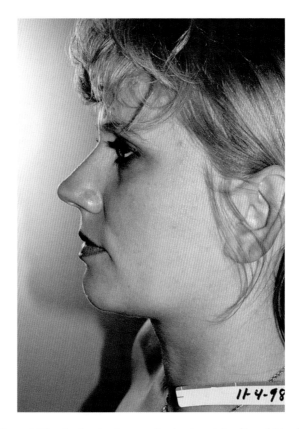

Figure 3-92   Pre-ultrasound view showing moderate skin laxity and prominent jowl, cheek, and neck fat, but no platysmal banding.

Figure 3-93   Contouring 2 years after treatment despite weight gain. Note the "clean" jaw line and regression of the nasolabial folds.

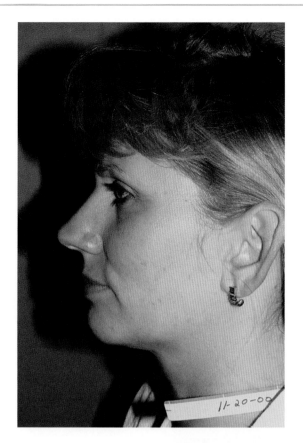
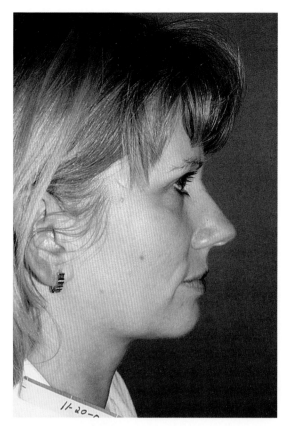
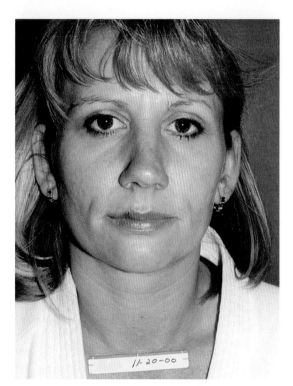

Figures 3-94 – 3-96   Facial contouring at 3 years, with early mid-cheek internal descent, but no recurrence of fat. nasolabial folds.

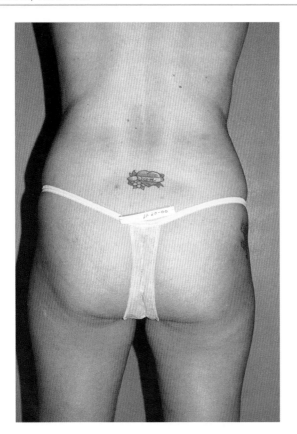
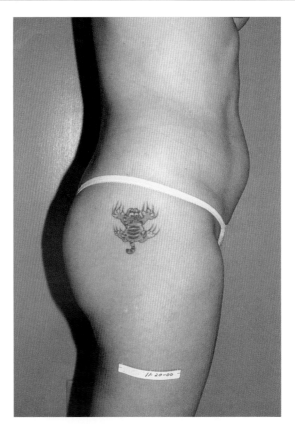
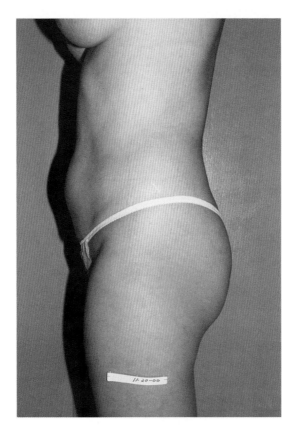

Figures 3-97 – 3-99   *Body contouring at 3 years despite weight gain reflected in the mid-abdomen. Note the smooth flank contour, which is unchanged. No fat was removed from the flanks, which were treated with ultrasound alone.*

Case in point—Continuing flank shrinkage after XUAL

The patient illustrated volunteered to have facial ultrasound without surgery while undergoing XUAL of her abdomen and arms. External ultrasound alone was used in her flank areas. Although she would have been considered a candidate for limited abdominoplasty, the musculature remained taut and the only concern was whether skin shrinkage would be sufficient (Figs. 3-100 to 3-102). A single application of ultrasound to the arms, flanks, abdomen, and face was performed during the surgical procedure. In October 1997, at nearly 3 months (see Fig. 3-100), shrinkage in the flank area was noticeable, but continuation of the shrinkage (see Figs. 3-103 and 3-104) at 1 year occurred despite weight gain. Paradoxically, her left arm increased in size during this time, whereas the right remained the same as postoperatively.

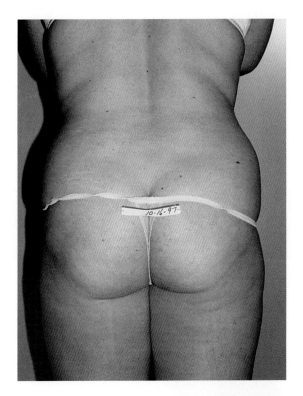
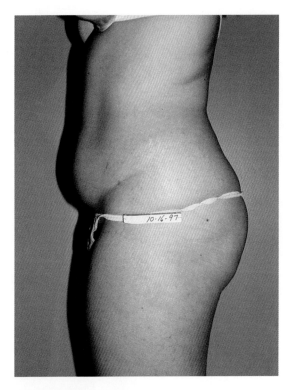
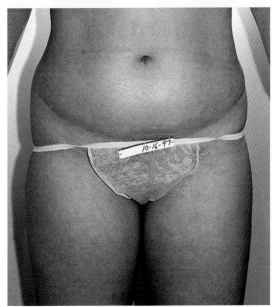

Figures 3-100 – 3-102   Preoperative view of the back and flanks to be treated intraoperatively with ultrasound, no fat removal.

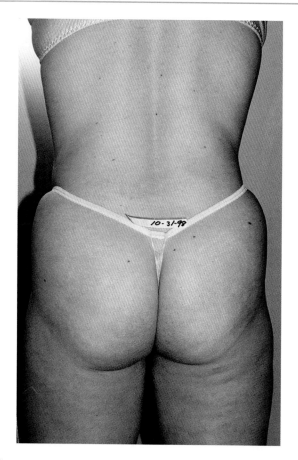 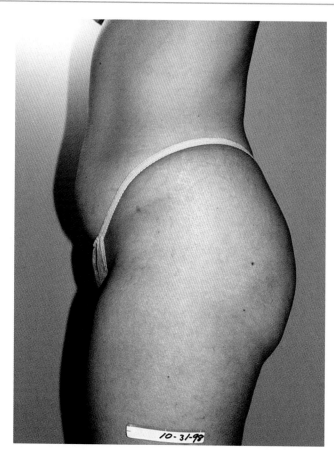

Figures 3-103 & 3-104   *Progressive shrinkage maintained without liposuction.*

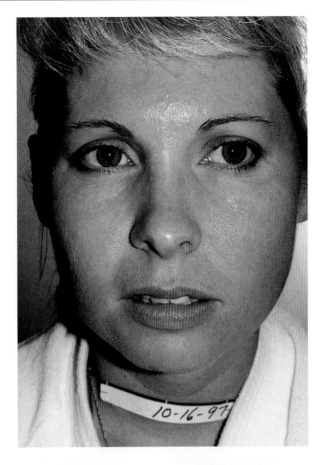

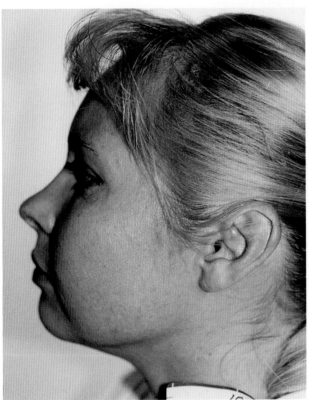
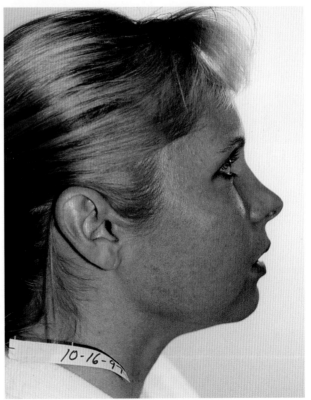

Figures 3-105 – 3-107   *"Moderate" jowl and neck fat and skin laxity before a single external ultrasound treatment.*

The facial photographs show the usual square-jawed full-cheeked individual who is often treated by liposuction and Bichat pad removal (see Figs. 3-105 to 3-107). In the 1-year photograph, despite weight gain, there is still noticeable fullness over the Bichat pad, but retraction of the jowl pads, flattening of the nasolabial fold, and a clear jowl line (see Figs. 3-108 to 3-110).

Many of the patients treated in the initial trials of external ultrasound reported continued shrinkage in XUAL-treated body areas. Facial patients, with and without facial surgery, reported that their faces looked "better" with defined cheek shadowing and cleaner jaw lines in comparison to 1-year photographs. Most patients were photographed for a period of 6 months, and then 1-year photographs were obtained and showed steady improvement, with most occurring in the first 3 months. It is still unclear whether this continuing effect is universal or occurs only in certain individuals, but it is easily documented in this series obtained during the 1997 evaluation period.

Comparison of SAL- and XUAL-derived fat grafts

A secondary face-lift with "double opposing rotations" to free the ear lobe and move hair-bearing scalp into the hairless temple also usually requires resuturing of the anterior and posterior platysma and the cheek SMAS. To achieve a "more natural" appearance, fat grafts play an important role. One such patient is shown (see Figs. 3-111 and 3-112) after several fat grafts to a nonexistent upper lip. The "lip roll" procedure was strongly recommended, but she chose a monthly fat graft approach, even with greater expense. An acceptable shape had been obtained (see Fig. 3-113) before she volunteered for our 1997 teaching seminar. The ultrasound-assisted secondary face-lift and final lip fat graft augmentation provided a pleasing rejuvenation with the lip size she had chosen (see Figs. 3-114 and 3-115). Ultrasound reduced the postsurgical edema, as well as the expected bruising at the fat donor site.

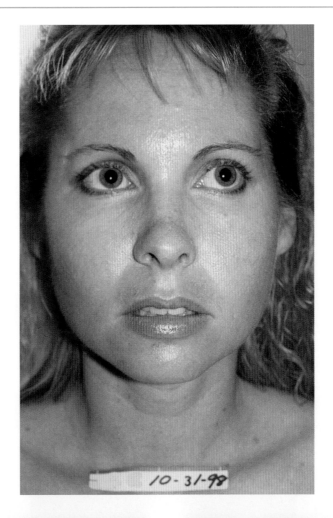

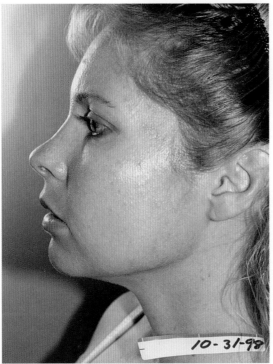

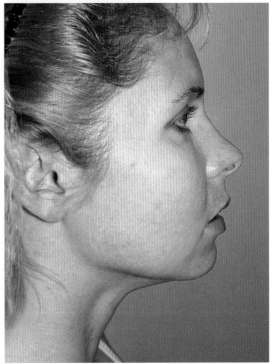

Figures 3-108 – 3-110   *"Improvement" in facial contouring with the noninvasive use of XUAL.*

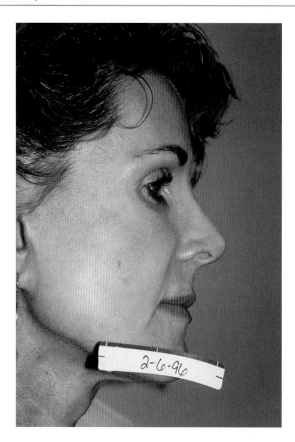
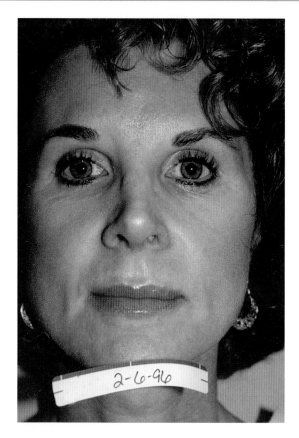

Figures 3-111 & 3-112   *This lady chose a series of autologous fat grafts to her lips and nasolabial folds as a partial correction of an unsatisfactory face-lift.*

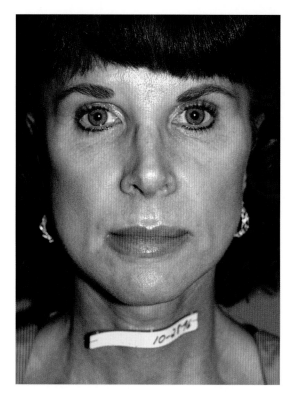

Figure 3-113   *Although the improved lip and depressed area contour are obvious, an XUAL secondary revision face-lift and XUAL-derived fat grafts were scheduled.*

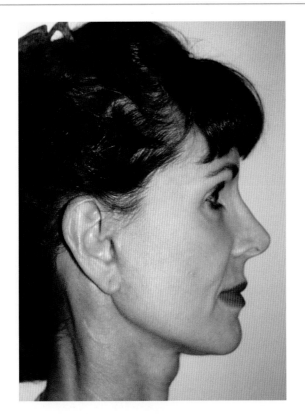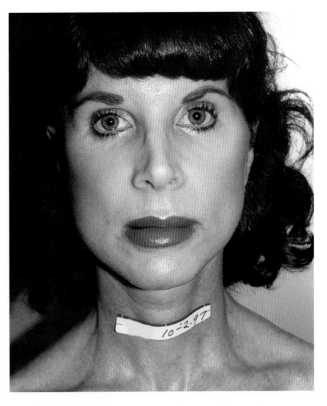

Figures 3-114 & 3-115   *"Double opposing" hair rotation above and behind the ears, along with plication and tailoring, gave this improvement, plus her personal choice of an above-average lip enhancement.*

Summary

All the technical aspects for ultrasound delivery from an external device are quite simple. Failure to observe the guidelines of pressure, timing, and the inevitable question of the appropriate power setting led certain surgeons to believe that XUAL played no role except in the resolution of postoperative edema. Further conversations and presentations in teaching courses by myself, Dr. Barry Silberg, Dr. Stephen Hoefflin, Dr. Gary Rosenberg, and others have convinced most active surgeons that ultrasound does play a role in rapid recovery by "softening" fat for less traumatic extraction by liposuction and assisting in the melting and dissolution of localized fatty deposits in what are termed transition zones. These are areas with little fat but some skin wrinkling, which one would not liposuction because the approach would result in more visible deformities as a result of further irregularity of the overlying skin. With XUAL, these areas have been contoured without surgical intervention as shown in this chapter. Although the plastic surgery community has been slow to accept this concept initially, enterprising surgeons such as W.R. Cook have reported successful application in the dermatologic literature,[19] and further reports appeared in news journals for both specialties.

After 5 years of experience, it can be stated without contradiction that XUAL does play a role in liposuction and, with proper training, skin burns can be avoided, even if one uses a combination of XUAL and PAL or a combination of all three modalities with XUAL used as a "pre-softener." This favorable result may be partly due to the increasing sophistication of delivery systems, as well as discussions in seminars and teaching courses. It will be interesting to see whether the combination of electrical stimulation with external ultrasound (used primarily as separate entities in the cosmetic skin care industries) will be effective in the surgical setting. In our preliminary work we are finding that there are certain advantages to more rapid resolution of facial contours with skin tightening, an effect previously attributed to electrical stimulation alone by the skin care community. We see the same dissolution of small jowl and nasolabial and malar pad fat deposits and perhaps more rapid shrinkage of facial skin.

POWER-ASSISTED LIPOSUCTION

Not every surgeon is an athlete who has not suffered any sports injuries or does not dread a large liposuction case. The advantage of PAL is reduced physical exertion, so the surgeon feels no obligation to hurry the procedure or to perhaps perform less extensive fat removal because of physical fatigue. The original power assist devices were heavier than standard cannulas and powered by a large cylindrical tank of gas. Though noisy, they found favor despite the inconvenience.

CLINICAL PEARL

PAL has improved considerably since the original devices were introduced. Surgeons objected to the weight of the handle and the necessity for moving a heavier instrument just as many times as a standard liposuction cannula, which was lightweight. Others objected to the noise, the bulk of the nitrogen canisters, the heavy cables, and the "general hassle" of getting it to work. The new generation is lightweight, and even disposable handles are a pleasure to use.

Enterprising surgeons in North and South America soon contacted local companies to provide less intrusive PAL devices that still conformed to the original concept of a moving cannula tip that required less physical pressure to advance or to harvest fat from fibrotic areas. This modality is made more acceptable with the development of lightweight handles powered by air pressure from remote pumps.

Surgeons who had been reluctant to use internal ultrasonic assistance for fibrotic and old previously liposuctioned areas soon found that the excursion of PAL allowed them to accomplish similar recontouring— and at a lesser cost! As with XUAL and UAL, the goal of finishing a carefully crafted liposuction procedure without any errors caused by exhaustion was achieved. Combining XUAL and PAL (see Fig. 3-116) has accomplished the goal of rapid and efficient body contouring, our current choice for lengthy procedures.

> **CLINICAL PEARL**
>
> Slow movements with PAL are best to avoid surgical catastrophes! When resistance is encountered, stop—then slowly advance. Let the motion do the work and "fine-tuning."

Although it is not recommended that PAL be used in areas such as the curve of the mandible, where the added trauma would be a disadvantage, PAL is currently in use with smaller cannulas for deeper resections, "fine-tuning," superficial liposculpture in the flank roll, gynecomastia, and previously liposuctioned body or extremity deformities.

> **CLINICAL PEARL**
>
> You may use PAL anywhere on the body where excess fat is present, but be very cautious along the mandibular border and in the cheek areas, where nerve injury or over-aspiration could result. When using PAL on the mandibular border, stay above the platysma and use very fine cannulas.

> **CLINICAL PEARL**
>
> **Gynecomastia with PAL**
>
> Power-assisted lipoplasty does not produce the same concerns regarding the effects of ultrasonic energy on breast tissue, and there is no generated heat that has been responsible for problems in the past. Dr. Leroy Young (plastic surgeon, St. Louis) says that PAL requires less physical exertion because the motion of the cannula powers it through tissue and fibrous bands. Young states the following: "Given my experience in treating gynecomastia, approximately two minutes of power per side is sufficient for aspirating about 120 cc of fat per side. The learning curve is minimal and the results appear to be equal to those of standard liposuction techniques."[20]

> **CLINICAL PEARL**
>
> You must keep the power setting with PAL at moderate levels at first and then work up slowly to higher settings when confidence is gained. There is definitely a learning curve!

Lightweight PAL Systems

The PAL system shown in these photographs is both quiet and lightweight and is powered by air and compression from the standing unit shown in Figure 3-116.

In Figure 3-117, the handpiece is disposable. An advantage is that the length of the excursion with this PAL unit is controlled by a dial system at the surgeon's fingertips. Another advantage of PAL is that the cannula can be curved as shown to reach difficult areas. The PSITEC system shown here incorporates a pressure delivery system for super wet infusion. The device will hold a single 1000-cc bag for smaller cases or a 3000-cc bag. The latter is chosen to avoid the delays of "change out" during an operative procedure.

PAL Liposuction on the Knee

With the nonoperative hand placed over the major knee pad, which may be anterior from the midline to the posterior curve, the knee is initially approached through a small stab wound just beyond the major fat pad (see Fig. 3-117). For smaller fat deposits, 3- or 4-mm PSITEC cannulas are used in a fan-like fashion to completely reduce the fatty deposit. In larger knee surgeries, a second posterior approach with a flat-bladed liposuction device is advantageous. The flat blade will separate more of the skin adhesions and thereby lead to more satisfactory knee shrinkage.

Procedure: How I Do It—Ralph Kloehn (Plastic Surgeon, Milwaukee)

Evolution of an ideal method of body contouring

As the first plastic surgeon in North America to use ultrasonic-assisted lipoplasty, I began my series in February 1990, with gradual progression to my current mode of operation. Since inception of the ultrasonic method, we have operated on 1450 patients, most of whom were female. The last 450 of these patients have undergone a combination of first applying XUAL sequenced by UAL, which produced excellent results but lacked the refining that can be attained with the final use of PAL instrumentation.

My final step, use of an electric reciprocating power cannula, allows for controllable, predictable, and precise fat extraction while being efficient and non-fatiguing. For the last approximately 100 patients in this series, I have combined the use of PAL with XUAL first, UAL secondarily, and last, use of the electric power cannula for the major portion of the debulking and refining.

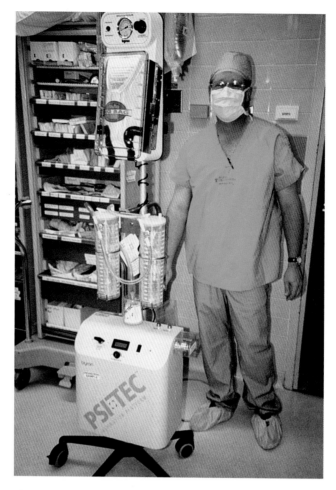

Figure 3-116 *The compact portable PSITEC system (Byron Medical) uses air pressure through a lightweight flexible hose to power a lightweight disposable PAL handle.*

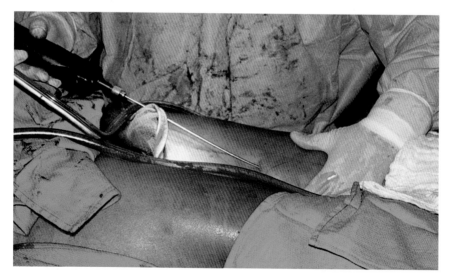

Figure 3-117 *With the nonoperative hand placed over the major knee pad, which may be anterior from the midline to the posterior curve, the knee is initially approached through a small stab wound just beyond the major fat pad. For smaller fat deposits, as in this illustration, 3- or 4-mm PSITEC cannulas are used in a fan-like fashion to completely reduce the fatty deposit. For larger knee surgeries, a second posterior approach with a flat-bladed liposuction device is advantageous. The flat blade will separate more of the skin adhesions, thereby leading to more satisfactory knee shrinkage.*

My first step, the use of a "super wet" infiltration of tumescent fluid, is followed by application of the Silberg XUAL device for a time sufficient to dissipate the local anesthetic and adrenaline. For example, UAL would be applied for 20 to 25 minutes to a moderately obese abdomen and hip rolls.

For my second step, after the XUAL device I briefly use a UAL cannula, usually applying first a solid cannula of the bullet-tipped variety and then a hollow bullet-tipped instrument, each for only minutes to one particular area. For example, we use each paddle for 8 to 10 minutes, or until passage is easy.

The third and final step consists of the use of a bullet-tipped PAL cannula to accomplish the end finishing and contouring. This step takes about 45 minutes of a $2^{1}/_{2}$-hour procedure and yields 75% of the total collected aspirate.

This three-step sequence has reduced my operating time to where I can now perform a major lipoplasty in 40% to 50% less time than it took for conventional lipoplasty techniques in the 1980s. The aspirate has a concentrated appearance with a lighter visual hematocrit than with UAL alone, and no transfusions are required. Postoperative comfort is high, with less bruising, but the most obvious difference is that normalization in contour and appearance is visible in weeks rather than months, thus making patient acceptance of this combination technique extremely high.

Liposuction of the inner thigh

Figure 3-118 shows a helpful technique in liposuction of the inner portion of the thigh, especially when using PAL. After preliminary liposuctioning of fat from the abdominoplasty incision and from the separate stab wound, it is helpful to compress the inner thigh fat with the opposite hand and suction from below. Note the entry point on the opposite leg. This entry point allows access to the pre-marked area of the knee, as well as the inner aspect of the thigh.

One of the advantages of PAL is that the cannula can be manually curved to fit the requirements of the particular case. In Figure 3-119, the cannula has been bent into a curve for access to the posterior portions of the inner part of the thigh. XUAL has been applied to the anterior of the thigh as well as the inner thigh and knee, thereby facilitating fat removal even more. In our experience, PAL and XUAL make the procedure less fatiguing, and as an added bonus, it is easier to gauge the amount of residual fat during sculpturing.

With the PAL cannula in its straight configuration, a portion of the knee fat is addressed in a fan-like pattern

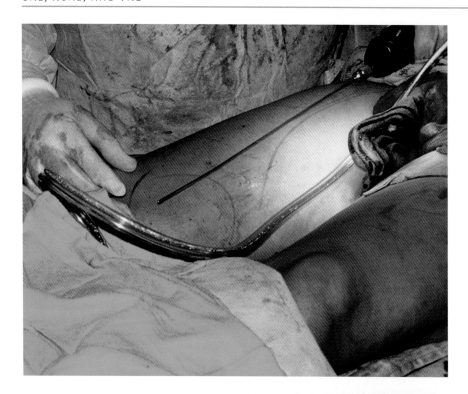

Figure 3-118 *Areas fibrotic from previous liposuction are marked. The PAL tip will be moved very slowly in these areas.*

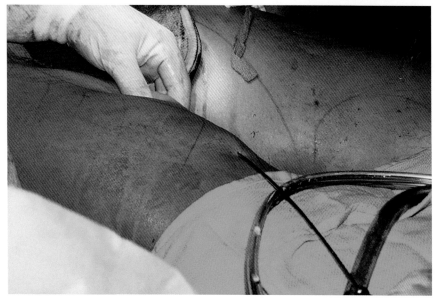

Figure 3-119 *Hand curving of PAL cannulas to this degree before insertion is a useful technique.*

through the entry point noted just above the cannula. Reversing the fan pattern is helpful for larger deposits on the inner aspect of the thigh.

VASER-assisted liposuction is a step-up from PAL in which grooves have been added to the end of the blunt probe to further disperse tip energy so that one encounters less resistance when tunneling through fibrotic fatty tissue. If the VASER is used instead of UAL, there is less likelihood of "end hits" or nerve damage. PAL is then used to remove the oil and complete the procedure. Comparing VASER-assisted liposuction with UAL, Dr. Simeon Wall (plastic surgeon, Shreveport) was

CLINICAL PEARL

A Plea for a Cautious Conservative Attitude
John Kelleher (plastic surgeon, Amarillo) has not had an infection, bleeding hematoma, or skin slough since 1983. He uses a "super wet" technique, 4-mm cannulas for the body, 3- and 4-mm cannulas for the arms, and 2-mm cannulas for the face and neck. His only experience with power assist was the MicroAire electric system. When asked for his opinion, he stated: "I thought the easier penetration was offset by the heavier weight of the handle and the vibration." Because it was not faster or easier and the $6000 cost was a factor, Dr. Kelleher declined use of the machine on subsequent cases.

unconvinced that VASER-assisted liposuction was an improvement in his hands and thought that it was not worth the cost and "learning curve."

Summary

Having served on the faculty of many national conferences that included presentations on improvement of liposuction, it is safe to say that many surgeons who discuss liposuction today include their experience with PAL. There are some concerns with the vibrating tip power assist, but little concern for additional complications with the various power devices that have been on the market for several years. The major improvement was in the surgeon's comfort. The earlier devices, and in fact many devices and many machines that are currently in use, are less popular because of the noise of their operation, the weight of the handle, and the impact on the surgeon, which may interrupt his concentration. Surgeons who began using the MicroAire device are still pleased with its performance, and the problems of noise and vibration are viewed by them as minimal inconveniences. Our experience has been with the newer air-powered machines as discussed in this chapter. Perhaps the most telling was a comment made in the operating room during our first trials of PAL: "Doctor, it doesn't look like you are even working hard; you haven't even broken a sweat!" That certainly was true. Although the disadvantage of PAL is that one cannot collect fatty tissue for re-injection, it is common practice to use syringe liposculpture to collect fat for re-injection into dimples and flat areas on the buttock and complete the procedure with PAL, not only for efficiency but also for speed in execution. As one of my colleagues pointed out to our local hospital staff, the savings in time allotted for liposuction, which reduces the overall cost per case, would more than offset the cost of purchase of the PAL machine.

Fine sculpturing, particularly in the face, requires a more delicate touch, and the lightweight syringe lipo-suctioning technique is the first choice. Pre-softening with XUAL is a valuable addition, and a combination of XUAL and PAL has been beneficial both to patients because of quicker recovery and to surgeons because of less fatigue. Although UAL devices are extremely expensive and require maintenance costs, PAL and XUAL seem to be exempt from these considerations.

References

1. Zocchi M: Ultrasonic liposuction. *Aesthetic Plastic Surgery,* 1992; 16:287-298.
2. Jewell ML, Fodor PB, DeSouza Pinto EB, Al Shammari MA: Clinical application of vaser-assisted lipoplasty: A pilot clinical study. *Aesthetic Plastic Surgery,.* 2002; 22:131-145.
3. Ellenbogen R: Cutting down the workout in liposuction. *Plastic Surgery Products,* 2003; 12:30.
4. Personal communication with Dr. Barry Silberg, 1997.
5. Kloehn RA: Liposuction with "sonic sculpture": Six years experience with more than 600 patients. *Aesthetic Plastic Surgery,* 1996; 16:123-128.
6. Kloehn RA: Rebuttal on ultrasonic liposuction [commentary]. *Technical Forum,* 1997;23:8.
7. Wilkinson T: Ultrasonic liposuction. *Technical Forum,* 1997; 22:2-4.
8. Innovative procedures and new technologies [panel discussion]. *Aesthetic Plastic Surgery,* 1995; 4-8.
9. Wilkinson TS: A simplified technique for obliteration of glabellar frown lines. *Annals of Plastic Surgery,* 1989; 3:341-344.
10. Wilkinson TS: Fat grafting. In: Wilkinson TS (ed): *Practical Procedures in Aesthetic Plastic Surgery.* New York, Springer-Verlag, 1994, pp 47-68.
11. Wilkinson TS: External ultrasound-assisted lipoplasty. *Aesthetic Surgery,* 1999; 19:124-129.
12. Wilkinson TS: New advances to improve outcome in cosmetic surgery. *Key Issues in Plastic Cosmetic Surgery,* 1999; 16:62-90.
13. Wilkinson TS: The role of XUAL in facial contouring. *Technical Forum,* 1998; 24:2-4.
14. Wilkinson TS: New perspectives in facial contouring using external ultrasonography. *New Directions in Plastic Surgery,* 2001; 28:703-718.
15. Wilkinson TS: Ultrasound for capsular contractures. *Technical Forum,* 1986; 9:5.
16. Belo V: Surgeon, patient reap rewards from liposculpture technique. *Cosmetic Surgery Times,* 2000; April:11.
17. Hoefflin SM: The future of liposuction and fat. *Plastic and Reconstructive Surgery,* 1998; 104:1585.
18. Hoefflin SM: Hypotonic pharmacological lipo-dissolution (HPL): A preliminary report and study model. *Perspectives in Plastic Surgery,* 1999; 13:67-84.
19. Cook WR: Utilizing ultrasonic energy to improve the results of tumescent liposculpture. *Dermatological Surgery,* 1997; 23:1207-1211.
20. Young V: Power-assisted lipoplasty. *Plastic and Reconstructive Surgery,* 2001; 108:1429-1432.

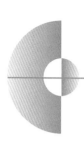

CHAPTER FOUR

Liposuction of the Trunk and Abdomen

Liposuction of the trunk includes the abdomen, the "high hip rolls," the flanks (which may have minimal fatty deposits or major "flank rolls" that extend into the back), and mid-sacral and buffalo hump fibrofatty deposits. Each area presents different challenges and requires different approaches.

The discussion with any patient involves regional anatomy and often whether liposuction should be used as an adjunct to abdominoplasty with skin removal and internal muscle tightening or whether liposuction should be used alone. Before the advent of ultrasonic assist, many patients were denied the latter simply because their skin would not contract. As will be illustrated, the various modalities of aftercare to improve skin contracture and reduce edema, including massage therapy, lymphatic drainage, and postoperative external ultrasound (XU), have allowed a choice for many patients who may benefit greatly from ultrasound-assisted liposuction (UAL) and yet may later choose to have a "flat tummy" that is afforded in their particular case only by abdominoplasty. This procedure has been modified in great detail since my 1975 presentations on the short-scar incision. Even with larger patients and larger fat deposits, the extensive use of liposuction of all types with abdominoplasty has reduced the need for extended incisions in most cases and has been used as an adjunct in achieving "aesthetic abdominoplasty." Liposuction is used to create the midline groove, re-create the lateral muscle depressions, and more importantly, reduce fatty tissues beyond the short incision to enhance contracture and smoothing.

It must be noted that with all procedures a certain number of patients will require "touchups." These touchups may include extra skin excisions after a period of 6 months, usually laterally, and secondary liposuction after abdominoplasty, as well as all cases in which patients have regained weight.

> **CLINICAL PEARL**
>
> Remember that the intra-abdominal fat that is routinely seen in males and near-menopausal women will contribute significantly to the appearance of the abdomen. This fat has a lower metabolic rate than subcutaneous fat does. It responds slowly to diet and exercise.

THE ABDOMEN

Patient Selection

The abdomen presents its own unique challenges. Contracture of the skin varies from individual to individual and is based on gender (men's abdomens contract to a greater degree), pregnancy (the severely damaged "stretch mark" skin of the lower part of the abdomen will contract very little), and the question of whether the patient's needs are best served by abdominal repair.

Liposuction of the abdomen has been the model for success in superficial liposuction and XUAL, both of which are designed to provide skin contracture to avoid the requirement of skin excision. Although many patients' skin will contract quite well, the *surgeon's decision and the patient's acceptance must include a careful analysis of all factors.* For patients requesting a completely flat abdomen, a limited abdominoplasty combined with liposuction is recommended. In patients with similar deformity but who for some reason reject the more extensive procedure, the addition of XUAL and UAL and/or superficial liposuction to reduce redundancy of the skin in the postoperative period will change the approach to the problem. *Patients who were once rejected for liposuction alone may achieve satisfactory results with the addition of these modalities.* Because the thickness of the panniculus varies, surgeons choose larger cannulas for the lower levels and 3- to 4-mm cannulas of various design for the upper levels and superficial liposuction, but only in certain individuals (see Figs. 4-1 to 4-3).

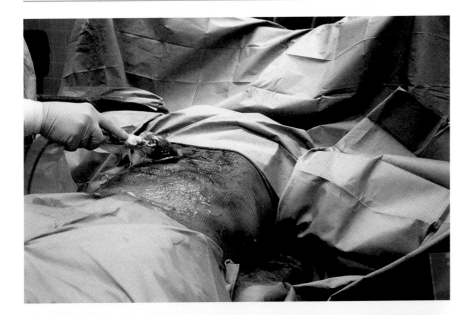

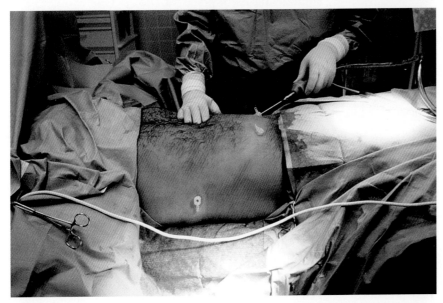

Figures 4-1 & 4-2 *Multidirectional liposuction using 4-, 5-, and even 6-mm cannulas reduces the midline bulk above the umbilicus, adding XUAL and UAL.*

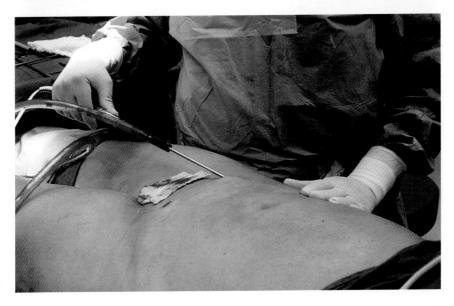

Figure 4-3 *Lateral skin and fat overhang areas respond well to deep and superficial liposculpture.*

As discussed in the chapter on superficial liposuction, this approach is fraught with danger and is certainly not to be universally applied. Separating the two procedures, abdominal repair and liposuction, may be in the best interest of certain patients, particularly those with larger fatty deposits or marginal health. Surgeons who accept patients for abdominal recontouring must be fully cognizant of the possibility of a hidden umbilical, spigelian, or ventral hernia, which would be perforated with disastrous consequences, as well as counseling of patients who mistakenly believe that a contoured abdomen will result from liposuction alone although *their anatomy dictates* the use of combined procedures.

CLINICAL PEARL

Dr. Yves-Gerard Illouz' suggestion of skin resection after liposuction of the abdomen is an easily misused concept. At a recent international meeting, a patient who really needed muscle repair underwent the Illouz skin resection with liposuction. Yes, there were big folds everywhere. If one must remove skin, use this as access for fascial plication! Remember that very few people have only a small amount of fatty tissue, no stretching of the underlying musculature, and only a small amount of excess skin in the lower part of the abdomen (see Figs. 4-4 and 4-5).

With our experience in performing XUAL, we are finding that laxity in the upper part of the abdomen will respond to a series of ultrasound sessions applied for 15 minutes to the abdomen in the operating room and for 10 minutes to the upper part of the abdomen on the second, third, and fourth days postoperatively. Such treatment eliminates the need for excessive stretch to smooth out the wrinkling above the umbilicus, as well as the need for separating and resetting the umbilicus.

Abdominal aesthetic units

Dr. Luiz Toledo, Dr. Alan Matarasso, and I have presented teaching courses on prevention of complications in abdominoplasty for about 15 years. In an effort to quantify and correlate anatomy with procedures, Dr. Matarasso has proposed that the abdomen be viewed as individual aesthetic units, especially in patients for whom liposuction is a better choice than liposuction combined with abdominal repair (see Fig. 4-6). Note that one must not neglect the mons, flank, or sacral fat deposits. The dorsal rolls ("flank" and "high hip roll") may regress with dieting in patients for whom lower abdominal fat is resistant to the effects of diet and exercise. Planning the liposuction with an overview of aesthetic units allows the surgeon to approach each individual in a calculated and careful manner.

Anesthesia

For healthy young adults who have failed to lose abdominal fat with diet and exercise, such as those shown in Figures 4-4 and 4-5, intravenous sedation is the safest, most convenient, and most cost-effective method of anesthesia for performing liposuction. With premedication and sedation, the anxiety and pain are eliminated or at least modified to a degree such that there is no longer hypertension, "emotional flashback," or more practically, the patient telling everyone in your city what a painful experience she underwent at the hands of a heartless brute! By using the current pump techniques, the abdomen and flank area can be infiltrated with "super wet" (1:1) solution in 2 to 3 minutes, which is the pain-free window of opportunity afforded by intravenous propofol, ketamine, or other short-acting barbiturates of choice. One should avoid heavy oral premedication because of the wide variation in individual response. A somnolent patient with depressed respiration is not desirable.

Instruments

For all but extremely large individuals, suction-assisted lipectomy (SAL) and XUAL with curved and straight 3- and 4-mm cannulas will effect deep and perhaps even superficial liposuction. Superficial suction should be avoided in all but ideal candidates—in other words, those with minimal excess skin, healthy young bodies, and a limited area of application, as well as the capacity to follow postoperative instructions to avoid excessive compression or damage to the more vulnerable superficial liposuction areas. For the deeper areas, where multihole cannulas are more efficient, open-tipped cannulas such as the "Mercedes" may be used. For final smoothing in certain areas, a flat-bladed cannula that breaks up more tissue adherence can be used, especially to create the midline "champagne groove." Entry through the umbilicus affords the development of a subcutaneous pocket from passage of the flat-bladed cannula with the suction hole downward. This technique can be performed with machine or syringe technology. To further create the visible mark, the cannula can then be turned upward and several passes made directly adjacent to the subcutaneous fat at the dermal level. This procedure would be unwise in other areas.

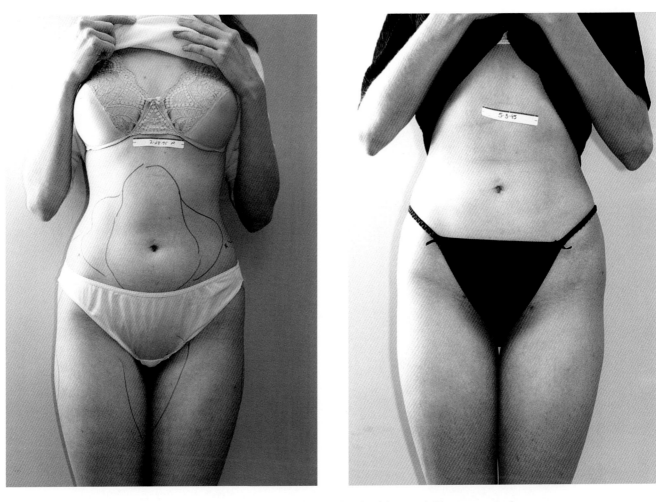

Figures 4-4 & 4-5 *The ideal liposuction patient is an athletic nulliparous female with natural skin contracture after surgery.*

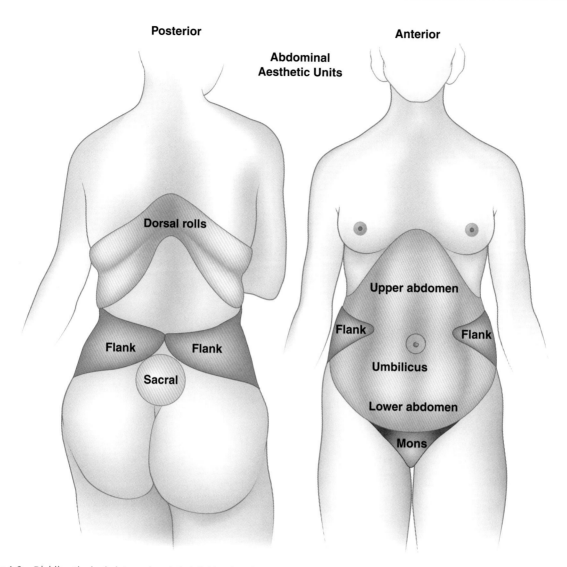

Figure 4-6 *Dividing the body into regions is helpful in planning procedures and in patient education, as in this composite prepared by Dr. Alan Matarasso.*

Lateral grooving can be created in the same way, but with a lesser degree of suctioning and without the component of subdermal suctioning. Fanning the flat-bladed cannula from within the umbilicus can be useful in recalcitrant midline deposits because it produces a degree of skin separation that is not afforded by standard round cannulas.

CLINICAL PEARL

The practice of liposuction on the West Coast is certainly different from that in the Midwest. John Emery (plastic surgeon, Sonoma) deals mainly with people who have "a bulge here or there rather than obese people." Correction is more exacting, but less fatiguing. Standard wet techniques with hand-held cannulas give him his best results. In the initial debulking, the full vacuum of the liposculpture syringe is used. For final refinement, however, one may increase or decrease the pressure of the syringe plunger, depending on whether the refinement requires more or less fat removal, by placing a thumb against the end of the syringe. Another advantage is that if overcorrection has occurred, it is possible to simply release the pressure and put the fat back into the depressed area. Light massage of the area with the left hand guides the redistribution.

Procedures

Staying out of trouble—Simon Fredricks, M.D. (plastic surgeon, Houston)

I think that the "super wet" technique magnifies the space to be aspirated of fat. Therefore, it is both mechanically easier to perform and less laborious, as well as a hedge against overcorrection leading to surgically created deformities. Whenever I see a *large* disproportionate hip, outer thigh, buttock, or belly accumulation, I counsel the patient that a two-staged procedure may be needed to allow overlying skin shrinkage to occur between stages. Furthermore, the possibility exists that secondary skin resection may be required.

CLINICAL PEARL

Pulmonary embolism is really rare, thank goodness, and it is always associated with large-volume SAL (over 2000 cc), hypovolemia, and inactivity.

As described by Rohrich, I believe that the zones of skin adherence where a minimal amount of deep fat is present should either never be entered or be entered very carefully with very small cannulas. These are the areas where surgically created deformities occur most frequently and are very difficult to correct. I think that awareness of these aesthetically problematic areas is a signal contribution to minimizing surgeon-created deformities.

"Thunder thighs" require circumferential suctioning, and the anterior of the thigh especially must be addressed with small cannulas from a port in the crease between the thigh and pubis. Gentle, slow strokes are required to avoid tearing the subdermal fat away.

I prefer to approach the calf and ankle from two ports on either side of the Achilles tendon with the patient prone, followed by appropriate and prolonged mild to intermediate compression. I believe that therapeutic postoperative spandex-type girdle compression for 6 weeks is beneficial in resolving operative edema and holds tissues in the proper relationship for aesthetic molding. Finally, I have no doubt that therapeutic postoperative ultrasound treatment reduces discomfort and edema and aids in molding the tissue to a smooth aesthetic contour.

CLINICAL PEARL

Remember that a liter of lactated Ringer's solution contains 24 fewer milliequivalents of sodium than a liter of normal saline solution does. In large-volume liposuction, this difference could be significant in avoiding overload.

Trunk liposuction with fat regrafting

A certain number of patients who would benefit from a lower or "limited" abdominoplasty decline this procedure because of cost, fear of complications, fear of pain, or time limitations for recovery. In planning these procedures, it is helpful to suggest that the mid-buttock depression be filled at the same time. Markings show the areas of thicker fat deposits in the mid-abdomen, extension into the flanks, lesser deposits in the upper part of the abdomen, and the typical inner thigh fat deposits that extend to the posterior aspect (see Figs. 4-7 to 4-10). Although she does not have a prominent "banana roll," a separate entry dot is marked in the lateral portion of the buttock fold for approach to the inner aspect of the thigh. These entry points are the same as those for "super wet" infiltration. Even if the entry points are small, they are *placed asymmetrically,* and an additional entry point is planned for the regrafting procedure, as well as entry into the high hip and thigh deposits.

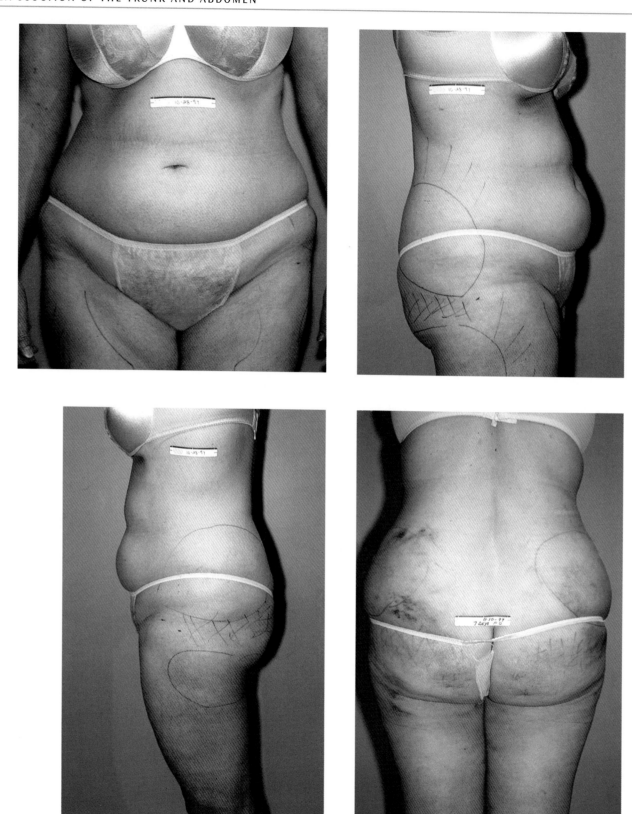

Figures 4-7 – 4-10 Typical middle-aged woman with skin irregularity and fat deposits who refuses abdominoplasty.

CLINICAL PEARL

In any patient, skin discoloration may persist at 4 months in the "banana roll" area if superficial liposuction was performed. In addition, a small amount of infolding may occur in this region as a result of edema. XUAL with massage will correct most of these cases if combined with "tincture of time." Skin bleaching creams may help. Consider secondary infiltration of the area, XUAL, and cannula removal of small amounts of residual fat if the problem is not corrected. In this patient, XUAL alone was applied to the pre-marked areas even though there was little, if any fat in these transition areas above the high hip rolls.

CLINICAL PEARL

According to a recent review of so-called ab-strengthening machines, if a patient has more than $1/8$ inch of fat on the abdomen, the natural rectus sheath "etching" depressions will be obscured. In addition, ordinary individuals cannot achieve this highly publicized abdominal contour unless they are genetically engineered to deposit fat elsewhere and are willing to use extreme dieting in conjunction with exercise. The article went on to say that the most effective exercise was the "bicycle maneuver," as well as "crunches." However, all the machines and attachments that are hawked on television infomercials are at best slightly better than standard exercise. We plastic surgeons know that *dieting and exercise are both important in our liposuction patients, yet we are willing to create etching shadows by superficial liposuctioning.* A flat-edged cannula with a relatively wide opening is first passed with the hole facing downward in the superficial subcutaneous fat and then upward to remove fatty tissue attached to the dermis and to the midline and the etching line. Because this maneuver is confined to the marked areas, there is little or no danger of interruption of the blood supply with its consequences.

Six months after the procedure, resolution of the postsurgical edema is apparent, particularly in the inner thigh and high hip rolls seen at 7 days; note especially the right high hip area that was not pretreated with ultrasound (see Fig. 4-10). Fat grafting has eliminated the shadows in the mid-buttock. Although there will be some continued resolution of the residuals in the mid-abdomen, this patient found the reduction in the fatty panniculus to be an adequate procedure for her and has not requested abdominoplasty for a "flat tummy" (see Figs. 4-11 to 4-13).

The guiding hand

Perhaps in no other area of the body is the guiding opposite hand so important. Fat deposits may extend above the rib margin, and the cannula must be torqued to get above the ribs. Using the flat of the hand to *press the ribs downward* allows free passage of cannulas from several directions. The opposite hand is also needed to *judge how much fatty tissue is left in place* (see Fig. 4-14). Over-resection is to be avoided at all costs, yet a too cautious undercorrection leads to justifiable patient anger and disappointment. Experienced surgeons can judge the degree of skin excess, assess muscle separation, and quantify the degree of contracture that can be achieved before advising the patient on the best course of action.

CLINICAL PEARL

Dr. Bruce Nadler (Smithtown), himself an amateur bodybuilder competitor, does the "abdominal etching" procedure in many of his patients. The umbilical and midline incisions are left unsutured to allow drainage and minimize scrotal swelling and ecchymosis in males. Other incisions are closed with 6-0 cat gut. A layered dressing with a pattern to fit the etching encourages enfolding of the skin. Within 6 to 12 weeks, the "defined look" becomes evident.

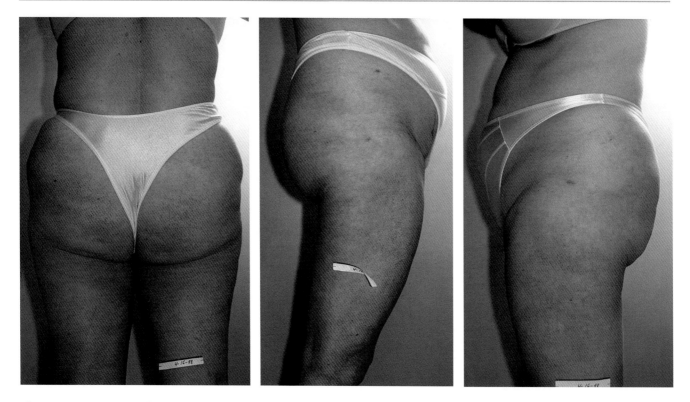

Figures 4-11 – 4-13   *XUAL-induced skin contracture in the suctioned areas and nonsuctioned upper back region.*

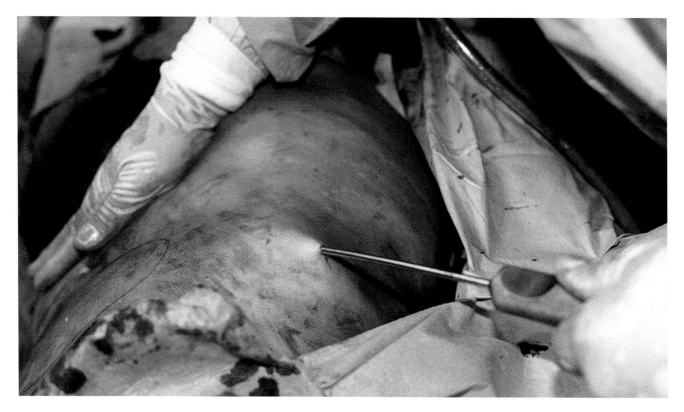

Figure 4-14   *Use of the curved "Mercedes"-tipped cannula and hand palpation to evaluate depth allows sculpture of the posterior of the hip without completely repositioning the patient on the operating room table.*

Helpful technical maneuvers to the bulky abdominal fat area

In Figure 4-15, note that the entry point has been made just below the *pre-marked high bulge* of the mid-abdominal fat pad. With the opposite hand in position and the "super wet" solution in place, suctioning from the midline proceeds in a *fan-like pattern both superficial and deep.* Note that the area has been coated with povidone-iodine (Betadine). This central area will also be approached from both sides to perform a triple crossing maneuver to reduce the fat with 3- and 4-mm cannulas.

Figure 4-16 shows the introduction of one such cannula through an umbilical incision placed in the upper portion under the umbilical overhang. This fan-like liposuctioning from the left across the center to the right is then extended downward into the flank to join the areas that will be approached through the marked spot shown in the lateral body fold.

Liposuction is completed by establishing the "champagne groove." The flat-bladed cannula is intro-duced through the umbilical incision and first advanced with the suction opening downward and then upward to reduce fat under the dermis.

Choosing liposuction rather than abdominoplasty with liposuction

The appeal of liposuction is the rapid recovery, the minimal and practically invisible pinhole incisions, and the eternal hope that once fatty deposits are removed, an exercise program will produce previously unobtainable results in abdominal wall tightening. Figures 4-17 to 4-19 show one of the initial volunteers who underwent XUAL of the abdomen and the high hip roll. Fat was regrafted in multiple levels into the flatter areas and the dimpling marked by "XX" in the buttock area. In addition, a relatively thick upper flank roll was desig-nated as a test zone for XUAL. *Fat was not physically removed in this area.* The face and upper part of the flank were treated with infiltration and a single application of XUAL.

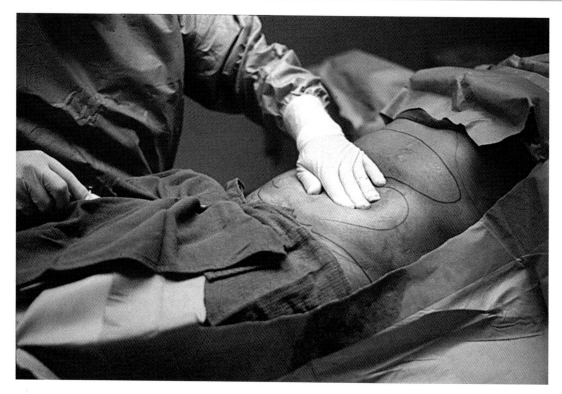

Figure 4-15   *Redirectional cannula placement from the opposite side for uniformity.*

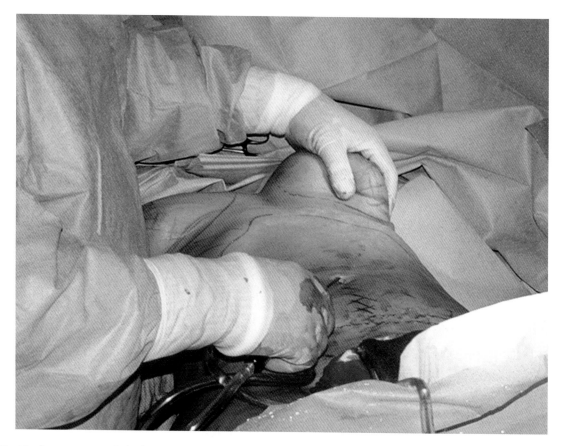

Figure 4-16   *The "super wet pump" via the umbilical stab wound is also used to develop the submammary space for breast augmentation. With the implant protected by the surgeon's hand on the breast, a cannula reduces the fat roll in the submammary fold.*

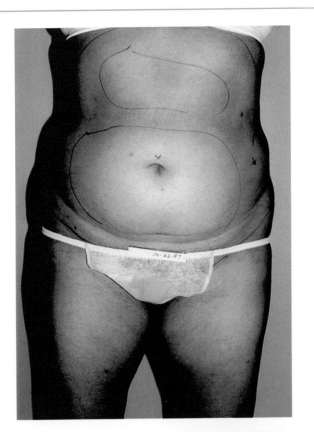
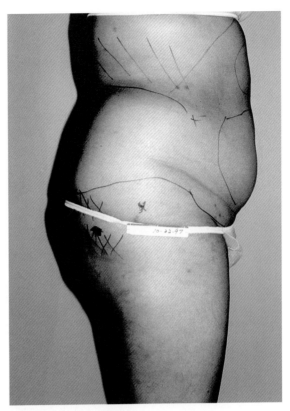
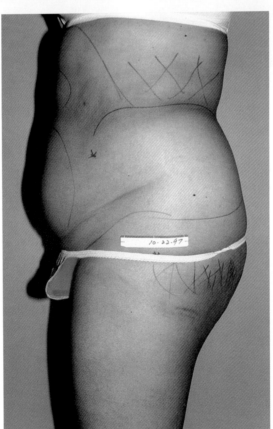

Figures 4-17 – 4-19   *Drawings delineate areas for XUAL (circles) and infiltration alone for external ultrasound with fluid infusion (XU) (vertical lines).*

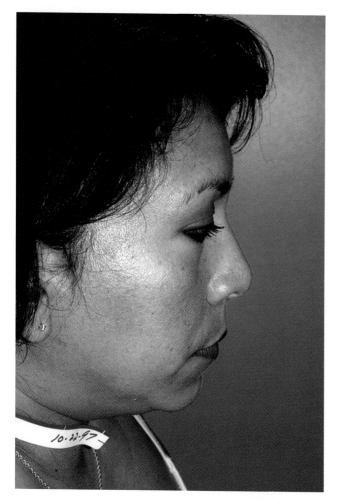

Figure 4-20 *This patient volunteered for ultrasound of the face and neck in preference to internal plication and skin excision.*

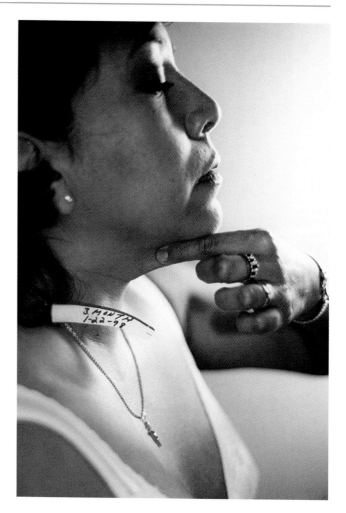

Figure 4-21 *The submental deep and superficial fat pads were dissolved with a single 6-minute facial surgery treatment.*

This patient exhibits the typical female problem of mid-abdominal fat 3 to 4 cm in thickness, a 2-cm upper abdominal fat pad, and gradual transition of lesser deposits in the mid-back. Her face showed the typical mid-face descent with fatty deposits above and below the platysma (see Fig. 4-20). Cost constraints led her to refuse facial surgery. She agreed to participate to see whether our initial evaluation of ultrasound was correct and could produce acceptable facial changes. The post-operative view (see Fig. 4-21) shows that although residual laxity is still present in the central portion of the neck, the mid-face has retracted. No fat is found on

a "pinch test" of the anterior part of the neck. The platysma is still prominent and can be addressed at a future date.

Postoperative photographs obtained at 3 months (see Figs. 4-22 to 4-25) show rapid resolution of the fatty rolls in the back, good contouring of the depressed areas of the buttocks (see Figs. 4-25 and 4-26), and improvement in the mid-abdomen. This improvement has been satisfactory, and the patient has not requested abdominoplasty for complete retightening and re-establishment of a waistline.

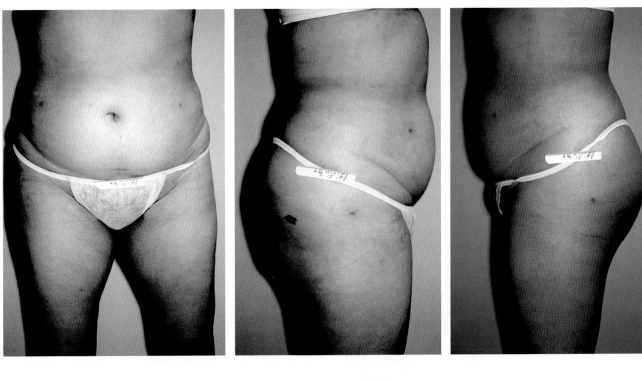

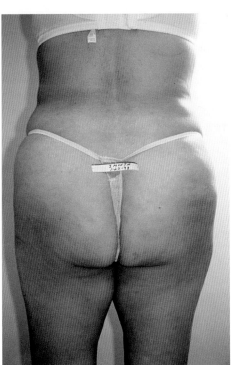
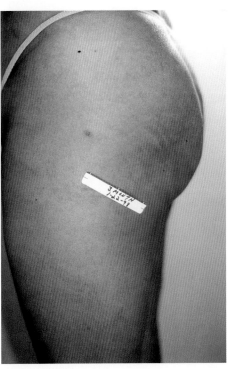

Figures 4-22 – 4-38 *Patients who truly believe that exercise can restore abdominal musculature benefit from XUAL alone. Note the XX markings for fat regrafting (Fig. 4-30) and the imperfect, but acceptable restoration of contour because of a limited quantity of available fat for regrafting.*

Liposuction as an alternative to limited abdominoplasty

This mid-40s patient desired only modest correction of her abdominolipodystrophy that included correction of the inner portion of her thighs, the outer hip area, and the high hip roll, as well as her abdominopanniculus (see Figs. 4-27 to 4-30). With the assistance of XUAL, liposuction was performed in these areas without repair of the abdominal musculature. Figures 4-31 to 4-34 show early contracture of the skin laxity 2 weeks after XUAL. *Fat that was grafted into the mid-buttock has restored the contour.* As one condition of her participation in the initial XUAL study, the left hip roll was removed with standard liposuction and all other areas were pretreated with XUAL. The bruising (and tenderness) shown in Figure 4-34 was in sharp contrast to the absence of significant bruising and general comfort on palpation of the opposite side (see Fig. 4-33). Photographs taken at 3 weeks (see Figs. 4-35 to 4-38) show further resolution with evidence of residual edema in the left high hip roll. Contracture of the skin over the abdomen has progressed and has thus provided *satisfactory correction with minimal recovery time.*

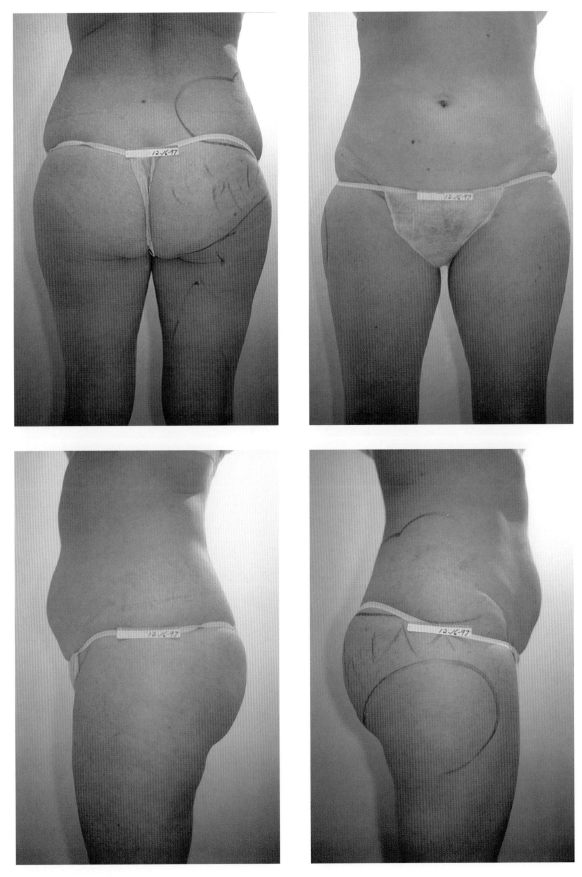

Figures 4-22 – 4-38 Continued

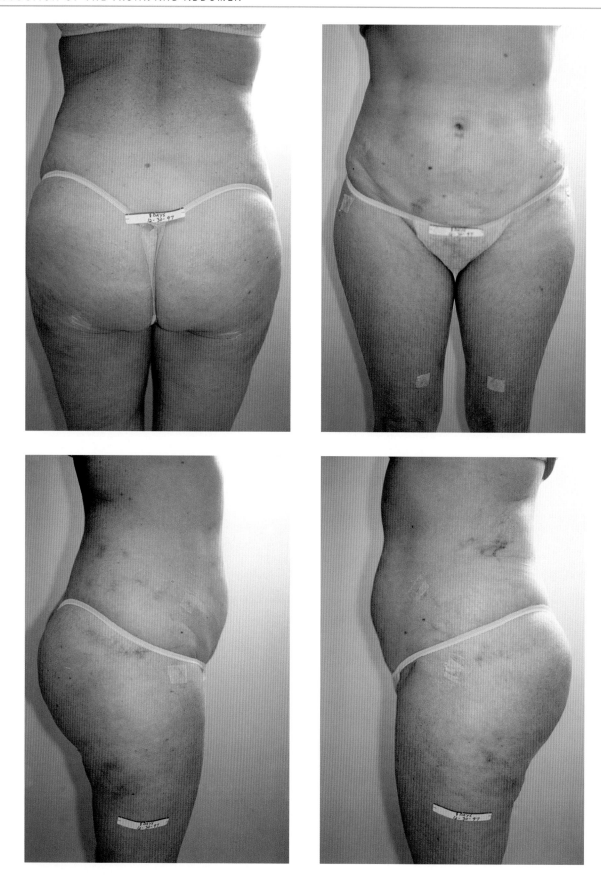

Figures 4-22 – 4-38   *Continued*

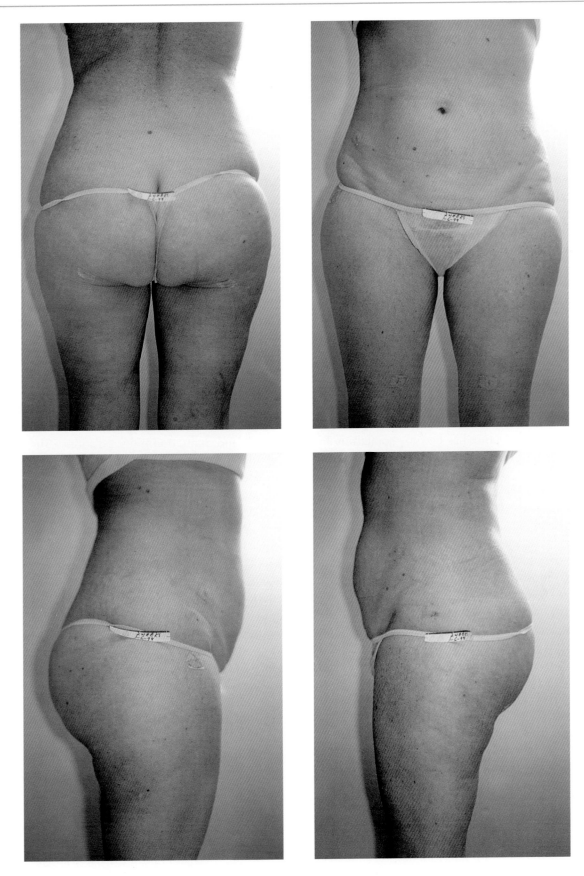

Figures 4-22 – 4-38 *Continued*

Revision of an abdominoplasty with liposuction

The patient in Figures 4-39 to 4-41 is pictured after weight gain that had increased the thickness of the abdominal panniculus and resulted in new fat deposits in her arms and the inner part of her thighs. In January 1998, the initial studies of the effect of XUAL were just beginning. It was proposed to this patient that we attempt to shrink the abdomen with XUAL and no skin excision. She was made aware of the failures of liposuction without excision in the past and that excision might be required in the future.

This patient was the first of many in whom we *avoided major skin excision by inducing skin shrinkage with an ultrasound assist*. After 15 minutes of XU, liposuction was performed in the red areas and then minor skin excision with the internal repair. The previous abdominoplasty, which had included standard liposuction, did not produce this effect. We were able to achieve satisfactory shrinkage by 3 months (see Figs. 4-42 to 4-44) that has been maintained to the present day.

Abdominal etching—Bruce J. Nadler, M.D. (cosmetic surgeon, Smithtown)

An athletic muscular body has become something for which both young men and women strive. One of the things that typifies that physique is the so-called six-pack or well-defined abdominal muscles. Yet many of these determined exercise buffs remain frustrated as they try to achieve this look. No matter how many sit-ups, crunches, or leg lifts they do, an adipose blanket over these areas hides the fruit of their hard labor.

Standard liposuction techniques uniformly remove the adipose tissue and can thin the fatty deposits over the abdomen but will not give the defined look that many seek. Enter the concept of abdominal etching. I have used it with equal success to achieve definition of the deltoid and latissimus dorsi muscles. The procedure has undergone a period of refinement. Although it was possible with standard liposuction cannulas, the advent of power-assisted liposuction (PAL) allows it to be performed with minimal scarring. I favor the MicroAire system because the excursion of reciprocation allows me to sculpt the inscriptions of the muscle from a distant site. In this manner, no scarring higher on the surface of the abdomen is necessary.

As with any liposuction procedure, the patient is marked in the standing position, with areas of lipomatous excess being outlined. From a seated position, additional areas of folding and fullness are marked. The patient is then instructed to lean to the left and right to discover any lateral folding of the trunk and then asked to contract the abdominal muscles, and the borders and inscriptions of the rectus muscle are marked in a contrasting color.

The surgery begins as a standard fluid injection. I use the skin fold over the rib cage as a guide to the end point thickness of the operated area. The thickness of this fold will vary with the body fat percentage of the patient. Use of this gauge allows for a uniform result in balance with the rest of the patient's body. Incisions are made in the upper part of the umbilicus, in the mid-pubis, and at the inferior aspects of the lateral rectus borders. If flank liposuction is also to be performed, additional incisions are made in the lateral-dorsal areas inferior to the posterior iliac crest.

The standard low-dose epinephrine-saline solution is infused into the areas to be suctioned. With use of the MicroAire handle and a 3.8-mm two-holed cannula, the entire abdominal area from the costal margin to the pubis is uniformly thinned to the predetermined thickness as noted earlier. I avoid use of the Mercedes cannula in this area to prevent over-thinning of the superficial fascia. If needed, a 3.8-mm Mercedes cannula is then used to treat the flanks with the patient in left and right decubitus positions. The Mercedes cannula can be used because of the greater thickness of the overlying skin. Attention is directed to highlighting the lateral sweep of the latissimus muscles.

The patient is then returned to the supine position, and a personally modified single-holed cannula is used with the reciprocating handle. The hole is directed against the inferior skin surface. *This process is similar to that used when creating gluteal creases.* By using the same incisions, the midline and lateral borders of the rectus muscles are highlighted. The controlled reciprocating nature of the power-assisted handle permits the inscriptions to be highlighted from the same entry points. I have seen other surgeons create additional incisions high in the abdomen to enable the use of standard cannulas for this task. These noticeable scars compromise the end result. The reciprocating tip of the MicroAire cannula can be controllably directed in segments along the inscriptions to allow the skin to gently fold into the muscle bellies. Care must be taken to not be too aggressive and allow adhesions that give an artificial appearance to the form. I have found that neither the standard cannula nor especially the ultrasonic one has the selectivity to accomplish this objective.

The umbilical and midline incisions, each measuring 4 mm, are left unsutured to allow drainage and minimize scrotal swelling and ecchymosis. Use of an open-crotch

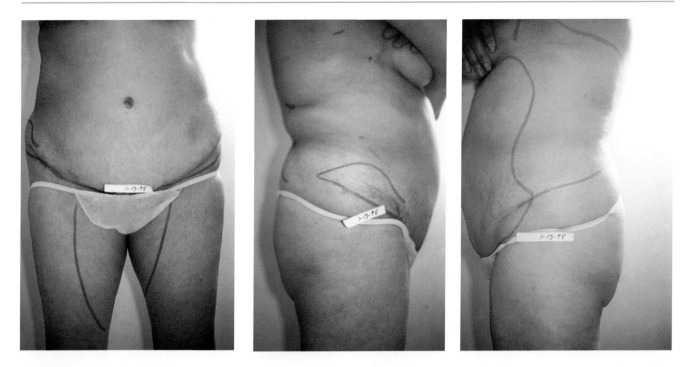

Figures 4-39 – 4-41   Repair of an abdominoplasty with an overly long incision involves repositioning the incision, as well as deep and superficial fat removal.

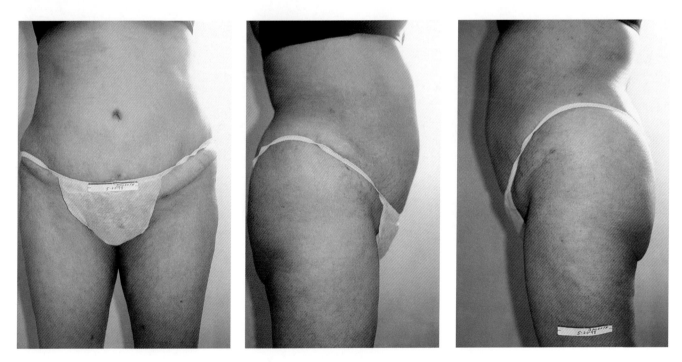

Figures 4-42 – 4-44   The restoration included lower abdominal wall resuturing.

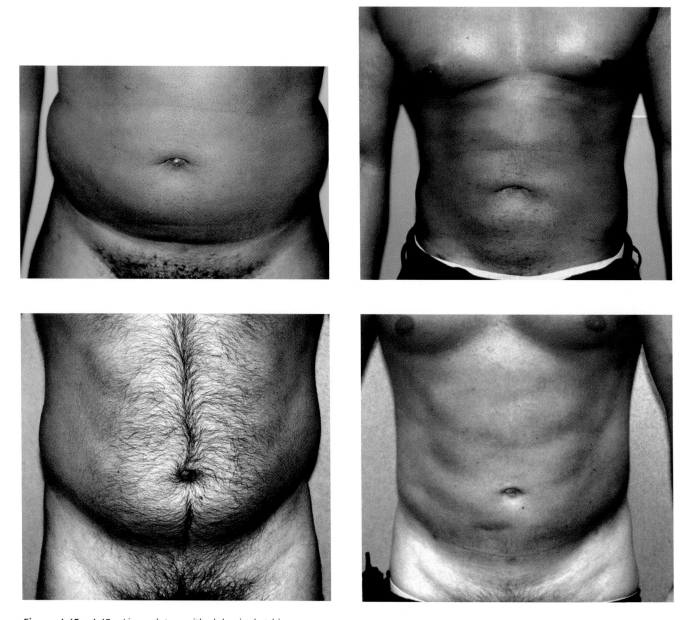

Figures 4-45 – 4-48 Liposculpture with abdominal etching.

postoperative compression garment tends to encourage this complication. The other incisions are sutured with 6-0 gut. The area is dressed with patterned absorbent pads in layers to encourage infolding of the skin. A compression garment is applied. The underlying bandages are removed at 3 to 4 days, and the compression garment is used for 3 weeks. The defined look is accomplished within 6 to 12 weeks of the surgery (see Figs. 4-45 to 4-48).

More on abdominal etching—Mark Gilliland, M.D. (plastic surgeon, Houston)

Athletes seeking detail in their abdominal musculature frequently fail with diet and exercise. Traditional abdominal lipoplasty involves the use of deep liposuction and generally leaves a subcutaneous pad of fatty tissue to cover any irregularities. This technique does not achieve the "washboard" aesthetic goal. Abdominal etching is a technique devised to enhance the appearance of rippled abdominal muscles by removing fat at variable levels.

Detailed preoperative markings are made over the *linea alba*, the *linea semilunaris*, and the *transverse tendinous intersections* with the rectus abdominis muscles. Retraction and flexion of the abdominal muscles assist in definition of the detailed musculature. Punctures are made in the pubic hairline, umbilicus, and either the upper midline or the anterior axillary line for the transverse intersections, depending on the amount of body hair. Either local or general anesthesia can be performed with the pressurized infusion technique of liposuction ("PIT" liposuction). In pre-marked areas requiring maximum retraction (linea alba, linea semilunaris, and transverse intersections), the peau d'orange appearance of the skin is beneficial before superficial liposuction. Multidirectional deep liposuction using a 2.4- to 3.0-mm Mercedes cannula is performed over the entire abdominal wall to create a 1.5- to 2-cm pinch test result. Superficial liposuction is performed over the linea alba and lateral to the semilunar line to enhance maximum retraction. The upper midline or axillary puncture sites are used to perform transverse superficial liposuction with an abrasive "etching" cannula in both the up and down position to create raw surfaces underneath the skin and over the transverse intersections. This "internal dermabrasion" creates adherence between the skin and rectus fascia. At the conclusion of the procedure, the grooves are stented and covered with Reston foam.

To date, follow-up has lasted from 6 to 12 months, and no major complications have occurred. Despite erythema of the "etched" area for several days, there have been no cases of skin necrosis. Patient satisfaction has been high. One patient gained weight and lost definition of two of the three transverse intersections. This procedure has minimal risk when detailed preoperative markings are made and the technical execution of superficial and deep liposuction is performed with precision. Appropriate patient selection is crucial because preexisting low body fat (less than 18%) and a long-term commitment to diet and exercise are critical.

By extrapolating the previous principles of deep and superficial liposuction, the concept of differential liposuction allows the lipoplasty surgeon to truly sculpt the body by creating smooth and retracted skin to enhance underlying muscle detail. Obviously, a large series with longer follow-up will be needed to determine the long-term efficacy of this procedure.

BACK AND FLANKS

"Buffalo humps," gynecomastia, and the "mid-sacral bulge" are fibrofatty areas. Although they can be reduced with pinhole incisions on opposite ends and cross-suctioning, UAL, PAL, and XUAL (see Figs. 4-1 to 4-3) are used primarily for ease of resection rather than as a requirement for skin contracture. Whereas compression of the lower back and gynecomastia area is easily achieved postoperatively, to facilitate skin contracture, the "buffalo hump" area fortunately responds well without continuous pressure. These areas do not return with weight gain.

> **CLINICAL PEARL**
> Liposuction is just that—it removes fat. Patients must recognize that "folds" or "rolls" are due to both fat and skin and that excess skin will not necessarily be improved with SAL. Patients should be advised to avoid thinking in terms of pounds or inches from liposuction surgery. It is an operation that contours fat. If pressed, Alan Matarasso (plastic surgeon, New York) tells them how many liters and grams were removed and that to lose the equivalent of 4.5 L of fat, they would have to burn 35,000 calories.

Compression is an important part of recovery in the hip and flank rolls and in the transition areas between the mid-back and the abdomen. Like the inner aspect of the thigh, these areas were considered difficult because of poor skin contracture. The addition of UAL and PAL not only facilitates liposuction of the folds, not the thin areas *between the folds*, but also promotes skin contracture. Early massage and intermittent compression during the edema phase of recovery begin within a few days of the actual surgical procedure. The upper flank roll, which joins to the posterior of the breast, is not easily compressed. Patients should be warned that this is the one area in the back that will bruise in almost every case and that recovery with resolution may be delayed.

Patient Selection

If every patient were in their twenties and physically active, we would not need XUAL, massage, or any postoperative care to achieve a 3-month follow-up as shown in the young woman in Figures 4-4 and 4-5. At 3 months, the entry points are still red, but contouring of the thighs and abdomen has proceeded without irregularity. In 1995, "super wet" infiltration accomplished during "brief twilight" intravenous sedation allowed us to achieve rapid resolution of edema with our *postsurgical programs of hydrotherapy and massage* at a faster pace than was observed in older patients undergoing similar surgeries. Older patients were often denied inner thigh liposuction because of the frequent complication of rippling and irregularities, a problem rarely encountered in younger individuals. With the use of XUAL for skin shrinkage, we no longer hesitate to perform liposuction on inner thighs and in patients in older age groups today.

Liposuction of the flank area is complicated by the *variety of tissues and their inherent resistance to removal of fat.* Many patients have a *small amount of fat and skin excess in the flank area above the "high hip roll."* Liposuction *in this area is not advisable.* Attempts to remove this small amount of fat even with small cannulas too often results in scarring, rippling, and distortion, as well as postsurgical suction defects. In other individuals, rolls of liposuction fat with excess skin extend almost to the midline of the back. These areas are typically more difficult to treat because of the dense *fibrous fat deposits.* The development of UAL, XUAL, and PAL was motivated by a desire to make removal of fat in these areas less arduous and accompanied by better results. Certain patients must still be advised that *skin rippling will persist* with the removal of fat. In the lower portion of the flank, or the "high hip roll," the fatty tissues are removed rather easily through a dual approach with small cannulas.

Because this procedure is so lengthy, body temperature is a major concern. Dr. Hunstad advises using the "Bair Hugger" over the patient's head and covering the upper part of the chest, the only area that is not being prepared for surgery. Many patients can lose the fat in this area with exercise, but they are frustrated by

CLINICAL PEARL

Circumferential skin removal, or a "belt lipectomy," is especially indicated for patients with massive weight loss. Removal of the skin and elevation will correct the buttock ptosis and give a degree of thigh-lift even though the incisions are higher. This massive operation is not one that we should be undertaking lightly. Technical points from Dr. Joe Hunstad (plastic surgeon, Charlotte) include infiltrating the "super wet" solution into the front of the patient, turning the patient prone for infiltration and posterior resection, and then turning the patient again for the abdominoplasty.

There is no undermining in the back, just excision of skin and subcutaneous tissue. Abdominoplasty is the last procedure because it is the more complex. It is performed after completing the back closure and liposuction.

Preoperatively, one can get a good idea of the amount of skin and subcutaneous tissue to be removed by performing the two-handed pinch test. Remember that the posterior midline just does not advance, so there must be conservative excision there and adjacent to the mid-back. Then the incision lines can extend in gullwing fashion just above the buttocks and in the upper portion of the back.

attempts to lose the fat in the central portion of the abdomen and the posterior breast and axillary fatty deposits.

Anesthesia

Infiltration in the flank and back is widespread because we want to induce shrinkage over the entire area, particularly areas that are not liposuctioned. This fluid remains in the tissue and is not removed by liposuction; therefore, when it is mobilized, there will be a prolonged period of hemodilution with a lowered hematocrit from the hemodilution, even though it is a site remote from the area used for obtaining blood samples.

Curved cannulas with a pressure pump to instill "super wet" dilutions are inserted through small incisions. These stab wounds are stretched with a hemostat to allow the entry of 3- or 4-mm cannulas. Obviously, the patient should not be in pain from these injections, thus again making the point for general anesthesia or intravenous sedation.

Instruments

To reach areas on the flank and back, the instruments must be curved with a hand placed underneath the patient. The entire procedure can be done with the patient in this supine position. Curved cannulas are then palpated as they cross from the visible to the hand area to ensure uniform resection of fat in these areas. Fan patterns and crisscrossing are required. It is often important to use an entry point high on the buttock, which was designed for fat regrafting, and pass a long thin cannula horizontally and in a fan fashion to do areas on the back. For larger areas, it is preferable to use the suction technique, but if a patient has little fat, the syringe technique allows regrafting. Using a syringe technique with a longer cannula allows one to withdraw the cannula to just below the surface, turn it, and pre-tunnel into the gluteus musculature and subcutaneous area for regrafting. Pre-tunneling opens a space in the already anesthetized area, and pressure is applied to gently deposit small columns of fat in a fan pattern in several layers.

Procedures

The posterior of the breast is liposuctioned during breast reduction surgery, as well as during liposuction resculpturing. The approach is from a small incision in the breast fold and usually a second incision for cross-sectioning above the axillary fold. This technique allows access to the anterior axillary fat pad, which must not be over-resected, and the axillary tail of Spence.

Placing the nonoperative hand above the area to be liposuctioned with curved cannulas (see Fig. 4-49) allows the operating surgeon to carefully estimate the amount

---

CLINICAL PEARL

Trunk Liposuction and Breast Implants
During the performance of breast implantation, it is sometimes helpful to contour the trunk, especially the area below the breasts and the subaxillary zone. The appearance of the breast implants is helped by making an umbilical incision and two paraspinal incisions to suction the lateral aspect of the chest below the breast, as well as the epigastrium and the lateral anterior portion of the chest. This is usually an uncommon procedure because very few patients require the combination of breast implants and liposuction; however, it is useful when performed (Adrien Aiache, plastic surgeon, Beverly Hills.)

---

of fatty tissue that will be left in the subcutaneous layer, particularly in areas toward the back (see Fig. 4-50). This technique allows a complete liposuction to be performed *with the patient lying in one position, supine.*

CLINICAL PEARL

For back liposuction, the most useful tool is a Robles open-ended cannula, according to Dr. Adrien Aiache (plastic surgeon, Beverly Hills). Its advantages consist of a cutting edge that severs the deep attachments of the skin, thus correcting the "waves" so prominent in the back. The second advantage lies in precise fat removal controlled by the hand of the operator, which leads to very superficial suction and allows skin retraction.

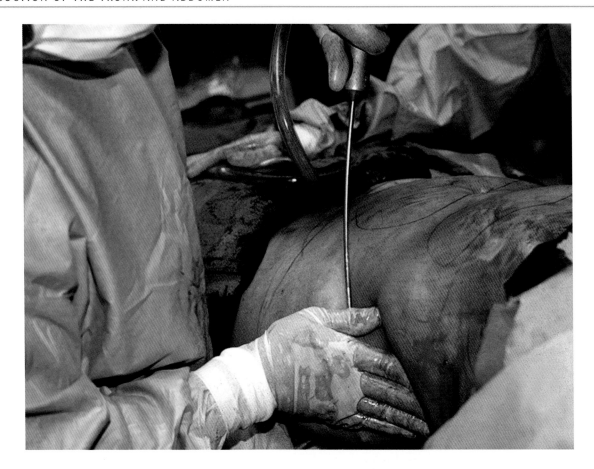

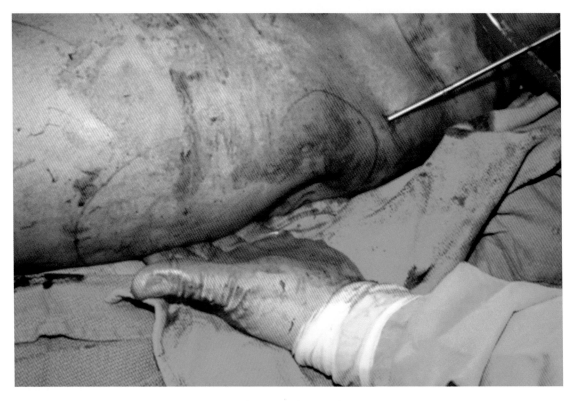

Figures 4-49 & 4-50 *Approaching flank fat deposits from a primary anterior entry is facilitated by lifting the back areas toward the cannula. This technique also gives the surgeon information about what fat is to be left in situ.*

Slow resolution of "love handles" in males

An over-30 male who is quite physically active participated in the initial trials of XUAL to reduce the typical "figure 8" mid-abdominal fat deposits and the "love handle" areas, which extended to the mid-back. The vertical lines indicate areas of transition beyond the liposuction zones that will be treated with ultrasound alone (see Figs. 4-51 to 4-53).

The problem in males has always been *slow resolution and incomplete reduction of the love handle area in many instances and, frequently, failure of the abdomen to flatten because of the thickness of the subcutaneous tissues.* See Figure 4-54. After preparatory counseling and discussions, the patient underwent the XUAL procedure with light sedation on an outpatient basis. He returned to his usual gymnasium routine and did 100 sit-ups the next day! He also reported that he had not taken any pain pills during the recovery phase and was very anxious to discontinue wearing the binder after the first 7 days. At 1 month (see Fig. 4-55), resolution of the abdomen is proceeding nicely, but visible bulges are still apparent in the love handle zone despite extensive deep and superficial liposuction in these areas. Fortunately, continued resolution improved his appearance in the photographs taken at 2 months (see Figs. 4-56 to 4-58). Although there was still edema in spots in the abdomen and flanks, he was advised to wait for an additional several months before contemplating a secondary procedure. It was not required because resolution continued at a steady rate.

This case illustrates the advantage of ultrasonic energy in difficult areas such as the "love handles" in physically active males and the advantages of ultrasonic energy in promoting skin shrinkage in the abdomen. Perhaps the rapid recovery was in part due to early physical activity and a pain-free period afforded by ultrasound dispersion of the "super wet" solution.

> **CLINICAL PEARL**
> UAL, PAL, and XUAL are adjunctive approaches that simplify removal of fat in the high flank area and, in the case of UAL and XUAL, induce a greater degree of skin contracture. In the early investigation of XUAL, we found that the transition area in which there is little fat could be adequately treated by the infusion of "super wet" fluid and a series of applications of XU at "full power"—3.0 W/cm².

How I do it: Tips on liposuction of the posterior trunk area—Dennis Barek (plastic surgeon, New York)

As liposuction became safe for large-volume removal, the areas being treated were no longer just saddlebags or the abdomen, but came to encompass the entire trunk. In fact, more and more patients are interested in sculpting the entire trunk in a single session. Even when feasible, one of the more difficult areas is the back, with its thick skin and rolls that cascade down to the flank and iliac deposits. This entire unit is also treated with the lateral aspect of the thorax and arm.

Proper evaluation of the tissues is necessary to avoid operating on an unfavorable patient. Those with thin, atrophic, ptotic tissues are, of course, poor candidates. However, some of these types of patients are frequently satisfied with fat removal without concern about loose skin.

Contour lines are drawn about the fat to be extracted, the patient is photographed, and then general anesthesia is used to put the patient to sleep. The patient is placed in the decubitus position with the arm extended over a padded Mayo stand to allow complete access to the target tissues.

"Super wet" infiltration is performed through convenient stab wounds, usually three, around the scapular area. Two are placed in each flank and hip roll area, plus one at the posterior axillary fold for the arm.

The cannula of choice for the scapula area must be able to cut through the dense fibrous fat under the thick dermis. For this I use Gram's "tiger-tip" cannula. It is not too long and I can etch the underside of this thick skin. The tip has sharp grooves that allow aggressive fat removal. The cannula is 3.8 mm in diameter.

For the flank and iliac area, I also try to remove as much fat as possible consistent with the type of skin, but preserve some fat in the area immediately below the dermis. Here, the standard "Mercedes" type of 4-mm cannula is used. In stubborn cases, I would use a "tiger-tip" cannula up to 5 mm in diameter. All the fibrous bands separating the rolls are aggressively lysed with the "tiger-tip" cannula.

The arm is approached with a single 3- or 4-mm "Mercedes" type of cannula, and the fat is removed in a more conservative fashion, mostly involving the dependent portion of the arm. Of course, appropriate measurements of the extracted fat are recorded and the contralateral side is done in a similar manner.

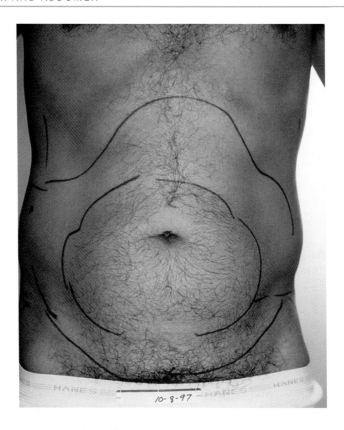

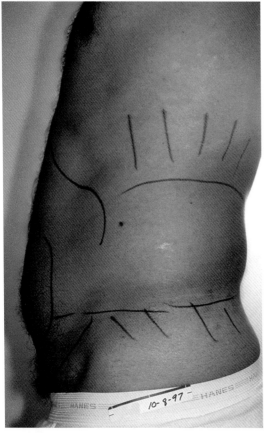

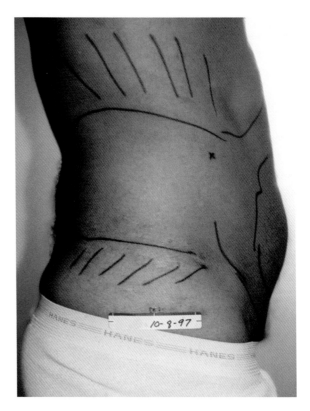

Figures 4-51 – 4-53   *The common resistant fat deposits in active males vary in width and thickness. Ultrasound alone is used above and below the "love handle" area for smoother contracture.*

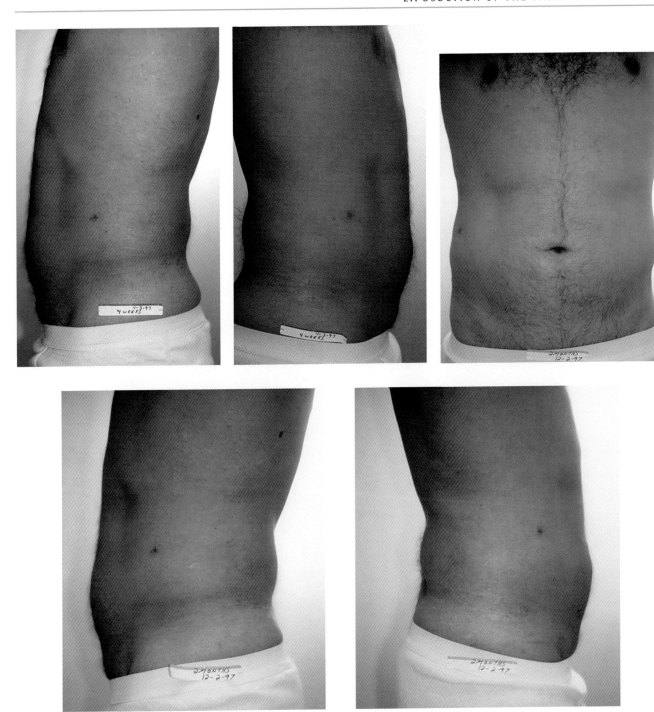

Figures 4-54 – 4-58   *Typically, the flank dermis is thickened and a completely flat contour cannot be achieved.*

The small stab wounds are left open. Compressive garments are worn for comfort for a week or two, but they are not needed unless the skin is pendulous. The results are quite gratifying, with marked changes in the way patients fit into their clothing (see Figs. 4-59 to 4-62).

Liposuction of the back and high hip region

In many patients the high hip roll is a major consideration, especially if it is associated with mid-buttock depression. The patient in Figures 4-63 to 4-65 has no depression, but her personal wishes were to reduce the height of the high hip roll, as well as the secondary rolls extending up to her back. This patient was treated with XUAL by passing cannulas *above and below the two prominent mid-back folds,* and external ultrasound was relied on to melt the transitional areas toward the midline. In the 10-week postoperative photographs, resolution is continuing (see Figs. 4-66 to 4-68). Reduction of the folds has been accomplished, and liposuction extending down to the mid-buttock elevation has produced satisfactory contouring in this area.

Fatty deposits in the supraclavicular area

Though less common than the "buffalo hump" deformity, fatty deposits in the supraclavicular fat pad may be noticeable, as in this patient (see Fig. 4-69). After infiltration, a 3-mm cannula is used to perform liposuction in a "spray pattern" to reduce the soft tissue deformity. This technique is the same as we use for lipomas. As in this case, an irregularity remains in the central area (see Fig. 4-70). Although this irregularity consists of only a half centimeter of fat, it must be removed as a secondary procedure, which can be accomplished nonsurgically by infiltration and application of XUAL or by local anesthesia and an adjustment liposuction of a minor nature.

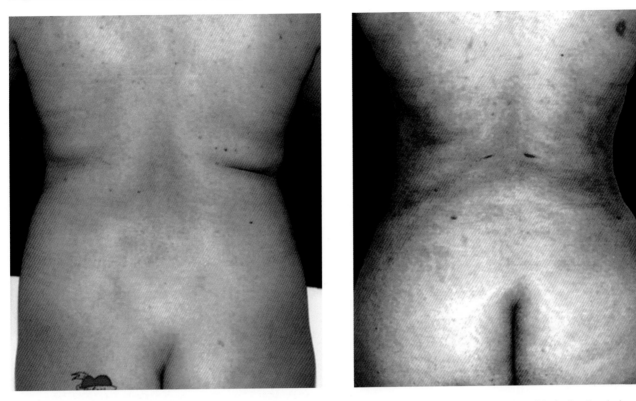

Figures 4-59 & 4-60 *Preoperative appearance of Dr. Barek's patient and postoperative flank and back contouring with the "wet" technique.*

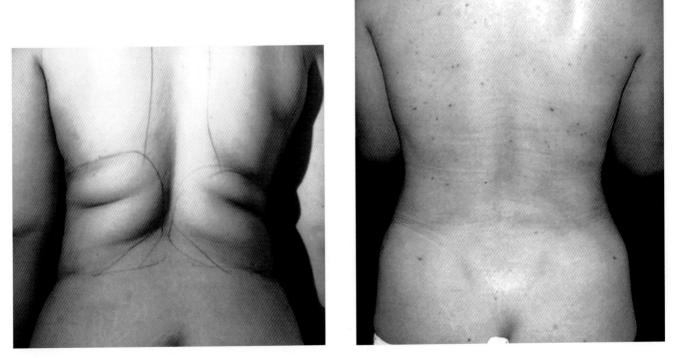

Figures 4-61 & 4-62 *Suctioning between skin folds and postoperative compression achieved Dr. Barek's restoration.*

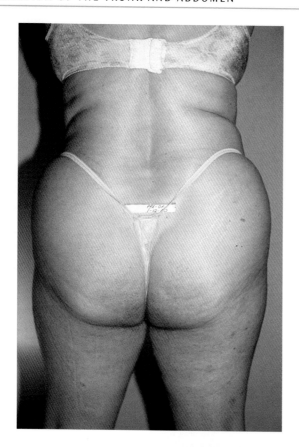
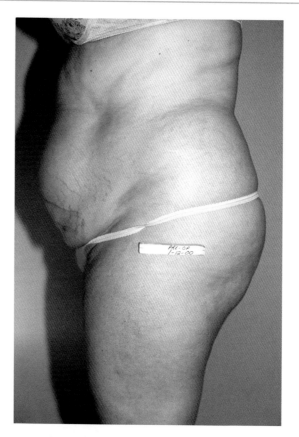
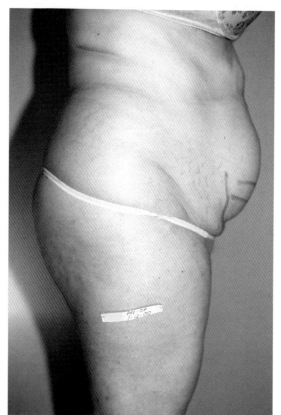

Figures 4-63 – 4-65 *Liposuction has been an essential component of abdominoplasty; it was originally confined to the abdomen but now includes the flanks.*

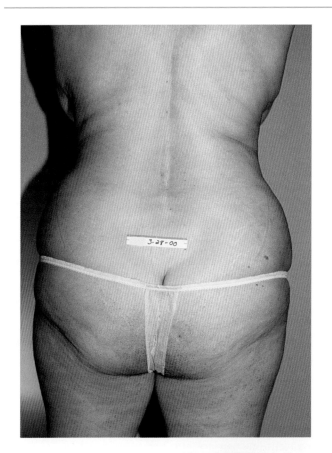
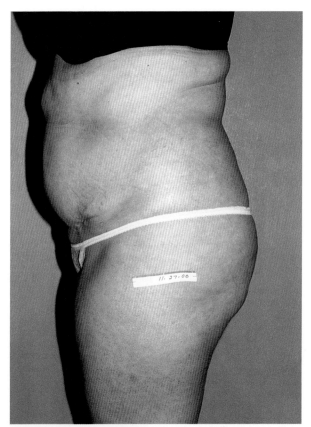
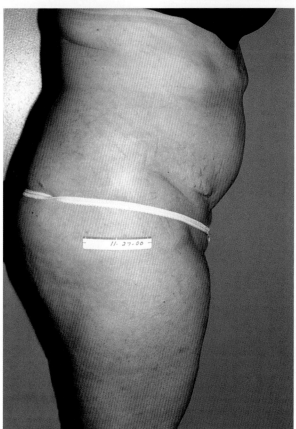

Figures 4-66 – 4-68   *Flank contouring adds to the restoration of contour in this category of heavy person.*

Liposuctioning the flank

Small stab wounds, as shown in these figures, allow the infiltration of "super wet" solution into the pre-marked folds of the flank and "high hip" rolls that have been marked previously, as well as the *depressions between these rolls, which will be elevated without suction.* Figure 4-71 shows the typical small cannula that is used for the lateral approach and, in this individual, for cross-suctioning of the mid-abdomen. Note that the skin is covered with Betadine during this procedure. This facilitates movement of the opposite hand over the area being suctioned to ascertain the depth of penetration and ensure sterility. The curve of the cannula shown in Figure 4-71 will be changed to a down curve for this part of the maneuver rather than the straight configuration used to go laterally. A second curve will be made in the cannula laterally to penetrate beyond the central area into the mid-thigh (see Fig. 4-72).

> **CLINICAL PEARL**
>
> Flank rolls should be approached from several directions, including placement of small cannulas in multiple levels vertically as well as horizontally. In the patient in Figure 4-73, preoperative markings distinguish the "areas of folding" and the extent of the liposuctioning to be performed.

XUAL in contouring of a fat-free abdomen

Patient D.R. was evaluated for an "internal bra" reconstruction of her breasts. These deformities, which are due to pregnancy, weight loss, rupture of the gel prosthesis, and the resulting contracture shown in Figure 4-74, are corrected by removal of the implant, high placement of a textured gel prosthesis, and internal muscle flap repair (the "internal bra" procedure) for a more natural breast with warmth and cleavage from the underlying muscle flaps. In addition, she volunteered as a demonstration subject for our seminar on XUAL. Although the defects were minimal, *buttock contouring was accomplished with a flat-bladed cannula from the buttock fold* and a two-directional 3-mm cannula laterally. All fat removed was regrafted into the marked dimples and flat areas to achieve successful recontouring.

The challenge in this patient was to improve the rippled contour of her abdomen. She has little loose skin and practically no subcutaneous fat (see Fig. 4-75).

The abdomen was infiltrated with "super wet" solution, and 12 minutes of XUAL was applied, followed by compression. Secondary ultrasound was applied as well to induce contracture of the rippled skin and to smooth the small amounts of irregular fat deposits (see Figs. 4-76 and 4-77). This patient was able to return to a strenuous professional schedule in 48 hours.

The postoperative photographs were taken during a convention trip to another city in which she was employed. Though not of professional quality, it is obvious that she has smoothing of the abdomen and restoration of contour without the irregularity and rippling shown in previous photographs.

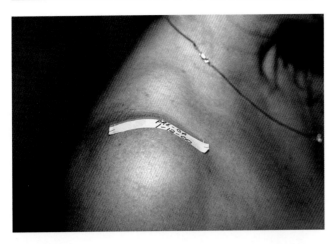
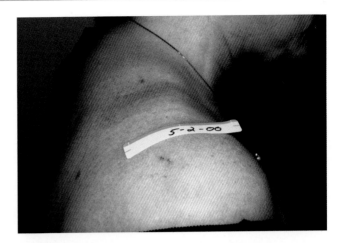

Figures 4-69 & 4-70   *Unusual fat deposits in the shoulder or "buffalo humps" respond well to infiltration and bidirectional fat extraction.*

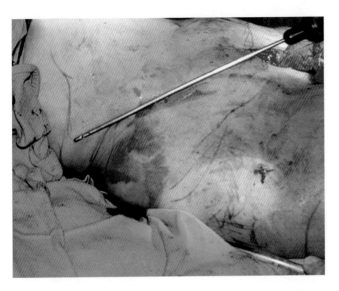
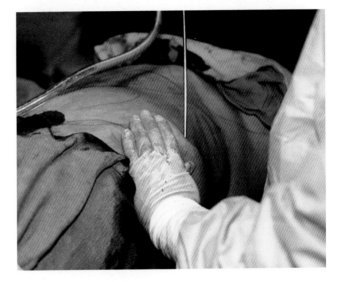

Figures 4-71 & 4-72   *Figure 4-71 shows the typical small cannula that is used for the lateral approach and, in this individual, for cross-suctioning of the mid-abdomen. The shape of the cannula will be bent to a down curve for this part of the maneuver rather than the straight configuration used to go laterally. Shown in Figure 4-72, a second greater curve will be made in the cannula laterally to penetrate beyond the central area into the mid-thigh.*

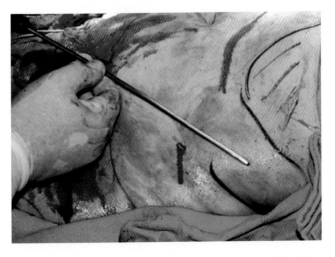

Figure 4-73   *Flank rolls should be approached from several directions, including the placement of small cannulas in multiple levels vertically as well as horizontally. In this patient, preoperative markings distinguish the "areas of folding" and the extent of the liposuctioning to be performed.*

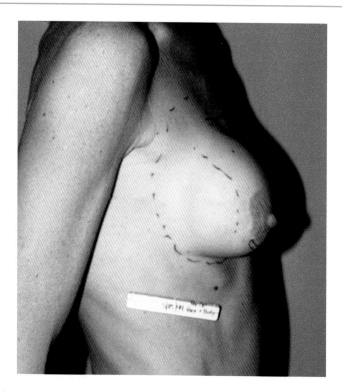
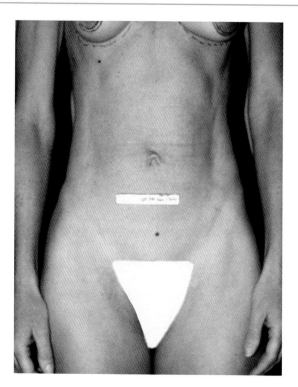

Figures 4-74 & 4-75   *While preparing for an "internal mastopexy" by way of her original periareolar incision and replacement with textured gel-silicone breast implants, a request was made for contouring of the abdomen. There is little fat and only fine rippling in this patient category.*

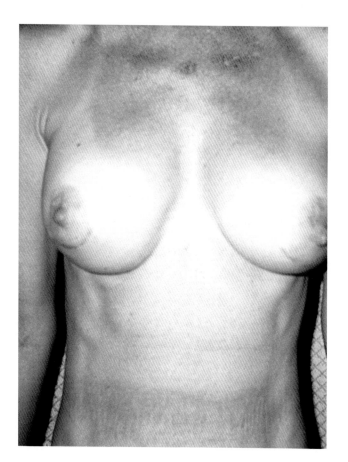
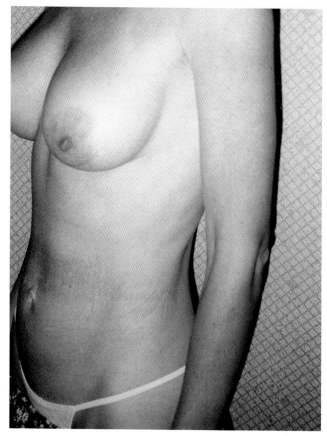

Figures 4-76 & 4-77   *Internal medially based muscle flaps and the fixed position of the new implant restored this patient's breast appearance. XUAL without fat removal re-created the smooth abdomen.*

SUMMARY

The flank and abdomen are sites of the most bizarre and often irreparable complications of liposuction. The primary culprit is over-resection or damage to the overlying dermis. When liposuction is used in conjunction with abdominoplasty, vigorous suction in the inflow areas laterally and superiorly will interrupt the blood supply to the flap. An additional problem is that the flanks, the abdomen, and the areas between these two separate zones of fat deposits are best addressed by curved cannulas. When UAL is used, the cannulas are straight, and separate larger skin openings are required. For many patients, this is a significant problem. More commonly, the flank area is simply rippled with small amounts of fat and loose skin. Liposuction in these areas would produce further rippling and the likelihood of permanent damage. The use of XUAL in these areas without invasion not only preserves the blood supply for the abdominoplasty but also induces smoothing of the skin contracture and dissolution of the small amounts of fat.

Flank rolls in the abdomen are unique in that there may be anchoring attachments between the individual rolls that are filled with fat as in gynecomastia. These anchoring tethers should be disrupted with a blunt cannula. The flat-bladed end without the application of suction is excellent for breakup. When the rolls themselves are reduced and pressure is applied with a garment of some type, these areas have a greater chance of smoothing. A dual approach is important in the midbody areas. Liposuction is performed with a fanning motion from several approaches via small stab wounds that can then be stretched with a small instrument to accommodate the entry of 3-, 4-, or 5-mm cannulas. As in the arms, compression is important because of the variability of these tissues and their resistance to contracture in certain individuals.

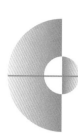

CHAPTER FIVE

Abdominoplasty

Abdominoplasty is a procedure once reserved for grossly distorted individuals in which stretching of the abdominal musculature was more of a health risk than a cosmetic problem. In 1975, I addressed patients who had lower abdominal muscle separation that did not respond to diet and exercise and who had skin folds. The "limited" short-scar or "smile" abdominoplasty was devised and published in 1985. It became apparent that if the incisions were shortened and closure of the panniculus was accomplished without tension, one could easily perform a complete abdominal repair and use liposuction to a much greater degree than I would have imagined being safe. Subsequently, I used external ultrasound-assisted liposuction (XUAL) and other modalities to perform the procedure and have changed the design of the incision to accommodate "French line" lingerie and bathing suit designs.

Despite teaching courses and textbook articles on this procedure, it is disturbing to see transverse abdominal incisions, skin sloughing from ultrasound-assisted liposuction (UAL) with its damaging effect on the sub-dermal plexus, and the "cookie cutter" approach of long incisions for all patients regardless of their requirements. This chapter will address patient selection, choice of the least visible and least problematic incisions, and various techniques of internal repair.

PRINCIPLES OF ABDOMINOPLASTY

Plastic surgeons in training in the late 1960s and 1970s were taught that abdominoplasty was a hip-to-hip incision, with full anterior repair and resetting of the umbilicus; fat removal from the panniculus was forbidden. The procedure was reserved for people who had true physical problems. The research that showed the

> **CLINICAL PEARL**
>
> How it's changed all over the world! Luiz Toledo (Brazil) reported in 1990 that he performed 83 abdominal lipo-suctions, 11 limited abdominoplasties, and only 2 "classic" abdominoplasties. Yet in 1981, most American surgeons performed only "classic" abdominoplasties. Some of us were already performing a variation of "limited" abdominoplasty on over 50% of our patients. Only a few Europeans were doing abdominal suction lipectomy.

improved cardiovascular status, relief of back and neck pain, and general overall well-being was in the future.

Within a year of leaving the university chairmanship for private practice, I was served with a lawsuit by a woman who had disrupted her incision during the influenza outbreak and objected to her very large mons veneris, which of course she had been unable to see previously. The initial review by an expert in another city stated that malpractice had been committed because the panniculus had been thinned with scissors dissection! Although the suit was abruptly dropped when the expert reversed his opinion, her comment about the large mons was a problem that we had not addressed. Before liposuction, manual defatting of the mons (which was accompanied by profuse bleeding) was added to the armamentarium.

> **CLINICAL PEARL**
>
> When you're explaining to patients the benefits of abdomino-plasty, use postoperative photographs to point out that the "after" pictures will inevitably show a more erect posture with no lordosis and reduced back pain. American Society of Plastic Surgeons statistics indicate a high percentage of patients who are completely relieved of back pain by anterior abdominal wall repair.

PATIENT SELECTION

The changing approach to abdominoplasty began when surgeons in Europe and the United States experimented with smaller incisions for a different category of patients: those who needed only low abdominal repair. It soon became apparent that the only satisfactory scars were those that followed incision lines placed in the natural fold of the lower part of the abdomen, the original "smile line procedure." Working with patients who had horizontal hysterectomy scars in 1975, I established a procedure called "limited abdominoplasty" in which much shorter incisions were used to reach to and beyond the umbilicus for plication (see Figs. 5-1 and 5-2). Leaving the umbilicus intact or "floating" it with manual defatting became accepted, as has today's approach of controlled liposuction in conjunction with abdominoplasty. When high-cut "French line" lingerie became popular, a patient who had a 45-degree lateral appendectomy scar underwent complete repair with the use of this scar and a small horizontal component. Now, "French line" procedures for both limited and "complete" abdominal repair are our standard approach. It was apparent that *incisions placed in these lines not only healed faster but also faded more rapidly.* Aftercare procedures such as lymph drainage, massage, oils, and creams facilitated this recovery, and complications were very few.

> **CLINICAL PEARL**
>
> Prompted by a presentation by an Egyptian colleague at an international meeting who said, "Egyptian women don't care about scars," in my 1996 review article,[1] as well as in commentaries in later seminars and instructional courses, the fact that American women do care was discussed. Changes from the flat-line abdominoplasty of the bikini era to the high-cut angled incision of the "French line" were also emphasized. "Remember the simple old days? All you had to do was make a smile line incision and curve the edges slightly upward and it would cover even the smallest bikini. Now we've got the French bathing suits and you've got to do all that angling so the scar stays within the material."[1]

ANESTHESIA

Requirements for anesthesia are tied to the degree of correction in abdominoplasty, not to the extent of liposuction that will be used as an adjunctive procedure. With an extremely large patient, it is difficult to obtain true muscle relaxation with intravenous sedation. General anesthesia is considered a wise choice for this category of patient, as well as those in less than optimal health, overly anxious younger patients, and even elderly patients who say, "I have just got to get rid of this abdomen so that I can get back on the tennis court." For these patients, general anesthesia and at least a 24-hour observation period by professionals in a "half-way house," outpatient overnight facility, or an office overnight facility are recommended.

For limited abdominoplasty, the use of intravenous sedation to allow "super wet" infusion is an excellent choice. The Hunstad formula of super wet infusion is placed in all areas, and then after the panniculus is elevated, the cannula is introduced within the rectus and oblique fascias to infuse anesthetics for comfort and to prevent spasm. Obviously, the confidence of the anesthesiologist in charge of the case is a factor. Many surgeons, however, believe that office sedation anesthesia with a nurse anesthetist or even a trained registered nurse is safe and sensible for limited abdominoplasty patients. As will be noted in this chapter, combining other procedures with abdominoplasty, which was once frowned on and considered unsafe, is no longer a concern in healthy patients. Although one would hesitate to perform a complex face-lift procedure with an abdominoplasty, a simpler face-lift procedure and/or breast augmentation with abdominoplasty keeps the patient in the ideal time frame of under 3 hours of general anesthesia. Because the secondary procedures are considered "bloodless," this is also acceptable. "Bloodless" procedures are those in which infusion of the super wet technique with a valacaine/epinephrine combination reduces bleeding to a minimum and also facilitates the liposuction phase of any of the procedures to be discussed.

> **CLINICAL PEARL**
>
> **Conscious Sedation for "Limited Abdominoplasty"**
> Use of the ketamine-diazepam (Valium) regimen championed by Dr. Charles Vinnik (plastic surgeon, Las Vegas) allowed our clinic to successfully perform limited or even complete abdominoplasties. We chose to use a lesser amount, 30 mg of ketamine, administered intravenously after intravenous Valium, which gave a sufficient pain-free window to allow infiltration of the abdomen and flanks in this individual. With the assistance of a nurse anesthetist for monitoring and subsequent additional intravenous sedation as needed, these procedures were accomplished with a minimum of delay and at a reasonable cost. Unfortunately, the rise in cost of nursing personnel, malpractice insurance, and operating facility fees has made this practice less financially rewarding and has led many surgeons to abandon office surgery procedures of this magnitude altogether.

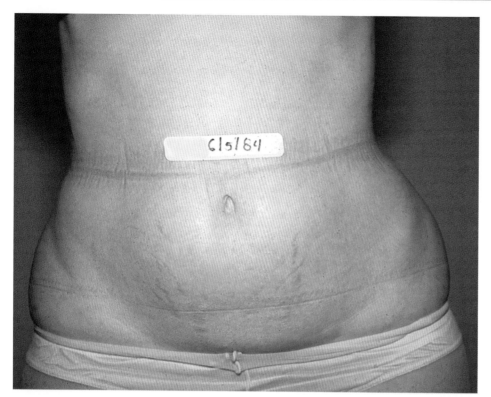

Figure 5-1 *What's wrong here? The unacceptable outcome of the old "tummy tuck" was a result of long incisions crossing the body folds, failure to defat laterally, and no liposuction!*

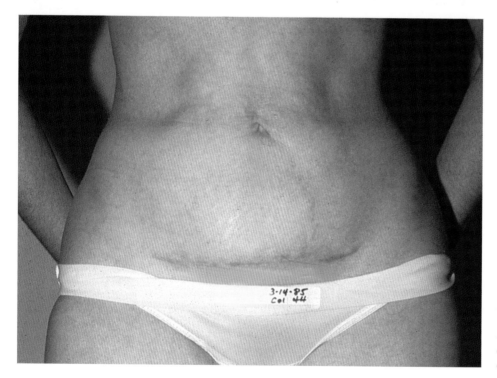

Figure 5-2 *Before liposuction, "limited" short-scar abdominoplasty results were not as "natural," and the area above the umbilicus was not debulked.*

The major complications of abdominoplasty are thromboembolism and pneumonia. Surgeons appreciated the need for early mobilization, compression stockings, deep-breathing exercises, and the like. Patients are kept overnight with intensive nursing care for the first 24 hours after "complete" abdominoplasty as a precaution.

I was one of the pioneers who stated that *liposuction was "an essential part of abdominoplasty."* In the mid-1980s, Drs. Matarasso and Toledo joined me in teaching a still popular course addressing complications in "aesthetic abdominoplasty." With combined experience, liposuction played an increasingly dominant role and in many cases eclipsed the use of incisional surgery altogether. Variations of the procedure include "floating the umbilicus," resetting it at a higher or lower level to allow access to the upper part of the abdomen, tension-free closure, and of course, categorization of patients. Today, most patients require lesser surgeries for lesser problems.

> **CLINICAL PEARL**
> To address the question of whether abdominoplasty may be safely combined with surgical procedures, Dr. Rod Hester (Atlanta) and his colleagues reported that in over 200 patients who underwent abdominoplasty with one or more major aesthetic procedures, obesity, not the complexity of the procedure, was the only risk factor that could be identified.[2]

In 1998, I introduced XUAL to our teaching course and demonstrated that this modality produced shrinkage of the upper abdominal skin, allowed sculpting of the lateral aspect of the flank without cannula invasion, and provided an increased degree of comfort beyond that afforded by the usual practice of injecting aesthetic solutions into the rectus sheath. With use of the pumps available for "super wet" anesthesia, it became common practice to *pump lidocaine (Xylocaine) solution into the obliques as well as the rectus fascia* and to place additional local anesthetic in the flanks at the end of the procedures. The decrease in bleeding with XUAL and super wet infusion made it acceptable to perform other procedures such as breast and face work at the same time as abdominoplasty. *Tension-free closure* and careful attention to postoperative management to avoid "girdle necrosis burns" reduced the complication rate even further.

An unexpected finding was the "wet recovery" of XUAL. The anesthetic solution that had been driven into the tissues by XUAL drained under the panniculus

in the postoperative period such that suction drains had to be left in place for 3 to 5 days or longer.

In this chapter we will explore the decisions that must be made regarding complete abdominal repair, limited abdominal repair, placement of incisions, and whether abdominal repair is required or optional for certain individuals.

INSTRUMENTS

Curved liposuction cannulas are useful in reaching flank areas that require suctioning, as are flat-bladed liposuction cannulas, which will be discussed as a helpful adjunct in defatting the area of potential "dog-ears." The abdominoplasty procedure (whether "limited or complete") requires long instruments and long retractors for full visualization. Although it is modern practice to clear only the area to be plicated, use of the common "sweetheart" retractor allows sutures to be placed above the umbilicus in complete safety by full visualization of even this minimally dissected area. Long-suture scissors are used for manual defatting on the final inspection and for removing any fatty tissue that may have been left on the fascia inadvertently. For abdominal etching, I prefer a narrow, flat-bladed cannula, which can be used with the hole upward in the midline and perhaps laterally and then with the hole downward to create a depression for this "skin shadow."

THE CHOICE OF PROCEDURE

Case in Point—Combining "Bloodless" Procedures with Abdominoplasty of the "Limited" Type

This patient requested face-lifting, blepharoplasty, "submental tuck," breast-lift, and "limited" abdominoplasty and liposuction (see Figs. 5-3 to 5-5). With light sedation anesthesia and XUAL to reduce edema and hemorrhage, this very healthy 60-year-old woman underwent the combined procedures with the usual expected rapid recovery. In 1985, this combination of procedures would have been considered too high risk to be performed simultaneously because of the anticipated blood loss and lengthy anesthesia. The "super wet" infusion plus the diffusion of epinephrine into soft tissues allowed us to complete these procedures with a minimum of blood loss.

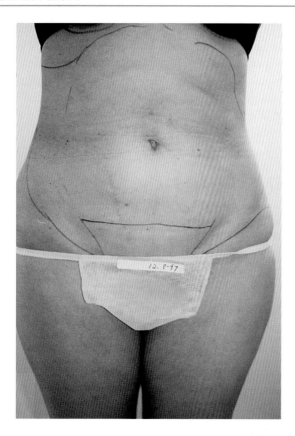
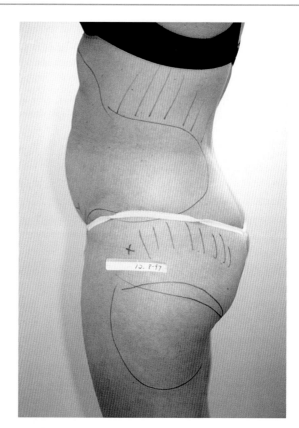
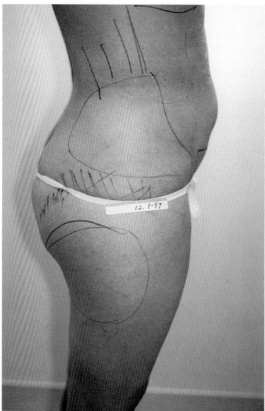

Figures 5-3 – 5-5   *The addition of XUAL, fat regrafting, and incisions limited to the width of the mons reduces operating time. Super wet infusion virtually eliminates blood loss. Patients may choose facial surgery as well as body sculpture if in good health and displaying the minimal deformities shown here.*

In the preoperative views, the extent of the abdomino-plasty incision is lengthened because of the width of her pelvis. Note the upward extension and minimal skin removal for a complete abdominal repair.

Also note the lateral view showing protrusion of the abdominal musculature to just above the umbilicus. In this "limited abdominoplasty," the umbilicus is not separated, a single figure-of-eight suture is placed above it, and then complete fascia plication is done from the umbilicus to the mons. The use of postoperative ultra-sound results in quicker resolution of edema in the lower part of the abdomen, edema that is still quite prominent in the 2-month postoperative photographs. The expected recovery time frame for resolution of the posterior hip area and completion of the contouring fat grafts is now 2 months (see Figs. 5-6 to 5-9). The edema noted in her face at 4 weeks (see Fig. 5-10) is responding to lymph drainage and intermittent ultrasound and ultimately resulted in the contoured and natural-appearing face-lift evident in the 1-year photograph (see Fig. 5-11). Fat grafting to the lips and nasolabial lines, with the incision hidden within the tragus by the tragal advancement sutures, a free lobule of the ear, and contouring of the jowl fat with XUAL produce a very natural and not overcorrected "operated" appearance.

Though not often the case, a combination of these repairs requested by an older patient in excellent health should be considered as an all-inclusive procedure with the assistance of XUAL and super wet infusion. Note the restored rounding of the hips from the autologous fat grafting, reduction of the high hip pads, and reduction of the upper part of the back, which was treated with ultrasound alone (see Figs. 5-12 to 5-15).

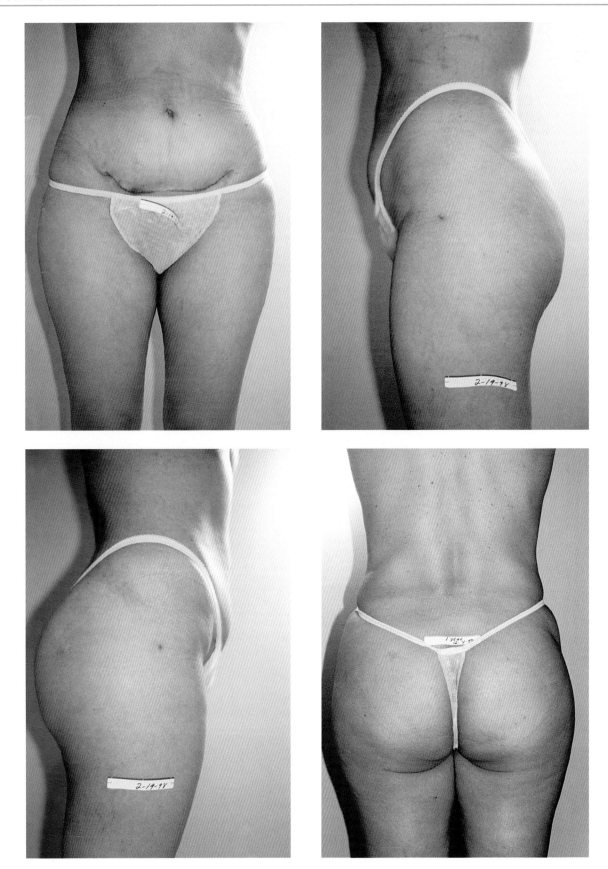

Figures 5-6 – 5-9   *At 2 months, edema persists above the "limited abdominoplasty" incision and will be treated with ultrasound. Note the contouring of the back treated by ultrasound with no fat extraction.*

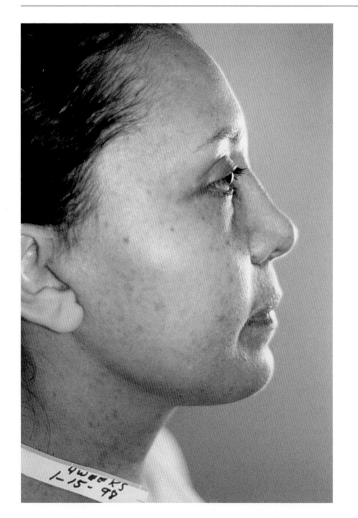
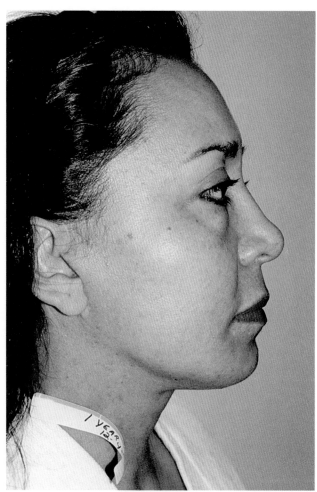

Figures 5-10 & 5-11 *Facial contouring from a mid-face–lift aided by ultrasound at 1 month. Further shrinkage continued, prolonging the effect seen here at 1 year.*

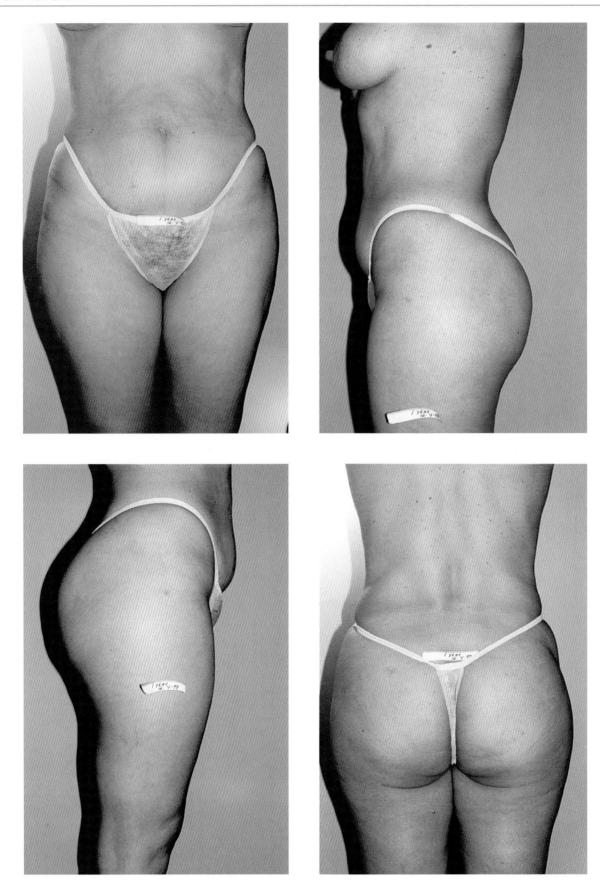

Figures 5-12 – 5-15 One-year results.

Case in Point—Traditional Abdominoplasty—Dr. Richard Heimberger (Plastic Surgeon, Jefferson City, Missouri)

This abdominoplasty design is a modification of Dr. Ted Lockwood's circumferential body reduction surgery, which is very similar to the 1970 standard for hip-to-hip liposuction. As shown in the illustrations, this patient underwent simultaneous breast reduction. Note the Bair Hugger on the lower part of the torso. Dr. Heimberger completes his mammaplasty first and then moves the Bair Hugger to the upper part of the torso for reprepartion and proceeds with the abdominoplasty. It is essential that the patient be marked preoperatively so that an agreement can be reached on the area of liposuction as well as the extent of the incision!

In a conversation with Dr. Heimberger, he told me that he begins the surgical procedure "…by elevating the upper abdominal skin by blunt and sharp dissection to above the costal margins. A lower abdominal incision is made just above the pubis and the groin elevated superiorly on top of the fascia to meet the other incision. With the panniculus elevated, imbrication is done to correct the diastasis. With the patient turned from side to side the posterior aspect of the flap is excised and closed during relocation of the umbilicus. I like to do this with an inverted V-incision and close it by incising the inferior aspect near its base and closing this with a running 5-0 nylon suture" (see Figs. 5-16 and 5-17).

In larger cases, Dr. Heimberger draws an autologous unit of blood before the procedure and inserts a Foley catheter at the beginning of surgery for overnight drainage. Intravenous and oral antibiotics are used as well as antibiotic irrigation during surgery.

Case in Point—Complete Abdominal Repair with Liposuction

The patient pictured in Figure 5-18 is typical of the mid-30s age group in which *diet and exercise have not reduced the fatty deposits* in the inner and outer aspects of the thighs and there is *early atrophy* in the mid-buttock. The lateral view shows the lower abdominal protrusion, which extends from the mons veneris to above the umbilicus (see Fig. 5-19). The umbilical float procedure with a small incision is ideally suited in this category of patient. By elevating the detachment of the umbilicus, *plication above the umbilicus* to a distance of 5 cm is facilitated, and only 2 to 3 cm of excess skin is resected. This is preceded by infiltration with the "super wet"

technique and liposuction in the areas noted. "Abdominal etching" has created the midline "champagne groove," as well as the lateral definitions at the new borders of the rectus abdominis musculature, which is sutured in the midline from just below the xyphoid to the pubis. The 10-day postoperative photograph (see Fig. 5-20) reveals only a moderate degree of bruising and edema in the lower part of the abdomen.

In 1994, this patient was instructed to wear compressive girdles for a period of 3 weeks. Self-massage in the treated areas began at 5 days, with the addition of lymph drainage procedures performed by clinic staff. Hydrotherapy with whirlpool baths and heat is initiated on the seventh day to increase the circulation and reduce edema. Today, these instructions are changed to a shorter time frame. This small incision, as noted in Figure 5-20, has been covered with paper tape and sealed with flexible collodion so that the patient may shower and bathe without fear of contamination.

Case in Point—Abdominoplasty and the Float Technique

Complete repair of the separation of the muscle fascia is accomplished from the xyphoid to the pubis. In the patient shown, the umbilicus was reset in its original position (see Fig. 5-21). Note that the incisions extend horizontally to the edge of the mons and then upward. This upward tailoring follows the natural lines of skin folds. Always "overcorrect upward" so that the incision will always remain within the "French line" of lingerie and bathing attire. All incisions tend to drift downward with time. Although *overcorrection with sutures fixing the mons and thigh skin to the abdominal fascia* produces visible tissue edema temporarily in the midline above the mons, resolution occurs with appropriate aftercare.

Case in Point—Limited Abdominoplasty at 11 Years

This young woman is shown in the original black and white photographs in 1989 when liposuction was used for her "banana roll" and upper hip fat deposits and a limited abdominoplasty short-scar procedure with liposuctioning was used for the abdomen. The preoperative photographs (see Figs. 5-22 and 5-23) show the deformities as well as bulging of the abdominal musculature from pregnancy, but only in the lower part of the abdomen. The shadowing of the abdomen is poorly defined.

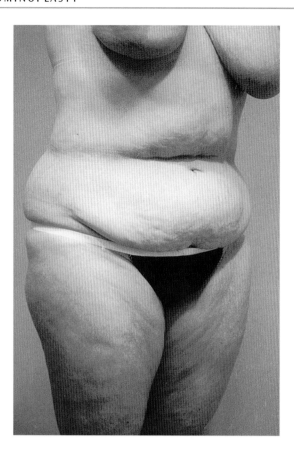
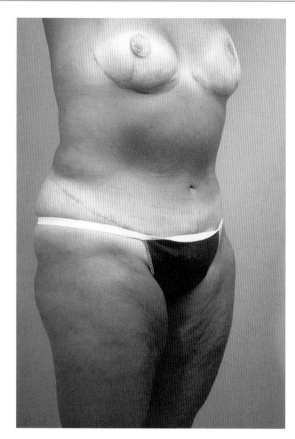

Figures 5-16 & 5-17   *"Standard" long-incision abdominoplasty with xiphoid-to-pubis repair and neo-umbilicoplasty. (Dr. Heimberger).*

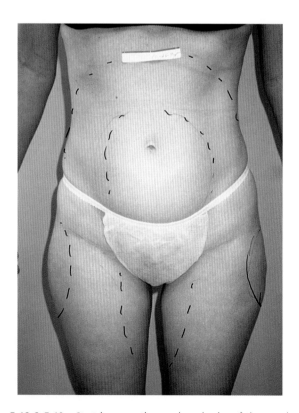
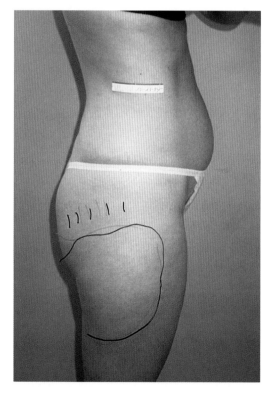

Figures 5-18 & 5-19   *Stretch, separation, and weakening of the anterior abdomen musculature. Plication repair will be assisted by liposculpture (suction-assisted lipectomy) with "super wet" infusion.*

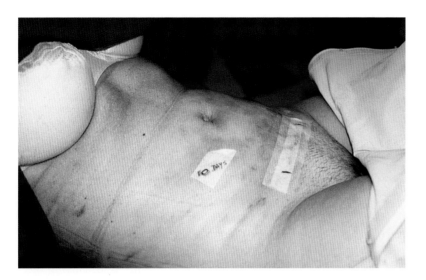

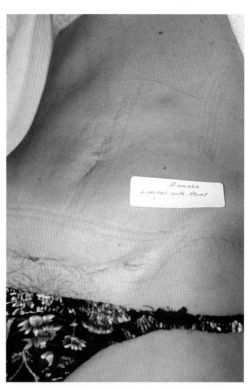

Figure 5-20 *The incision is protected by waterproofed tape dressing after drain removal. Minimal ecchymoses developed.*

Figure 5-21 *The change from straight "bikini" incisions to "French line" up curves is dictated by a change in lingerie design.*

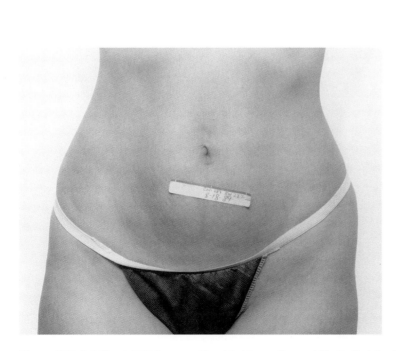

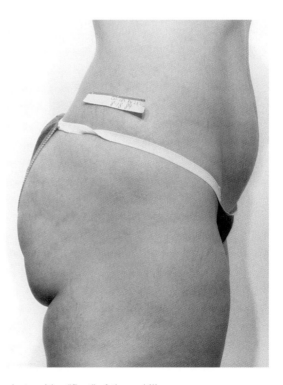

Figures 5-22 & 5-23 *A 1989 "super wet" assisted liposuction and "limited" abdominoplasty, with a "float" of the umbilicus.*

In the postoperative photographs, taken when the patient was preparing for an internal mastopexy with replacement of an old prosthesis, the mature scar is shown in the "French line" configuration (see Figs. 5-24 and 5-25). The effect of abdominal liposuction is to create the central and lateral shadowing "risk free" with a careful tension-free closure for a more acceptable appearance.

THE UMBILICUS

Reducing Tension on the Incision Line with Umbilical Relocation

When the umbilical stalk is stretched and there is an excess of upper abdominal skin, the use of liposuction is recommended if the closure is without tension (see Figs. 5-26 and 5-27). The "umbilical site closure technique" shown here keeps the new lower panniculus intact, with only a small amount of skin resected. In Figure 5-28, the new umbilicus has been set 13 cm above the incision line, which is covered by her "French line" lingerie. *The old umbilical site is closed vertically* in the midline with an additional 4 cm of length left so that closure to the fixed position of the mons is without tension.

Setting the Umbilicus

Once the position of the umbilicus is determined, a simple technique for bringing the stalk through the skin is the "modified Grazer" technique (see Fig. 5-29). Before determining the position, the mons veneris is elevated and sutured directly into the abdominal fascia at the preferred position. The flap is then tailored and measurement made for a new midline position, usually 13 cm above the closure line. Shown is a simple elliptical excision, although an open V may be preferable so that the upper portion of the skin can curl over to make a more natural appearance. A nylon suture is first placed through the umbilical stalk (see Fig. 5-30) and then into the fascia to hold the stalk in its preferred position. With the abdominal flap elevated, the suture is lifted out and passed through subcutaneous tissue (see Fig. 5-31), back through the fascia, and then out through the skin of the stalk (see Figs. 5-32 and 5-33). Once the final tailoring is complete, these two sutures are tied down to anchor the stalk and surrounding skin. Additional sutures are easily placed; see Figure 5-34. Having only two sutures to deal with in the closure is an advantage, and inversion of the skin edges creates a more natural umbilicus.

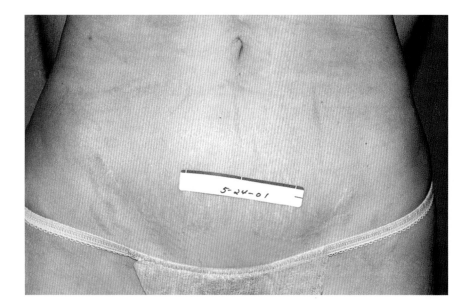

Figure 5-24 *Eleven-year appearance of a "Victoria's Secret" French line incision.*

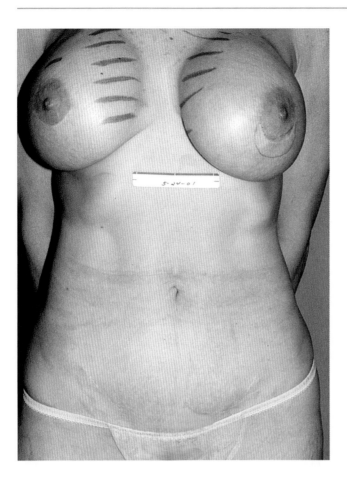

Figure 5-25 *Note the lateral and midline liposculpture shadows and markings for a replacement internal lift/repair of the breasts via the original periareolar incision.*

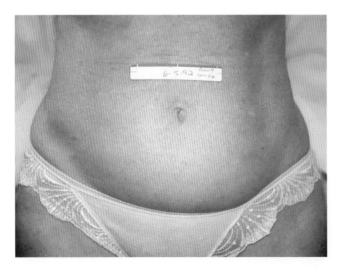 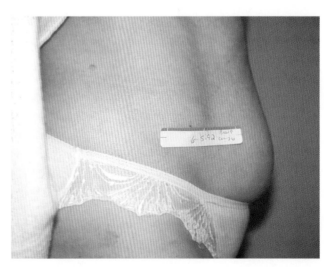

Figures 5-26 & 5-27 *When the umbilical stalk has stretched, repositioning is required along with a full "diastasis-ventral hernia" repair.*

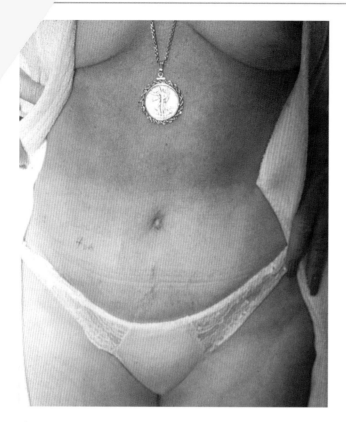

Figure 5-28 *At 4 weeks, the incision is concealed, the midline vertical closure of the old umbilical site is fading, and the new umbilicus is in the proper position.*

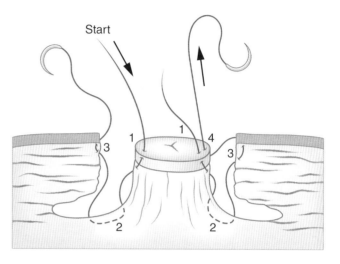

Figure 5-29 *"Two suture–four suture" umbilicoplasty. The top and bottom sutures of 2-0 nylon pass from the umbilicus to the fascia, then subcutaneously at the new site, and then back to be tied at the stalk later in the procedure. Side sutures are then added.*

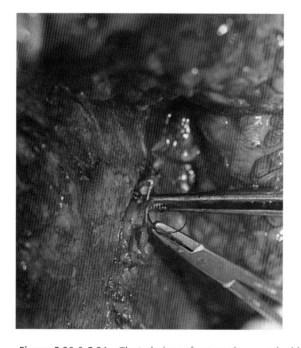

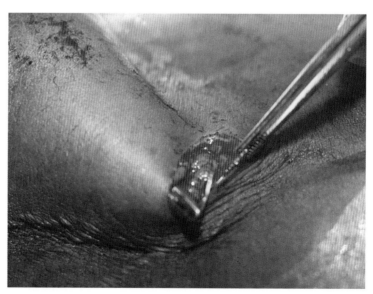

Figures 5-30 & 5-31 *The technique of suture placement in this simplified method of umbilical positioning.*

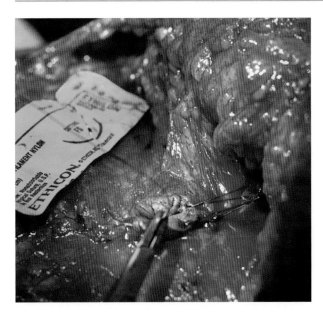

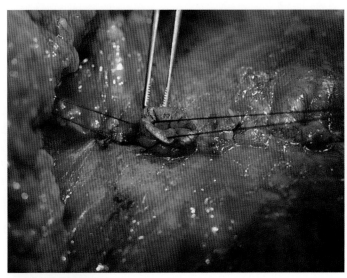

Figure 5-32 *Only two nylons sutures, top and bottom, are placed before closing the incision.*

Figure 5-33 *The tension of the closure will leave a mark, so the knot is tied on the stalk.*

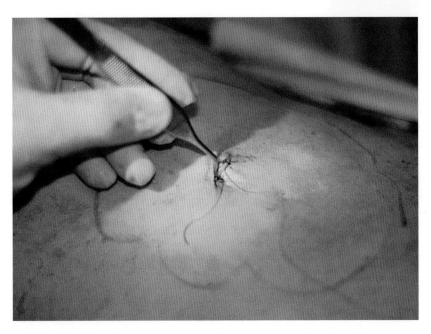

Figure 5-34 *Overlap of the new umbilicus gives a more natural appearance.*

THE FRENCH LINE INCISION

French Line Small-Incision Abdominoplasty with XUAL and Nonsurgical Facial Contouring

In the initial evaluation of XUAL, there were concerns about possible damage to the facial nerve at the crossing of the jowl line area and damage to blood supply of the midportion of the abdominal flap in abdominoplasty. This patient underwent simultaneous procedures that included a single 6-minute application of XUAL to the infiltrated jowl, submental triangle, and neck. As shown in Figure 5-37, there is minimal internal descent and minimal banding of the platysma. The early jowl changes place her in the category of a younger female patient who desires changes without the expense or recovery time of a mid–face-lift. This physically active woman was the only one of our original group who actually lost weight during the first year of follow-up, which was thought to be the reason for the continued improvement between the 2-month and 5-month postoperative photographs (see Figs. 5-38 and 5-39). Our subsequent experience revealed that this is an ongoing effect of XUAL because it occurred in *all* of our evaluation group. The contrast is even more marked when the 15-month postoperative photographs are compared with the preoperative status (see Figs. 5-40 and 5-41). The contrast was not as marked in a comparison of the frontal view preoperatively (see Fig. 5-42) and the 1-year photograph (see Fig. 5-43) in terms of resolution of the jowl fat and shaping of the neck.

Shaping the Umbilicus

Believe it or not, some physicians have spent a great deal of time investigating the shape of the umbilicus. Whereas most are vertical, there is a surgical advantage to making the umbilicus horizontal, particularly if the umbilical stalk is being used as a tether to stretch upper abdominal skin downward to relieve tension on the lower panniculus flap. This, however, is not the most natural umbilicus, as noted in photographs from 1975 (see Figs. 5-35 and 5-36). If one excises the skin and simply uses half-buried mattress sutures, a recessed inverted vertical umbilicus is created. One technique is to excise abdominal skin as a "V" and remove a pie section of the umbilicus so that the V-flap can be brought over it and create a hooded contour. Half-buried mattress sutures are used. In the "modified Grazer" procedure, mattress sutures are passed through the abdominal fascia to prevent stretching of the umbilical stalk. By tying the sutures on the stalk, one avoids visible hatch marks. It is certainly permissible to place a few tacking stitches on either side of the overhanging V-flap. As the flap contracts, it will tuck under and create the hood overhang, which should extend across the entire upper portion of the umbilicus and produce a more natural curve with a downward extension on either side. It's the little things that matter.

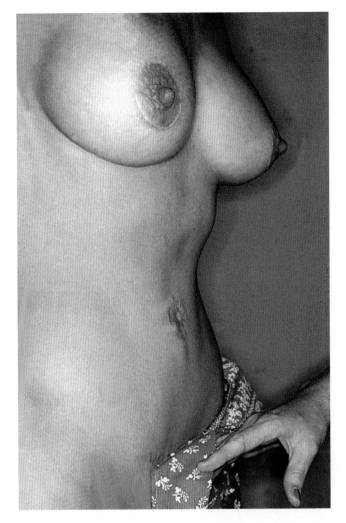

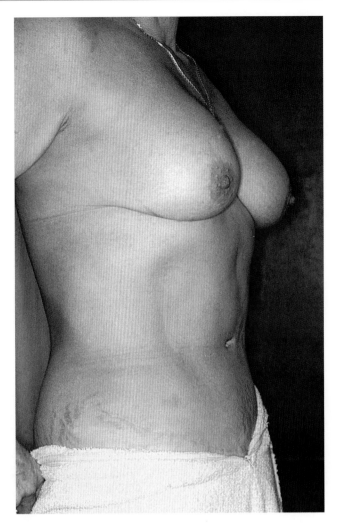

Figure 5-35 *Overstretch of the neo-umbilicoplasty requiring revision.*

Figure 5-36 *Ideally, the stalk–abdominal skin junction is below the surface.*

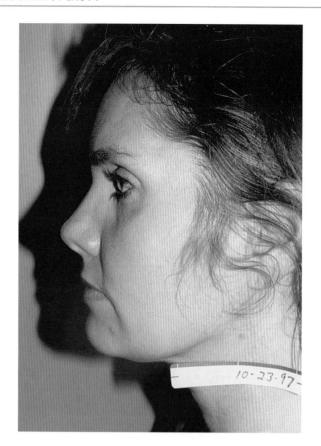

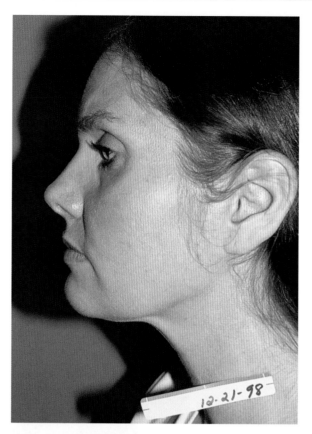

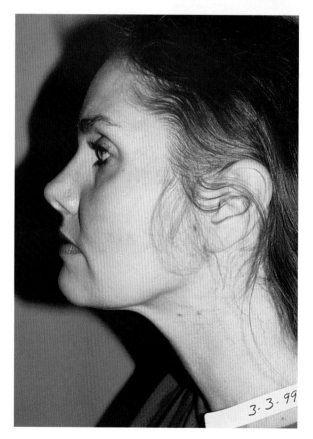

Figures 5-37 – 5-39 *Preoperative 9- and 15-month facial recontouring by ultrasound (XU) alone, applied while undergoing limited abdominoplasty.*

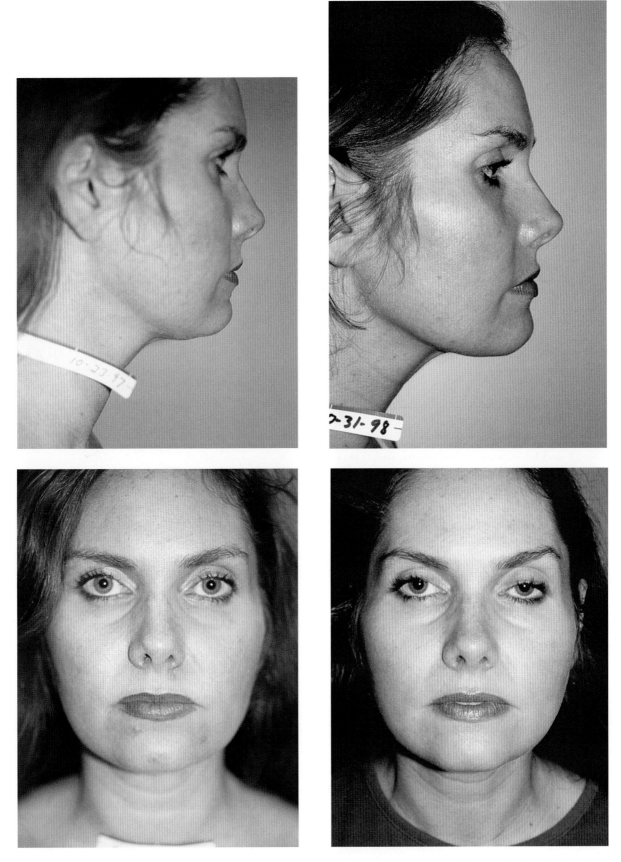

Figures 5-40 – 5-43 *Contouring with the single XU treatment nearly completed the transition at 12 months. Note the clean jaw line, but further improvement was seen in the 15-month photograph (see Figs. 5-39 and 5-43). Weight has remained stable.*

Shrinkage of the inner aspect of the thighs without rippling and contouring of the anterior of the thighs with ultrasound alone show the marked contrast between the preoperative view of the body (see Fig. 5-44) and a postoperative view at over 17 months (see Fig. 5-45). The change in the waistline is a result of the interior plication. Removal of a small amount of skin for access with a float of the umbilicus allowed complete plication from the xyphoid to the pubis, and XU was freely used in areas outside the triangle drawn above the mons.

As will be discussed in further detail, XU induced shrinkage of the flank areas without direct invasion of the liposuction cannula and gave a better contour in the flanks, as well as the upper lateral portions of the abdomen, in abdominoplasty patients who required a "complete" anterior repair of a central hernia with diastasis.

Complete Abdominoplasty with Extensive Liposuction

One of the most difficult problems in abdominoplasty and liposuction is folding in the mid-abdomen, often an area resistant to liposuction even with the assistance of shrinkage and facilitators such as XUAL and UAL. In the patient in Figure 5-46, the mid-abdomen ptosis is accompanied by thickening of the flanks and fat deposits in the inner aspect of the thighs. Conventional wisdom would be to ignore the back, thighs, and flanks because of fear of embarrassment of the blood supply (see Figs. 5-47 to 5-49). The infiltration solution was placed from the midline to the mid-back, and direct liposuctioning after XUAL was performed in the central folds as well as the high hip roll. The area between these zones was treated with XU alone, and XU was used alone beyond these areas both above and below the flanks. The fatty deposits in the inner part of the thighs were approached from the abdominoplasty incision and through a separate stab wound posteriorly to allow reduction of the "saddlebag" deformity.

A total of 4000 cc of the Hunstad formula was used. For the larger liposuctions, a single 50-cc vial of 1% lidocaine with 1:100,000 epinephrine is added to each liter. For smaller liposuction procedures, it is perfectly safe to add two such vials to obtain a more prolonged anesthetic effect. The diluted epinephrine of either combination is effective. The 5-month postoperative photographs show that the "French line" extension of the abdominoplasty is a smooth contour because of the lateral defatting (see Figs. 5-50 to 5-53). The umbilicus has been reset with the "modified Grazer" technique for suturing. The mons, inner aspect of the thighs, and hips were liposuctioned with 3- and 4-mm cannulas. Liposuction was performed across the midline from several directions with 6-mm cannulas in the deeper areas and progressed to superficial liposculpture with 3-mm cannulas. Postoperative ultrasound is applied to only these areas, including the abdominal flap, 24 hours after the operation. The remodeling will continue, especially because young individuals who are able to exercise will embrace a healthy lifestyle that includes exercise.

Although the weight loss associated with surgery may have contributed, remodeling of the facial fat deposits and jowl descent (see Figs. 5-54 to 5-56) was accomplished by infiltration and application of XUAL without liposuction. The platysma had not bowed or banded, so a clean jowl line was obtained with retraction of the mid-cheek and progressive smoothing of the nasolabial folds (see Figs. 5-57 to 5-59) long after her weight had stabilized.

CLINICAL PEARL

Should Anyone Ever Use UAL with Abdominoplasty?
Teaching courses rarely discuss this question. In my opinion, there is far too great a risk of interrupting the blood supply, even in experienced hands. Perhaps it should be used for a really, really fat abdomen! The surgeon will not tire as easily.

Dr. Gabriel Alvarado (plastic surgeon, Bogotá) agrees that UAL is helpful in abdominoplasty, but he will use it only in the hip area outside the main tension zone.

The effect of sound waves and the heat generated extends beyond the tip, thus making it essential that UAL be used carefully with abdominoplasty. UAL patients have a risk of necrosis of the flap, even if it is closed without tension and placed in the proper position.

Experienced UAL surgeon Dr. Joe Hunstad (plastic surgeon, Charlotte), an advocate of UAL, no longer uses UAL in any abdominoplasty area whatsoever. Furthermore, even with the use of low power, Dr. Hunstad has encountered internal burns and dysesthesias that last over 6 months in other areas as well. Needless to say, this dampens one's enthusiasm.

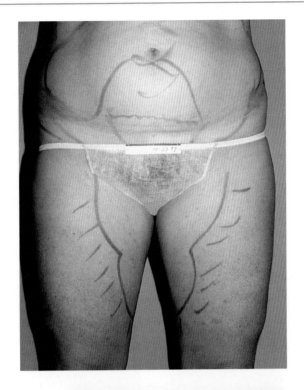

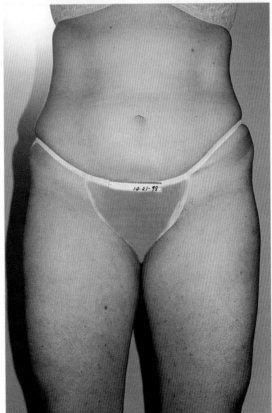

Figures 5-44 & 5-45   *By contrast, the improvement in the thigh XUAL areas was complete at 3 months. Limited abdominoplasty typically produces edema above the short "trapping fluid" incision, with final scar resolution typically, as shown, after 1 year.*

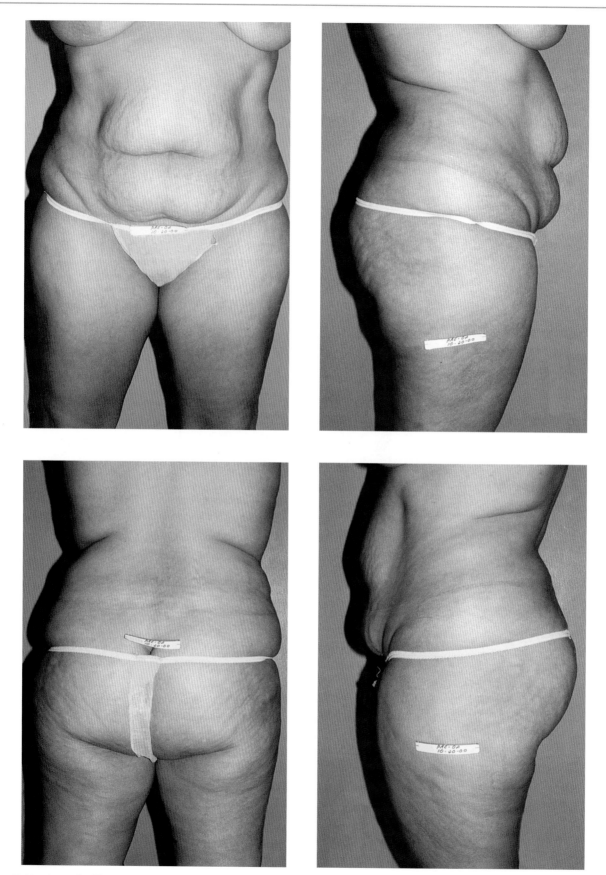

Figures 5-46 – 5-49 *"Full" abdominoplasty requires an extended-incision ("French line") abdominoplasty. Extension of the incision is required when major skin folds are present. XUAL will be directed at the flanks, back, hips, and thighs.*

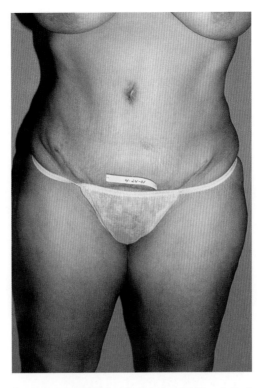

Figure 5-50 *The design of the extended "French line" and neo-umbilicoplasty places scars in natural fold lines.*

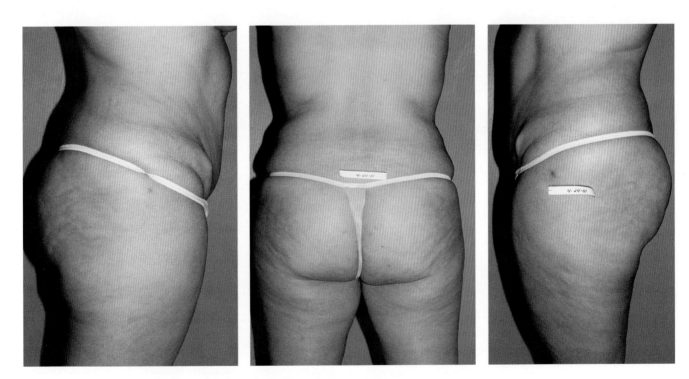

Figures 5-51 – 5-53 *Remodeling assisted by XUAL intraoperatively and postoperatively.*

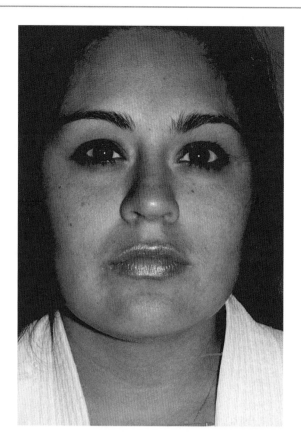

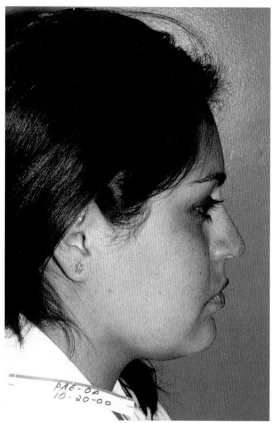
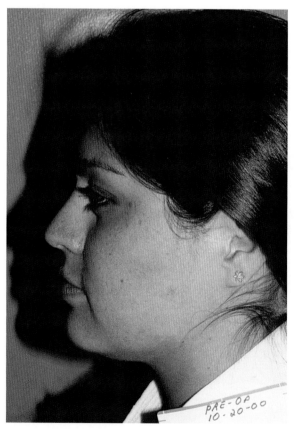

Figures 5-54 – 5-56   *Facial contouring: weight loss or ultrasound? Infiltration and XU of the face add little operating time and are greatly appreciated by "jowly" young adults whose facial fullness does not respond to diet and exercise.*

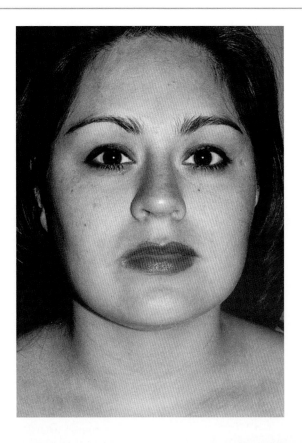

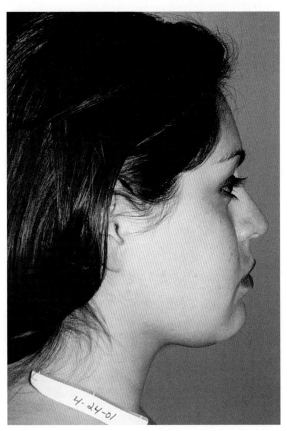
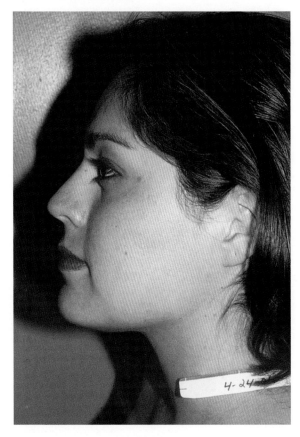

Figures 5-57 – 5-59   *Facial contouring continued to develop long after surgical recovery and weight stability, thus indicating that XU played a role.*

How Much Should Be Trimmed?

With extremely damaged abdominal skin, the lateral limbs of the abdominoplasty incision are lengthened so that *undamaged thigh skin can be moved upward* and a greater degree of damaged abdominal skin can be resected. In Figure 5-60, an operative photograph, the initial incision has been made but no decision has been reached regarding how much soft tissue will be removed. After the umbilical float has been completed, the skin will be stretched downward to the lifted and anchored lateral limbs and mons and then be trimmed appropriately.

CLINICAL PEARL

Avoid the Horseshoe!

In early attempts to limit the incision of abdominoplasty, Elbaz and others described an abdominoplasty in which a horseshoe incision was made around the mons veneris and extended downward but with no lateral extension. American surgeons have been unable to achieve the smoothness that was reported, and the operation fell into disfavor a decade ago. Unfortunately, bad ideas tend to resurface, and the newest version—the Mouffrage procedure—is no exception. Patient dissatisfaction leading to lawsuits was unfair to plastic surgeons who did not have the experience or know the development of these procedures. Natural body lines extend *upward* at the edge of the mons, which is the reason for the "French line" short-scar incision.

STAYING OUT OF TROUBLE

CLINICAL PEARL

Dr. Malcom Paul (plastic surgeon, Newport Beach), the past president of the American Society for Aesthetic Plastic Surgery, discussed the most dreaded complication of abdominoplasty—fatal pulmonary embolism. Although fatal pulmonary embolism is extremely rare, surgeons take all necessary precautions. Such precautions may include low-dose heparin in patients at risk, compression devices, early ambulation, and other measures. A once often overlooked problem is dehydration and constipation, which of course is compounded by narcotics. As a gastroenterologist pointed out, when a patient is in the flex position, a heavy colon will be lying against the pelvic veins. With positive-pressure ventilation there is an environment for stasis because of the weight of the colon. The recommendation is for a preoperative liquid diet, which may include the use of laxatives for a "clean out" of some sort before abdominoplasty. This practice has the additional benefit of avoiding postoperative constipation.

Correction of Endoscopic "Abdominoplasty"

This patient was referred for correction of her lips after an ill-advised attempt to achieve lip fullness with a dermis graft after lip roll failure resulted in transcutaneous perforation. She had undergone what was described as a lengthy endoscopic abdominoplasty but still exhibited laxity of the abdominal wall and irregularities of the fatty tissues (see Fig. 5-61). For unknown reasons, the dermis graft was taken from an area high above the mons line, and a visible scar was left.

Endoscopic abdominoplasty is rarely the procedure of choice. The avoidance of a scar is its primary advantage.

In the correction, a new incision was made at the level of the mons and then angled upward. Removal of 3 cm of skin between the old and new incisions was adequate for complete visualization and repositioning of the scar to an acceptable position in the "French line" (see Figs. 5-62 and 5-63). The procedure was preceded by XUAL. With the limited incision and "no-tension" closure, more aggressive liposuction, including the "champagne groove," and lateral liposuctioning from the original incision could be safely performed. The incision line has been lowered into a more acceptable position, and the entire abdominal contour has improved (see Fig. 5-64). It continued to improve despite weight gain (see Figs. 5-65 and 5-66), with fading of the incision into natural crease lines above the mons veneris (see Fig. 5-67).

Small incisions allow full visualization up to and beyond the umbilicus. In this case, the umbilicus was separated, "floated," reattached after plication in the upper part of the abdomen, and then reattached at the original level. XUAL provided the additional shrinkage of the upper abdominal liposuctioned areas.

CLINICAL PEARL

Endoscopic Abdominoplasty

The role of endoscopic abdominoplasty is limited to patients who have good skin tone not requiring excision and a rectus muscle diastasis near the xyphoid that cannot be corrected by conventional measures (i.e., long fiberoptic instruments). Patients should realize that there are many different surgical options for abdominal contour surgery—and for that matter for the breasts, the face, and any area. Some leave smaller scars, but the results are not interchangeable. If they were, there would be only one operation.

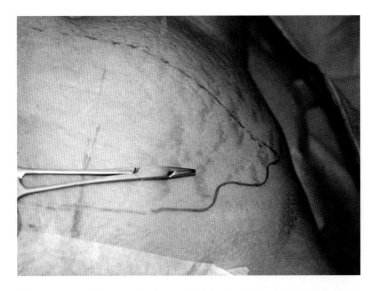

Figure 5-60 *With extremely damaged abdominal skin, the lateral limbs of the abdominoplasty incision are lengthened so that undamaged thigh skin can be moved upward and a greater degree of damaged abdominal skin can be resected. In this operative photograph, the initial incision has been made, but no decision about how much soft tissue will be removed. After the umbilical float has been completed, the skin will be stretched downward to the lifted lateral limbs and mons and then be trimmed appropriately.*

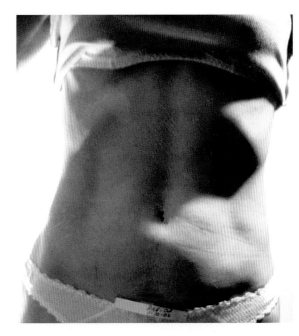

Figure 5-61 *Failed endoscopic abdominoplasty. "Shadow" photographs taken in addition to standard views emphasize the folding of incomplete fascial repair, excess skin, and residual fat after a failed procedure.*

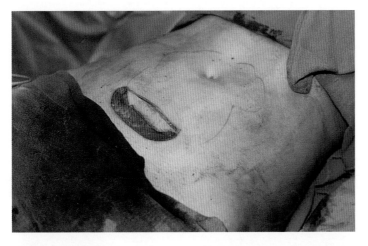

Figure 5-62 *An unrelated scar above the French line incision is included in our skin removal.*

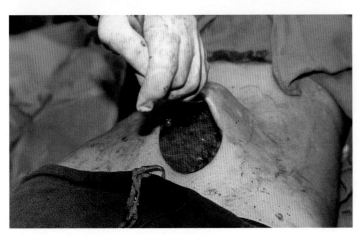

Figure 5-63 *With an "umbilical float," the entire central abdominal wall is easily exposed for precise fascial repair.*

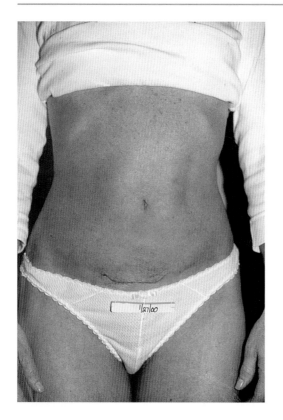
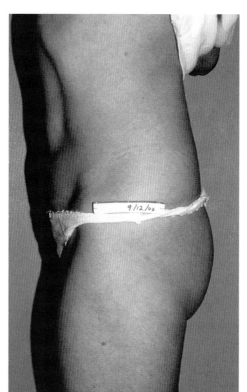
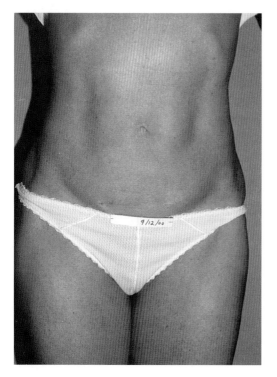

Figures 5-64 – 5-66 *XUAL, plication from the xiphoid to the pubis, and a low "French line" incision.*

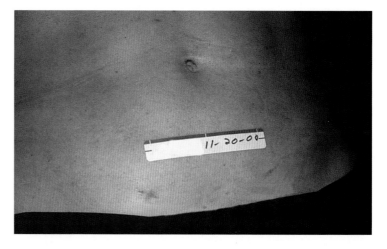

Figure 5-67 *Progressive improvement in appearance of the incision from oils and massage.*

Liposuction and Scar Elevation in Secondary Abdominoplasty

Although fat deposits can certainly recur after abdominoplasty, the extension of the incision shown in the patient in Figures 5-68 and 5-69 did not give her the smooth contour of the abdomen that was desired, presumably because the surgeon was reluctant to invade the flanks and hip rolls at the time of abdominoplasty.

Fashion changes to "French line" lingerie and bathing attire brought this patient to our clinic for revision surgery. One can certainly be more aggressive in lipo-suctioning a patient in whom only the lateral aspects of the incision line will be redone. With advancement of the unmarked high hip skin onto the abdomen and resection of a triangle above the original incision, as well as deep and superficial liposuction, restoration of contour is achieved (see Figs. 5-70 and 5-71). Moving the lateral scar and fixation to the underlying fascia allow her to wear high-cut lingerie with total conceal-ment of the incision (see Fig. 5-72).

She Almost Required a Second Abdominoplasty

The patient in Figures 5-73 to 5-75 had the typical lower abdominal stretch extending 4 cm above the umbilicus with only a moderate amount of fat deposits. Our plan was to include the right hip scar in the procedure so that we could move it into a French line position. During the limited abdominoplasty the umbilicus was lifted, plication was performed in multiple layers, and the right hip scar was advanced upward 3 cm and fixed. At 3 months, the patient had an excellent contour and the scar was beginning to fade. However, she immediately became very lax with her exercise and diet and presented with the problems shown in Figures 5-76 to 5-78, lower abdominal stretch.

Certain patients will maintain the full abdominal repair regardless of exercise habits and will deposit the gained weight in other places. Most will deposit the gained weight in the central portion of the abdomen. Fat cells are thought to have "first choice" in dietary fat.

In most patients, stretching of the repair requires secondary intervention. However, this case ended happily. She began a vigorous spa program, with diet and massage, abdominal crunches, and other exercises, and completely restored her abdomen to the original flat position that we had observed 3 months earlier. More often, a second liposuction procedure is required.

The Unsatisfactory Abdominoplasty

One problem that we have in south Texas that may be unique is "across the border" cosmetic surgery. Although many surgeons in our neighboring country are excellent, those who are not quite so accomplished tend to gravitate to the border towns where they offer face-lifts, abdominoplasty, liposuction, and other operations at less than the cost of our operating rooms here in the States. All of us in practice in San Antonio have been faced with the dilemma of redoing poorly performed surgery. Some patients are so embarrassed that they will not return for follow-up, especially if you have removed umbilical sutures 6 months after the original surgery. Others are ready to have something done to accomplish their goals. The problems are as follows:

1. The umbilicus is too large, too low, and off center.
2. Despite what our national seminars may say, patients are not happy with long incisions. Even folded lateral skin can be undermined and liposuctioned without extending the scar.
3. The scars are flat and long, hypertrophic, and crosshatched. (See Figure 5-89.)

What are your plans at this point? The initial step is to plan an extensive liposuction and resetting of the umbi-licus. Because the flap has been elevated before, lipo-suction can be more aggressive. In addition, there will be a tension-free closure, and the blood supply is already established. I elevate the entire panniculus after liposuction and stretch it downward after first resetting the mons. The mons is sutured directly into the deep fascia with No. 1 Dexon sutures so that it cannot ride upward or be a drag weight when the flap is laid in place after internal retightening of the rectus abdominis fascia. After flexing the table 20 degrees, the panniculus is trimmed so that it just touches the new position of the mons veneris. Plans include temporary tissue expanders on the hips and secondary advancement of these scars from the "bikini" position to the "French line" position. This technique has been especially useful for patients whose original stretch marks extend down-ward below the anterior iliac spine. Removing this damaged skin and rotating the normal hip-side skin upward is a good thought, especially in large persons.

However, if we simply remove everything from the old umbilicus down, the closure would be tight. This is a good spot for the "umbilical closure technique." First, separate the umbilicus from the panniculus. Second, working from below, place 2-0 Dexon sutures in the deep dermis and through the underlying fat and tie

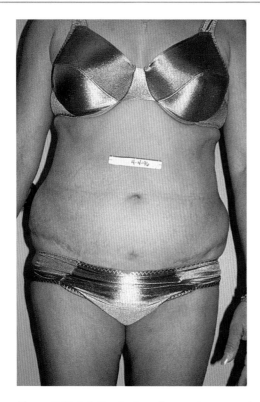
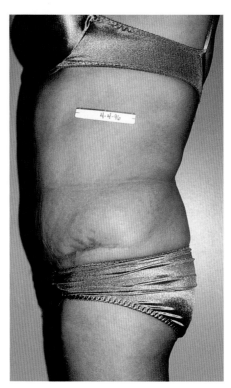

Figures 5-68 & 5-69   *Patients do care about scars. Secondary abdominoplasty usually involves liposculpture, defatting laterally, and replacing and retightening fascial sutures.*

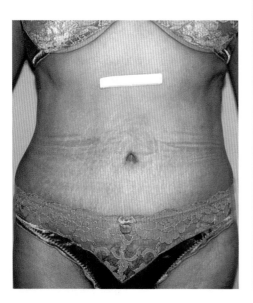
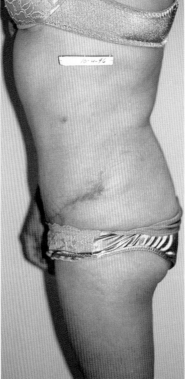
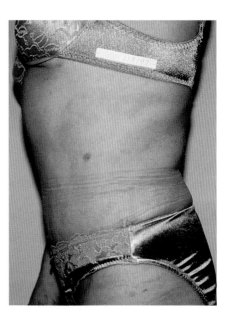

Figures 5-70 – 5-72   *In these cases, moving the lateral incision upward to be covered by "French line" lingerie was a priority.*

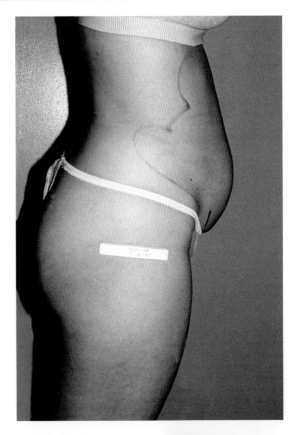

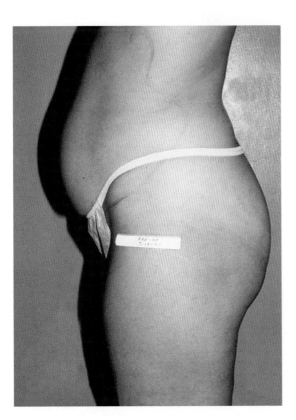

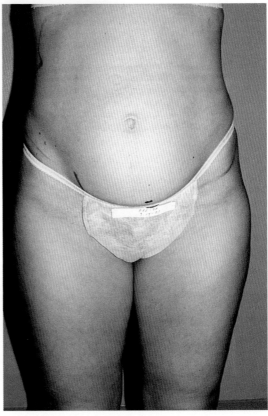

Figures 5-73 – 5-75   *Persistence of lower abdominal protrusion. With moderately thick abdominal fat, a xiphoid-to-pubis diastasis, and lateral folds requiring extension of the incision, there is no indication that this patient would require a secondary procedure in less than 6 months.*

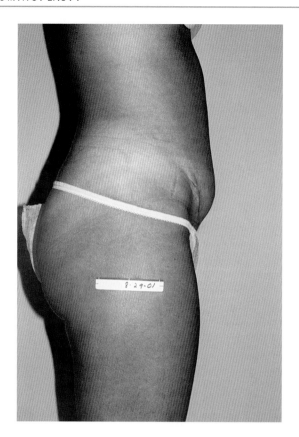
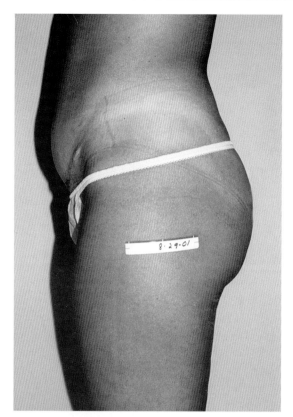
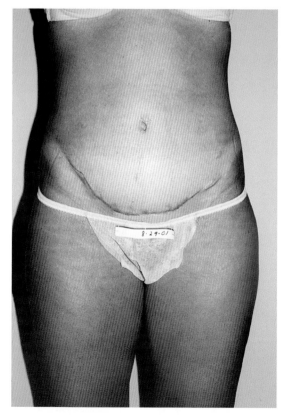

Figures 5-76 – 5-78   *Examination will reveal when weak musculature or lack of exercise has distorted the previously flat lower abdominal wall or whether simple XUAL will suffice for restoration after weight gain. More often than not, secondary plication plus liposculpture by XUAL is indicated. Fortunately, diet and exercise prevailed in this case.*

them without tension. This closes the soft tissue underneath the old umbilicus and converts it to a vertical slit. The umbilicus stalk can be brought through at the appropriate position.

Redoing the scar is a matter of outlining running W-plasties, closing underneath without tension, and ending with subcuticular sutures, preferably those that dissolve. (However, if you are performing a thigh-lift, it is probably better to use heavy nylon because there is more tension on these sutures with everyday activities.)

> **CLINICAL PEARL**
> When revising an unsatisfactory abdominoplasty, liposuction may be more aggressive because the flap has been elevated in the past. The revision is accomplished without tension on the flap. Typically, long lateral scars are advanced upward to bring undamaged thigh skin onto the abdomen so that the incision is no longer outside the lingerie line. Triangular excision above the original scar line is planned, but actual removal of the skin is not executed until the advancement has been completed. Resetting the umbilicus as a "tether" to the upper abdominal skin further reduces tension on the midline. In such patients, the mons must be elevated and resutured to its natural position, thus reducing tension further.

A Learning Experience

Seromas after abdominoplasty are unusual with modern techniques of gentle postoperative compression, prolonged drainage, povidone-iodine (Betadine) flush, and other measures. An infected seroma is even rarer, especially if one did not suspect that there was a seroma to begin with. In two recent cases, the source of the infection was a breakdown in the umbilical repair in patients who had no physical evidence of fluid formation. In each patient copious amounts of foul-smelling fluid developed under the lower abdominal area. One was treated by opening the entire incision and daily painful packing of the subpannicular area, and the other patient was treated by simple drainage and irrigation. In the first case, a woman who had been seen several days earlier and was at full activity, the patient was admitted to a hospital by a colleague to lift the flap for drainage. Apparently, this was a life-threatening or flap-threatening infection. On the advice of an infectious disease consultant, the patient was admitted for intravenous antibiotics. The entire incision was open and packing was placed. The pain of packing changes led the patient to consult an attorney.

> **CLINICAL PEARL**
> Dr. Edward Melmed (plastic surgeon, Dallas) highly recommends the Stryker epidural pump for post-abdominoplasty pain. The two fine catheter lines are passed through the abdominal wall, and the pump will then instill bupivacaine for 48 hours. After the pain has subsided, the lines are simply pulled out, and no marks are left. The pump unit may be carried in a bag on the hip, which is all supplied in a unit by the Stryker Corporation. We now use several manufacturers' pain pumps for all of our abdominoplasties. Patients tell us, "It was worth it."
>
> It has become common practice to use the "super wet" pump to instill the dilute solution intramuscularly, through incisions in the rectus and oblique fascia, and to inject bupivacaine (Marcaine) into the rectus fascia after the blockade has been complete. Although some surgeons may wish to avoid an additional variable, use of the "On-Q," "Scarlato," or new Byron Medical pump is a useful adjunct in pain control that permits pain-free deep-breathing exercises and more extensive easy ambulation.

Three years later, a police officer who was recovering well from abdominoplasty and breast surgery and had returned to her full police duties noticed that her gun belt was rubbing on the umbilicus. When she appeared at our office 3 days later, copious amounts of fluid were palpable beneath the flap. Because her insurance would not help, I drew on my experience in controlling superficial fluid infections in breast surgery. A far simpler approach was taken and was successful. The mid-flap was opened and drainage instituted. Irrigation with peroxide and Betadine was continued daily until fluid had ceased to form. A Jackson-Pratt drain was placed through the umbilical separation and left in place for several more days. After removal of the drain, healing progressed with only a single complication, an irregular umbilical scar.

One's first thoughts are that admitting the first patient was a careful conservative decision by physicians unfamiliar with a rare problem. She had noticed the drainage while she was taking a shower at a motel where she was spending the last few days in our city before her final checkup on Monday. The conservatism of infectious disease consultants (who still cannot grasp that an infection around a breast prosthesis can be controlled successfully in over 80% of cases by only temporary removal of the prosthesis to allow irrigation before immediate replacement), led to the decision to institute aggressive treatment. This was also based on the aggressive nature of this rare complication.

THE BURIED "EIGHT" KNOT

Originally published in *Technical Forum* in 1979,[3] this technique of burying the knot of the nonabsorbable suture not only simplifies the procedure by requiring fewer sutures but is a reliable method of closing the anterior fascia. An open-weave suture such as Mersilene is preferred because tissue ingrowth will further stabilize the repair. A running smooth nylon closure may disrupt and unravel, as noted in several of the cases of secondary abdominoplasty presented in this chapter. This was a major cause of the postsurgical protrusion. Once the deep nonabsorbable suture has been buried with the figure 8, an additional layer of erupted sutures of an absorbable material such as Vicryl may be used for further tightening and as an insurance repair. See Figure 5-79.

MORE WAYS TO STAY OUT OF TROUBLE: A CASE BY CASE REVIEW

Case in Point—Abdominoplasty with Liposuction—The Early Years

The patient shown in the 1985 black and white photograph in Figure 5-80 would have been treated differently today, but in my 1985 series, liposuction was used conservatively and primarily in the midline.[4] Many surgeons reacted with dismay. This was radical and unheard of! Because of concerns of blood supply, the past and present prescription of liposuction in the lateral upper portion of the abdomen is still wise. However, even with time and exercise, rippling and irregularity still remained in the areas that were not addressed. With the advent of XUAL without suctioning, shrinkage in lateral upper aspect of the abdomen was achieved without disturbance of the incoming blood supply.

This case also illustrates a heroic attempt to move an irregular vertical midline scar to a lower position by resetting the umbilicus. When the panniculus is separated and the umbilicus is reset in its normal position, most of the scar can be moved. Closure is performed with a running "W-plasty" using subcuticular and subcutaneous sutures. At 2 months (see Fig. 5-81), "dog-ears" from the shortened incision are evident, yet by today's standard, this incision is longer than required. Liposuction would have been performed in the lower lateral portion of the abdomen, plus defatting in the area covered by the distal 3 cm of the incision.

Lengthening the abdominoplasty scar does not necessarily eliminate "dog-ears." Defatting plus subcutaneous freeing of soft tissues is a better solution.

In time, the midline scar has faded nicely, the "dog-ears" have disappeared, but the fatty deposits and irregularities lateral to the rectus musculature still remain; today, these deposits and irregularities would have been addressed by XUAL (see Fig. 5-82). In addition, there is tissue reaction around the umbilicus. In 1985, fascia closure was done with Mersilene suture. To our dismay, Mersilene suture eroded through the umbilical stalk, which was thought to be safely at a distance of 1 cm. Eight years after the abdominoplasty, the resulting low-grade infection gave the appearance exhibited in Figure 5-82. Fascial sutures that are close to the umbilicus should be an absorbable type.

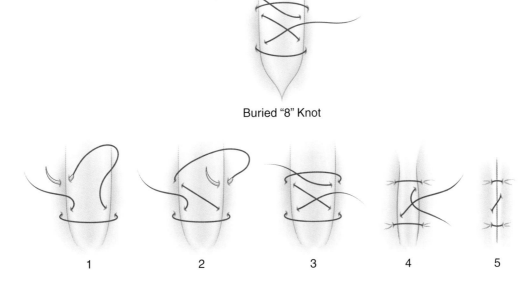

Buried "8" Knot

1   2   3   4   5

Figure 5-79   *Keeping it simple. A two-layered repair of the diastasis/ventral hernia should be rapid—using the "buried knot" figure-of-eight technique for the nonabsorbable first layer. My choice is No. 1 Mersilene and "O" Vicryl for the superficial layer.*

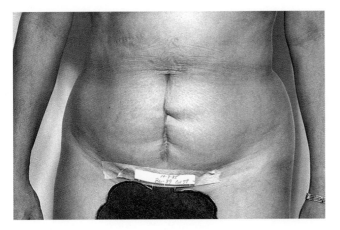

Figure 5-80   *Secondary liposuction after a difficult "complete" abdominoplasty. Correction will include W-plasty and Z-plasty of the vertical scar, relocation of the umbilicus, and suction-assisted lipectomy.*

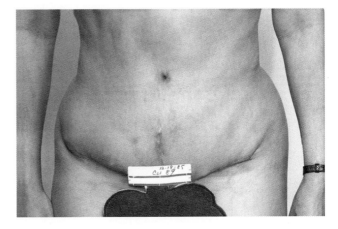

Figure 5-81   *Resistant "permanent" edema above the extended incision.*

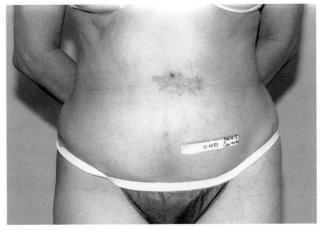

Figure 5-82   *The result at 8 years includes the benefit of being able to exercise. The rash is from an extruding umbilical suture.*

Case in Point—Elliptical Excision of Wrinkled Supraumbilical Skin

This patient had complications from old breast prostheses consisting of ptosis, capsular contracture, and distortion and required "internal mastopexy" with a textured gel prostheses to reconfigure the breast. Her second complaint was the laxity of her abdominal wall complicated by an extremely wrinkled "starburst" around the umbilicus (see Fig. 5-83). Simultaneous procedures were performed to correct the breast problem (see Fig. 5-84), as well as the abdomen, with the "super wet" pump technique used for dissection of the breast capsules as well as infiltration of the abdominal wall.

In patients of this category, removing a circle of skin around the umbilicus during the procedure plus enclosing it with an internal double-circle advancement suture is a good alternative. The surrounding tissue beyond the excision is brought inward and anchored to the umbilical stalk, which is left in its original position (see Fig. 5-85). The short-scar incision in the postoperative photograph shows persistence of tissue edema above the incision, which happens on occasion. Such edema is treated by instillation of local anesthetics and XUAL, often with the addition of superficial liposuction with a small cannula. Breast repair done with an internal lift has given a pleasing contour to the entire torso (see Fig. 5-86).

CLINICAL PEARL

A word of warning: when operating on patients who have had massive weight loss from such procedures as gastric bypass or extreme will power, remember that almost all of them have midline hernias. Be careful; they are very difficult to detect, and rupturing them with pre-suctioning in abdominoplasty can be dangerous.

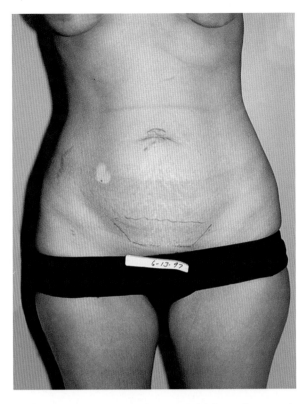

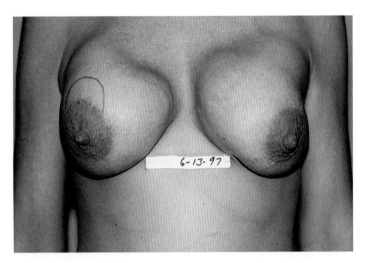

Figure 5-83 *Limited abdominoplasty with liposculpture and periumbilical excision. Individuals with lower abdominal diastasis complicated by circular wrinkling at the umbilicus are treated by excision and shortening of the umbilical stalk.*

Figure 5-84 *With XUAL's minimal blood loss, additional problems such as "internal mastopexy" are corrected simultaneously.*

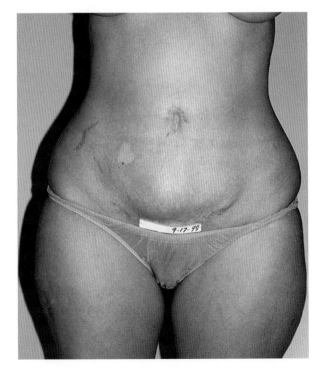

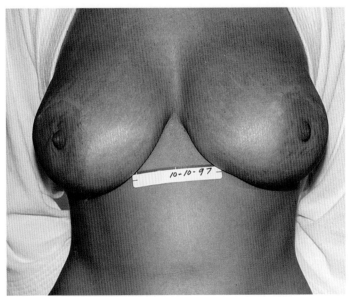

Figures 5-85 – 5-86 *Short-incision abdominoplasty with subumbilical repair and liposuction for contouring.*

Case in Point—Lateral Liposuction during Abdominoplasty

With short-incision surgery and tension-free closure, liposuction may be used to a greater degree in abdominoplasty than previously. The high hip roll is approached from an umbilical incision, from a mid-flank stab incision (see Fig. 5-87), and through the abdominoplasty incision by using a standard 3- or 4-mm cannula. Superficial suction may be safely performed laterally in the pre-marked areas. Fat removed from these areas will be immediately transferred for regrafting into the hip depression marked with the X's.

To avoid bulking and "dog-ear" formation lateral to the incision, this area is defatted manually during the abdominoplasty. The addition of liposuction is helpful as well. Figure 5-88 shows the introduction of a flat-bladed cannula passed superficially with the aperture pointing downward to completely flatten the area in a fan pattern beyond the incision.

The same flat blade is used with the aperture directed both up and down to create the "champagne groove" as shown in Figure 5-89. Entrance through the umbilicus is achieved with a small stab wound that is spread with a hemostab and allowed to stay open postoperatively for drainage and contracture of the incision.

CLINICAL PEARL

Remember that hernias in the midline can occur even in patients who have not had previous abdominal surgery. Be very cautious in liposuctioning a large person for that reason; although most of these hernias contain only fat, intra-abdominal bleeding can occur. There are also cases in which an abdominal viscus has been perforated, especially with UAL. The surgeons reported that they did not get the sensation that anything other than standard resistance was being encountered.

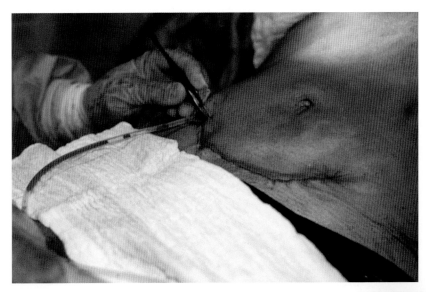

Figure 5-87 Fat deposits may extend into the thigh. They are removed through the abdominoplasty incision or a separate entry.

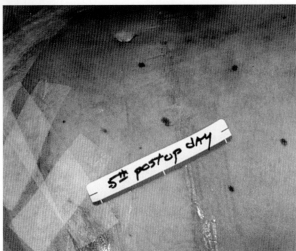

Figure 5-88 Prevention of "dog-ear" edema includes thinning the fat layer beyond the incision.

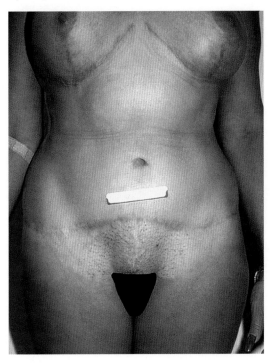

Figure 5-89 Long scar breast and abdomen surgery without more fixation can be improved upon with high advancement XUAL, and resetting of the flap.

Case in Point—Male Abdominoplasty with Umbilical Hernia

In a small minority of male patients, factors other than general health will affect the ability to control the anterior abdominal wall. The patient shown here has little subcutaneous fat, although liposuction in the flanks will be useful. Distortion of the abdominal wall and the presence of an umbilical hernia are easily diagnosed in this case, but in more obese patients, a high degree of suspicion of umbilical hernia is essential to avoid damage to the internal organs during liposuction.

Despite exercise and dieting, there is no improvement in the body contouring of these males (see Figs. 5-90 and 5-91). The same separation in the midline as in a postpartum female is to be expected. The plan of attack includes preliminary liposuction in the upper part of the abdomen and flanks, careful isolation of the expanded umbilicus, and conservative removal of skin and subcutaneous tissue after a "full" abdominal wall repair.

The incision around the site of the umbilicus allows placement of a finger to dissect and join the dissection from below. This avoids damaging the umbilical hernia invaginated by the index finger (see Fig. 5-92). It is closed during the plication process. Defatting of the lower abdominal flap is accomplished under direct vision for safety and efficiency. With one hand on the outside and the panniculus inverted, flat-bladed scissors are used to level the fatty tissue, including the predictable bulging fat on either side of the original umbilical site.

While the panniculus is everted, deep sutures are placed with inverted knots to close the original site of the umbilicus. The new site is set at 13 cm, in this case just slightly above the original site. At that point, abdominal "etching" proceeds with a flat-bladed cannula (see Fig. 5-93). Small entry points are made at one end of the pre-marked lines. Because the panniculus will be closed without tension in the recumbent position with only 30 degrees of elevation, etching can be performed during these abdominoplasties with safety. The cannula is first introduced with the hole down and then, as shown, withdrawn with the hole upward. This technique created a groove of the rectus sheath simulating that achieved by exercise.

Closure of the incision is begun in a lateral-to-medial direction, with shortening and elevation of the incision, which appears to be longer in the operative photograph because of tissue relaxation. Overcorrection is essential even in men who are increasingly vocal about their preference for high-cut "French line" bathing attire and thong underwear.

CLINICAL PEARL

Preventing and Treating Seromas

In the teaching course that Dr. Alan Matarasso, Dr. Luiz Toledo, and I have presented for the past 15 years on avoiding complications in abdominoplasty, seromas are always addressed with regard to both prevention and treatment. Few surgeons have embraced the "quilting procedure" in which the flap is anchored to the underlying soft tissue. It is not as effective as was hoped. With the advent of ultrasound liposculpture, however, the greater degree of tissue fluid release gives a "wet recovery." The use of light pressure and restrictive garments is more important than surgical technique, assuming that there is no bleeding postoperatively. Seromas can occur from suture tears in the postoperative period, as well as from traumatic disruption of the adhesion between the flap and the underlying fascial repair.

One year during the teaching course I stated that seromas were unheard of in my practice, but the next year I reported five! No change was made in technique—just the "gods of surgery" had stopped smiling.

Seromas are treated by aspiration and compression. After a period of time, if a true pseudobursa forms, open excision is mandatory. Lesser seromas are treated with liposuction, which will also reduce the bulkiness of the overlying soft tissue.

Although aspiration on a daily basis is usually effective, the device in Figure 5-94 is an improvement. The blunt-tipped seroma catheter is left in place for continuous suctioning. Certain surgeons will instill antiseptics or antibiotics in the belief that seromas may be the result of contamination. Certain antibiotics such as tetracycline will produce fibrosis. A far simpler approach is to maintain surface pressure and continuous aspiration.

CLINICAL PEARL

Remember that abdominoplasty, by the nature of the operation, eliminates the direct blood supply to the subscarpal abdominal fat; consequently, it is more prone to necrosis because the only oxygenation is now coming from the intercostals, which is another good reason to remove this fat with sharp or blunt dissection (see Fig. 5-95). Experienced surgeons believe that they can easily perform lower abdominal contouring with scissors dissection rather than liposuction, but the opposite is true of upper abdominal contouring.

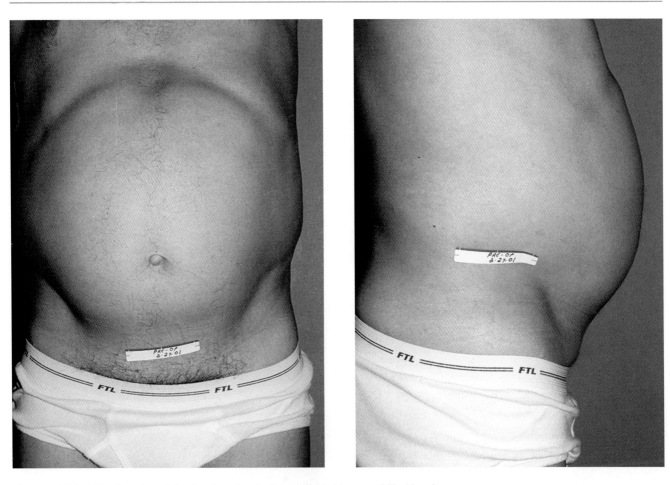

Figures 5-90 & 5-91   *Complete abdominoplasty in a male complicated by an umbilical hernia.*

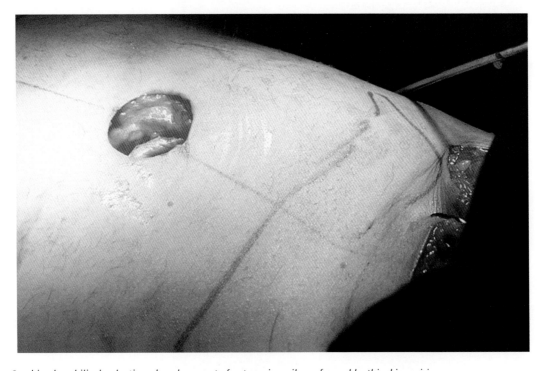

Figure 5-92   *Combined umbilical reduction plus placement of sutures is easily performed by this skin excision.*

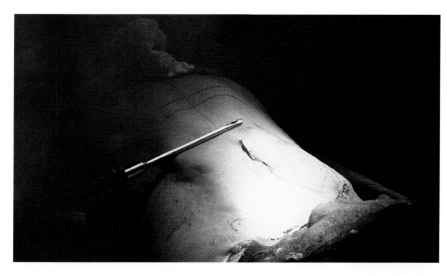

Figure 5-93 *Cross-suctioning of residual fullness at the completion of an abdominoplasty procedure.*

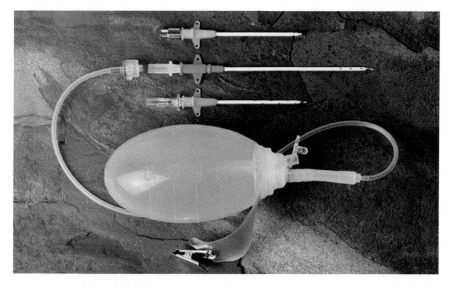

Figure 5-94 *One drawback of ultrasonic liposuction is the prolonged "wet recovery" of abdominoplasty. Despite leaving suction drains in place for 5 days, seromas may form. A simple treatment is the "Seroma-Cath" device, aided by antiseptic flushing of the cavity.*

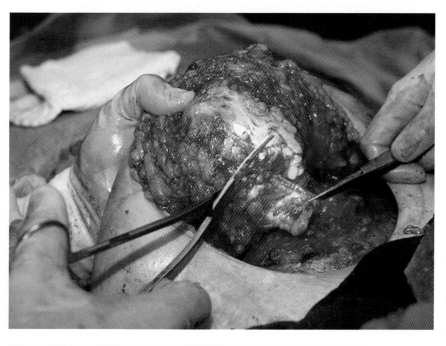

Figure 5-95 *Remember that by nature of the operation, abdominoplasty eliminates the direct blood supply to the subscarpal abdominal fat, which means that it is more prone to necrosis because the only oxygenation is now coming from the intercostals—another good reason to remove this fat with sharp or blunt dissection. Experienced surgeons believe that that they can easily contour the lower abdomen with scissors dissection rather than liposuction, but the opposite is true of the upper abdomen.*

CONCLUSION

As stated in a recent presentation at our local plastic surgery conference, a visiting professor said quite clearly, "liposuction is the standard of care in abdominoplasty." Those of us who have been involved with the development of liposuction certainly agree and have often stated, dating back to publications in the mid-1980s, that liposuction is a "essential part" of abdominoplasty. Obviously, over-resection of the panniculus is dangerous and unwarranted, but etching and sculpturing and the use of XUAL in the lateral flank areas to reduce rippling are advances in recent years.

The most common mistake of an inexperienced surgeon is to offer a patient only liposuction when the major problem is the abdominal wall. The second mistake is to assume that there are no paraspinous, umbilical, or fragile ventral herniations beneath the thick panniculus that might be injured by pre-suctioning. For this reason, liposuction should be performed in safe areas only; the abdominal wall should be identified before any manual or liposuction thinning of the panniculus is performed on more difficult patients. We also emphasize that the panniculus must be kept at a greater thickness than a liposuctioned abdominal area to maintain the blood supply, and closure without tension is a valuable adjunct in preventing ischemic necrosis.

References

1. Wilkinson TS: Abdominoplasty. *Advances in Plastic and Reconstructive Surgery,*. 1996; 12:173-205.
2. Hester TR, Baird W, Bostwick J, Nahai F, Cukic J: Abdominoplasty combined with other major surgical procedures: Safe or sorry? *Plastic and Reconstructive Surgery,* 1989; 83:997-1004.
3. Wilkinson TS: Abdominoplasty and figure-8 closure. *Technical Forum,* 1979; 3:7-9.
4. Wilkinson TS, Swartz BE: Individual modifications in body contour surgery: The "limited" abdominoplasty. *Plastic and Reconstructive Surgery,* 1986; 77:779-784.

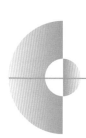

CHAPTER SIX

Liposuction of the Legs, Calves, and Arms

Although surgeons were pleased with the results of standard pre-liposuction arm, thigh, and calf reduction, patients were appalled by the resulting scars and discomfort. Even clear preoperative consultation was not effective when patients were faced with this dilemma postoperatively. In certain patients skin reduction is still required, but the various techniques of thigh-lift, with avoidance of a vertical scar, and reduction of the arm to a degree that is acceptable, even in extreme cases, or without skin excision are advantages.

In my practice, most arm and thigh reductions are performed with tiny incisions for external ultrasound-assisted liposuction (XUAL). Even patients who are offered the choice of skin excision may reject it and will be pleased with the result of ultrasound-assisted liposuction (UAL). A secondary XUAL procedure has been performed on a number of these individuals' arms and inner thighs, with the usual postsurgical massage, ultrasound, and other modalities, and has induced secondary skin contracture, which made the final appearance more satisfactory.

Liposuction of the calves and ankles has evolved into a useful procedure for a small subgroup of patients. Patient selection is important, and the technique is extremely difficult. This chapter will include advice from experts who have mastered the intricacies of these seemingly innocuous procedures to reduce complications and enhance patient satisfaction.

The extremities offer various challenges for liposuction and require different approaches, different cannulas, and different aftercare. They have a higher risk for pulmonary embolism unless ambulation, compression, and fluid balance issues are addressed.

PATIENT SELECTION

In no other area is patient selection so critical. Because the ankles and calves are the most dependent parts of the body that are addressed, one question is whether the patient will cooperate with compression garments and early ambulation to avoid the common complications of extremity surgery. Preoperative counseling should stress prevention of pulmonary embolism. In addition, these patients must be made fully aware that much of the bulk of the ankles and calves is not fatty. These areas cannot be reduced by any known means. A "thick-ankled" individual will have wider bone structure and fascia than normal and must be aware preoperatively of the limitations of liposculpture. The same applies to the calf zone, where an overdeveloped gastrocnemius and wide bone structure may be the only problem. These areas are not correctable. The use of fine cannulas, as will be described by Dr. Mladick in a later section of this chapter, with curved approaches is a technical detail that is of utmost importance in achieving good contouring in these areas. Rather than open-tipped cannulas, which may inadvertently remove the fat nearest to the skin in these minimally enlarged areas, a "standard" cannula with a single downward-facing hole may be a better choice.

Because the skin of the calf will contract well, ultrasound does not play an important role as it does in patient selection of the arms. Most arm deformities are fat in the lower third of the upper part of the arm with minimal fat in the upper, outer two thirds. These patients were formerly offered only skin resection, and despite our best efforts, the scarring was not only symptomatic but also highly visible. The application of UAL and XUAL to these areas brings another category of patient for evaluation.

In a true "bat wing deformity," liposuction plays a role in contouring after skin excision. Such skin excision, beginning at the elbow and extending to the axilla, may be the only choice for these individuals. A lesser skin excision extending partially from the axilla with a Y extension may be a good selection as well. However, given the choice in counseling, patient will choose to have a lesser procedure such as XUAL if it will achieve their goals.

In most patients whom I have counseled, a completely smooth, contracted upper arm is an ideal that cannot be achieved with these lesser means. These patients often express their desire to rid themselves of bulk, and they are not overly concerned with the irregularity that may result from incomplete contracture as shown in the presurgical counseling. These individuals were quite pleased to undergo arm reduction by XUAL, and often to our surprise, the contours were "good" to "extremely good."

In an effort to improve these results, several patients agreed to undergo a trial of a second XUAL. As in the first treatment, ultrasound is applied circumferentially and compression is continued for 6 to 8 weeks postoperatively. The secondary procedures yielded very little fat, but there was a surprisingly good increase in overall contour from circumferential shrinkage that was attributed to the effect of ultrasound on the deep dermis.

There is a "tradeoff" between accomplishing a procedure and making the arm veins off limits for postoperative blood analysis. When compression garments or wraps are applied to the upper part of the arms, the patient must be made aware that the hands and forearm will remain swollen for up to 72 hours. The same applies to the feet and ankles when calf liposuction is performed. In these instances, if an additional "blood loss" procedure has been performed concomitantly and the surgeon desires to have information regarding blood loss, a finger or toe stick is still out of the question. An arterial sample or an earlobe stick will reflect only the hemodilution of the original procedure, which generally stabilizes at 48 hours.

As Dr. Fodor and others discussed in an analysis of fluid balance in the late 1980s, blood loss is judged by the amount of liposuction and not by peripheral blood

analysis because of these hemodilution factors. The additional factor of XUAL hemodilution is that the areas that are infiltrated are not aspirated. This additional fluid enters the bloodstream, and with compression of the arms or calves, centers in the feet and hands. It all equalizes after a while, and the danger of skin loss from compression is eliminated by periodic release of the compression bandages.

Empirically, we have advised arm and calf reduction patients to wear compression garments for weeks longer than body reduction liposuction patients do. The difference in small amounts of shrinkage is quite visible, and the additional compression certainly plays a role.

CLINICAL PEARL

Beware of Snug Binders and Girdles

It is important when measuring patients for postsurgical garments to make sure that the "fit" is snug, but not tight. The use of these garments must be intermittent to avoid complications. It is helpful to remind patients of media reports of pulmonary embolism after transatlantic airplane flights. The problem is immobility with the knees flexed.

As Alan Matarasso (plastic surgeon, New York) comments, "All patients should be appropriately screened before surgery, especially for hereditary thrombophilias, such as protein C or protein S deficiency, factor 5 mutation, or prothrombin 21202A mutations." More important than detecting these rare bleeding disorders (which should have been reported by patient complaints to primary care physicians) is sufficient hydration. One may disagree with Dr. Matarasso's prohibition of "all female hormones" and the recommendation for systemic steroids as prophylaxis, but there is no question that patients who have been in good health and never experienced surgery should have at least basic screening tests for liver function and blood-clotting ability.

The "banana roll," a roll of fatty tissue under the buttock fold, resists improvement unless the subcutaneous tissue is separated by liposuction. Cannulas are turned both toward the skin and away. *This is one area where tape compression may be used today as it was in the early 1980s.* The buttock itself is part of the problem and may be addressed by fat grafting into dimpling with or without liposuction across the entire area or in selected spots. The "banana roll" fat may blend into the area generally called the hip and thigh, or the deposits may be separate. The lateral area traditionally responds well to liposuction, but the inner aspect of the thigh has always been an enigma. *Liposuction of the inner part of the thigh was often discouraged because of the high incidence of rippling and irregularity.* The advent of ultrasound has changed this practice considerably by making the results of inner thigh liposuction acceptable for older age groups.

CLINICAL PEARL

Liposuction of the Inner Thigh

Preoperative assessment and consultation are essential when addressing fatty deposits in the inner aspect of the thighs. Although these deposits occur primarily in women, men may also list this as an area for resection. Perhaps some of the improvement that is obtained is due to the fact that these individuals can now exercise, including power walking and use of the treadmill, without the discomfort in the inner thigh fatty areas.

Until recently, it was advised that inner thigh liposuction be avoided in all but young women with good skin tone. Rippling occurs naturally at a certain age in many individuals, and this rippling was accentuated when the fat was removed despite efforts at massage, taping, compression, and other modalities. Inner thigh skin contracture is a major benefit of XUAL, but it is certainly limited. For older individuals, only an improvement in bulk but not appearance should be the goal of the surgeon and accepted as a goal by the individual patient. In the intermediate group, older women and most men, the rippling that is apparent after fat removal can be improved dramatically by XUAL skin contracture. It is essential that ultrasound, massage, lymph drainage, and exercise be included in the postoperative recovery period.

The knee with its softer fat has always responded well to liposuction. Good results are obtained in the 70+ age group, in which one would not expect this degree of tissue contracture. Ankles and calves are always approached with some trepidation, but with the pioneering effort of many surgeons, the technicalities of liposuction of the inner aspect of the calves have been addressed successfully.

CLINICAL PEARL

The inner knee fat has been said to be softer and a better graft material for facial defects, although this point is impossible to prove. One fact is apparent, however: it is very easy to over-resect fat on the inner portion of the knee.

Although fat grafting in the hands is often performed in the elderly in conjunction with chemical peeling, it is advisable to avoid the "hand-lift" once enthusiastically endorsed by Mexican surgeons. Excision of skin on the hand is fraught with the same complications as thigh-lift excisions: stretching scars, taut skin inhibiting normal motion, and a generally unsatisfactory scar in a very visible area.

I have often stated that "surgical thigh lift and surgical arm reduction are unsatisfactory operations performed for an unsatisfactory condition in an unsatisfactory location." Modifications of the arm reduction, such as incisions with shorter scars, are still required for certain "bat wing" deformities. These procedures *must* be performed in conjunction with liposuction. Even short incisions may be avoided with the skin contracture achieved after the application of ultrasound with liposuction. Although certain patients may accept the problems inherent in thigh-lift incisions, such as scar migration and hypertrophy, few patients will accept even properly performed inner excision with W-plasty closure. With increasing experience, arm reductions are rarely performed in my practice, which admittedly rarely includes the severe "bat wing" deformity.

ANESTHESIA

The extremities lend themselves to regional block or spinal anesthesia, which are preferred by many surgeons. The old technique of filling the venous system with anesthetic while a tourniquet compresses the upper part of the arm has fallen into disfavor, but regional blocks in the axilla may still be preferable. Unfortunately, most arm liposuction procedures include the anterior and posterior axillary fat pads. My preference in healthy patients is intravenous sedation to avoid the consequences of pain with injection and "super wet" infusion in the entire circumference. If one is performing suction-assisted lipectomy (SAL) or UAL, it is necessary to infuse only the area that will be suctioned. Adding the additional fluid to this circumference will of course hemodilute any blood samples drawn from that extremity to a greater degree, but this consideration is not valid when evaluating one's choice of anesthesia.

Because the extremities are easy to infuse and the patient is comfortable during the liposuction phase, one preference is the use of a posterior pharyngeal balloon, which is chosen because it avoids intratracheal intubation. It gives the anesthesiologist control of the airway and delivers the anesthetic gases into the respiratory system. Only when the area for secondary liposuction is small should one use local anesthesia alone. As noted in earlier chapters, the pain factor with its systemic effect far outweighs any other considerations for liposuction, except in the smallest areas. One should defer to the judgment of the anesthesiologist, who evaluates all factors with the surgeon, including patient health, the position of the arms, blood loss, and such.

INSTRUMENTS

Smaller cannulas are chosen for liposuction of the extremities for several reasons. In the typical patient who asks for arm reduction, there is a fine line between over-resection and adequate resection. A dual approach with 4- and 5-mm single-hole cannulas is a conservative, but effective way to approach these previously outlined areas that have been infiltrated. For larger deposits in the thigh or hip area, multiholed 5- and 6-mm cannulas are often used in the deeper fatty layers with a change to a curved cannula to reach as many areas of the extremity as possible with the fewest incisions. This technique will be discussed by Dr. Mladick. Smaller-diameter cannulas are certainly helpful in contouring the areas of transition between fat that must be removed and areas where fat should not be removed. One must remember that even small cannulas can damage the deep dermis and thereby result in inoperable, uncorrectable scarring and deformity.

CLINICAL PEARL

Multihole or Single-Hole Cannula?
Complaining to me that no one seemed to be interested in the certainly not earth-shattering discussion of whether cannulas with a single or multiple holes are preferable, Dr. Carson Lewis (plastic surgeon, La Jolla) related that he realized that the diameter of the cannula was more important than the number of openings. With a smaller diameter, fat can be removed more rapidly, but a lesser effect is achieved in contouring. Initial concerns of a "rasp" effect (scraping between the two openings that might injure blood vessels or cause soft tissue damage) have not materialized. Double-hole and triple-hole cannulas were originally promoted by Dr. Pierre Fournier (Paris). The additional holes do speed up the process, especially if one chooses smaller-diameter cannulas.
All in all, it comes down to experience. For a larger area, go ahead and listen to that persistent cannula salesman and use a multihole 5- or 6-mm instrument. For "superficial" suction closer to the surface, a multihole or single-hole 3-mm cannula is an excellent instrument for final contouring and avoiding damage to the overlying dermis and blood supply.

LIPOSUCTION OF THE THIGHS

Case in Point

This patient exhibits the *typical lower abdominal fatty deposits, which include much of the lower part of the buttock; the "transition zones," in which there is little fat above the major lower buttock accumulation; and the usual "banana roll" and inner and outer thigh zones,* which are seen more commonly as an isolated occurrence. Figures 6-1 to 6-4 indicate the areas for liposuction. Liposuction will not be performed on the inner part of the thigh. In patients with minimal fatty deposits in this area, furrowing and irregularity are common. In this patient the interior thigh and upper buttock area was treated with XUAL only, a 10-minute application for the legs and 10 minutes for the upper portion of the buttock after full "super wet" infiltration. The diagrams for XUAL and external ultrasound alone (XU) are shown in Figures 6-5 to 6-8.

Some 4 months previously during surgery for a breast-related problem, this patient underwent standard liposuction (SAL) for the hip, thigh, and high hip roll. Significant weight gain was responsible for the second surgery about 4 months later. The fat grafts that had been placed in the buttock fold (see Figs. 6-3 and 6-4) had stabilized and did not have to be repeated. However, these photographs before her second surgery show an increase in fatty tissue not only in the original suction area but also in the lower part of the buttocks.

External ultrasound assist was used in the surgery, and the results shown in Figures 6-9 to 6-12 confirm rapid resolution of the problem. This patient was asked to compare the two procedures. In her opinion, the external ultrasound procedure, even though it covered a more extensive area, resulted in less discomfort, very rapid return to full normal activity, and accelerated regression of the deformity.

This patient illustrates our impression that the use of external ultrasound preoperatively and in postsurgical treatment makes recovery faster for these individuals with less discomfort and less bruising. Serving as her own control made her observations valid. In the subsequent 4 years, she has not regained the fat and has maintained the correction shown in the last photograph.

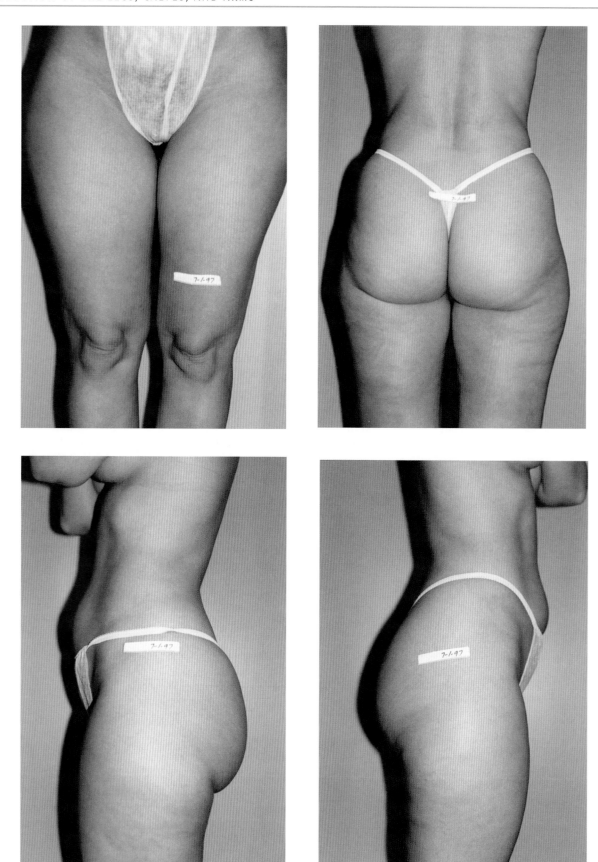

Figures 6-1 – 6-4   *The surgeon is expected to evaluate all areas of concern and point out areas amenable to correction.*

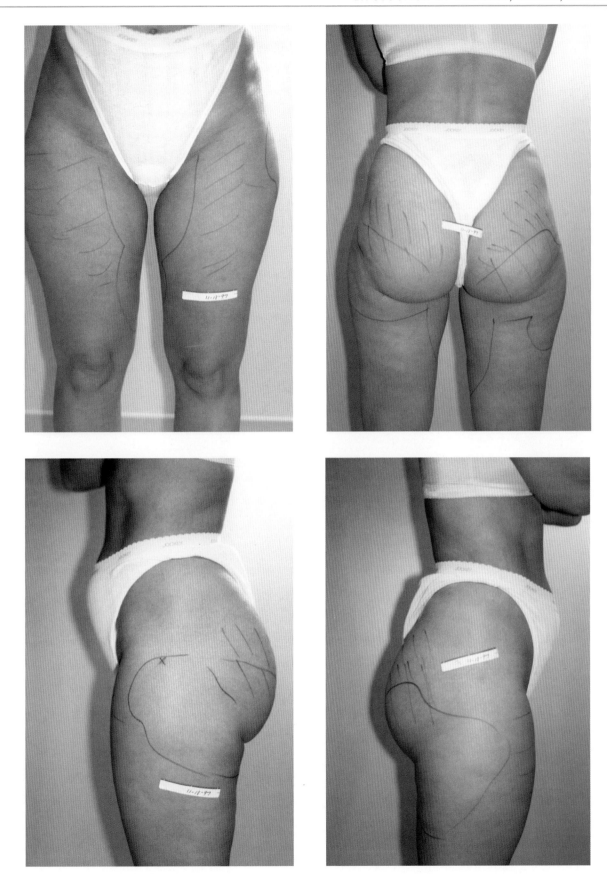

Figures 6-5 – 6-8   *At the first examination, a plan is drawn with washable ink that should be reinspected by the patient later that day. In this case, XUAL of the inner aspect of the thighs and hips was performed, as well as autologous fat grafting across the buttocks.*

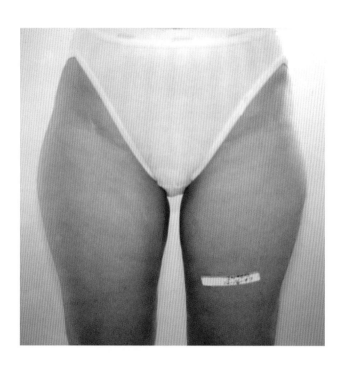
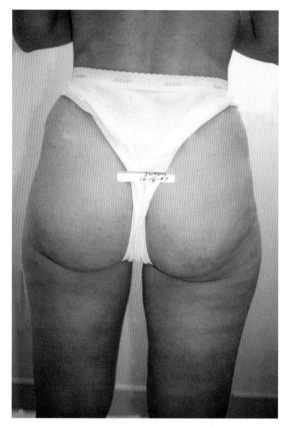
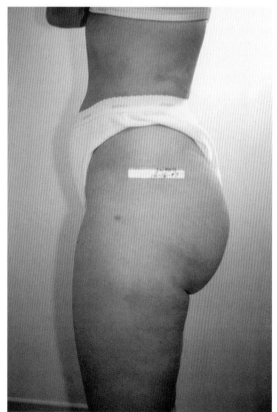
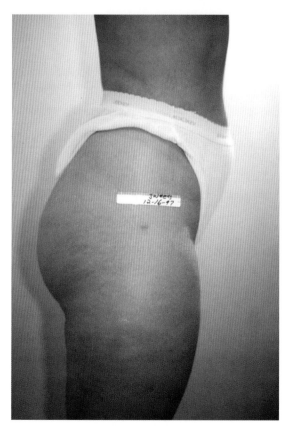

Figures 6-9 – 6-12   *While XUAL resolution continues, the results seen at 30 days are equal to the expected result of standard liposuction between the third and fifth month.*

Over-resection

A patient who had undergone liposuction under general anesthesia in 1990 asked for help in 1992 in correcting the deep over-resection areas, as well as a mixture of under-resection, scars, dimples, and "pockmarks" (see Figs. 6-13 to 6-16). Fortunately, interior thigh fat was available for "donor fat."

To correct problems of this nature, all the marked depressions, including the large central one, are undermined completely with a "pickle fork" or in a tunneling fashion. Fat is then removed from the under-resected areas with 3-mm cannulas after local infiltration. This fat is immediately transferred after concentration with the drainage "Telfa pad technique." For more superficial depressions, a pickle fork frees the dermis, and the fat is laid beneath the area with a blunt-tipped 14-gauge cannula. For smaller areas, the tip of a 16-gauge needle is used to release the banding, and small fat grafts are placed directly under the skin. If sufficient fat is available (and it was in limited supply in this patient in 1992), crisscross filling is done in the central buttock depression in several levels, including intramuscularly.

After 6 years and some weight gain, the patient presented for further repair in 1998 (see Figs. 6-17 to 6-20). Ultrasound was then used in areas outside the remaining fat zones. Continued atrophy of the buttock area left the depressions noted especially in Figure 6-20, but there had been little recurrence in the inner and anterior thigh areas that had been liposuctioned earlier. Fortunately, a high hip roll donor site was present bilaterally, and the resulting depressions in the mid-buttock were not as deep as in 1992. Small-cannula resection of fat superficially in the circled areas gave sufficient donor fat to fill the depressed areas. Ultrasound pretreatment enhanced skin contracture, as seen in the postoperative photographs (see Figs. 6-21 and 6-22).

As noted in the discussions in this chapter, over-resection should be avoided at all cost. It is certainly simpler to take more fat later with a small 3-mm cannula in a "touchup procedure" for under-resection than it is to attempt such a repair.

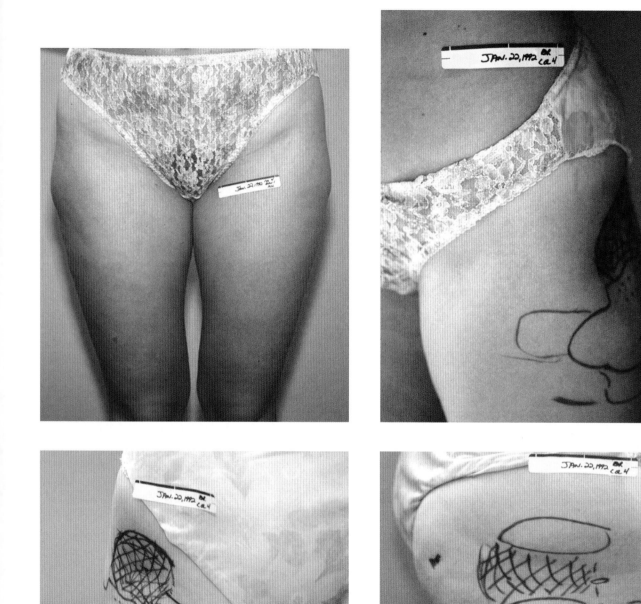

Figures 6-13 – 6-16 *Poorly performed liposuction leaves gross irregularities complicated by scar tissue and adherence of skin to muscle.*

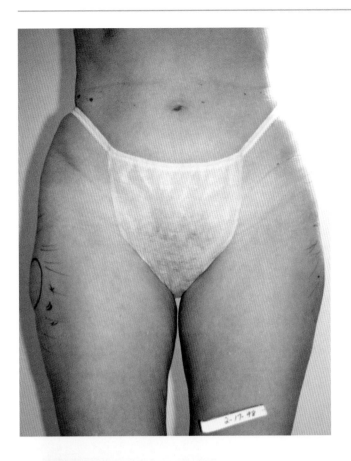
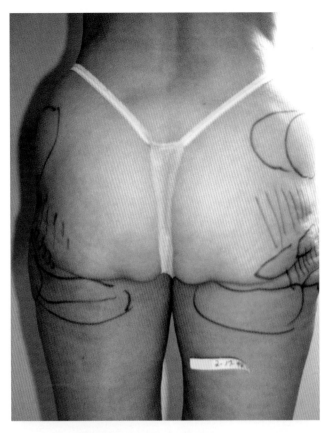
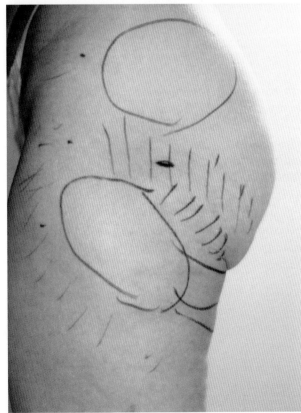
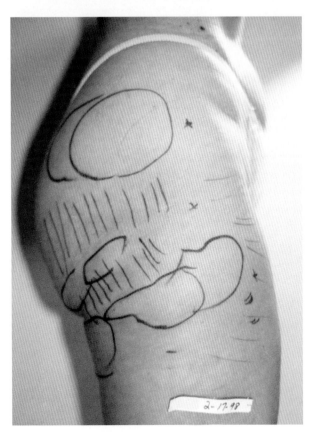

Figures 6-17 – 6-20 *After a staged first procedure with selective liposuction, scar separation, and fat regrafting, plans are drawn for the second procedure that will be facilitated by operative and postoperative XUAL to continue the improvement.*

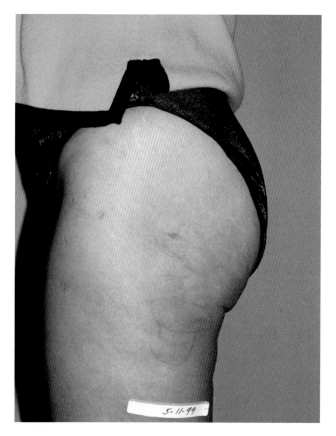 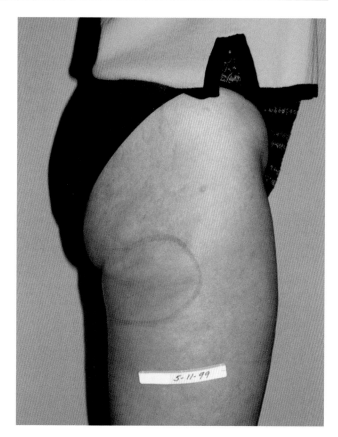

Figures 6-21 & 6-22   *Ultrasound facilitates liposuction, contributes to overall shrinkage and remodeling of the area, and reduces bruising in these difficult, but preventable corrections.*

The Inner Thigh: Over-resection or Under-resection

Four months after XUAL of the abdomen, hips, and thighs with mid-buttock regrafting and two-directional liposuction of the inner aspect of the thigh, the irregularities shown in Figure 6-24 raise questions. How could this irregularity occur when the standard approach was used on both inner thighs? One answer is that the *affected thigh was larger*, with bulkier fat deposits (see Figs. 6-23 and 6-24). Then one must ask whether the

circled areas were under-resected or whether the area between was over-resected.

In many cases it is a combination of both, but in this illustration, the central area has a normal fat component equal to that on the opposite side. The patient's concern is the thickness of fat in the circled areas (see Figs 6-24). Small elevations are treated with local anesthetic infusion and ultrasound (Figs. 6-27 to 6-31). Larger elevations are treated with infusion, again in the clinic setting, and small suction cannulas to remove the central fat.

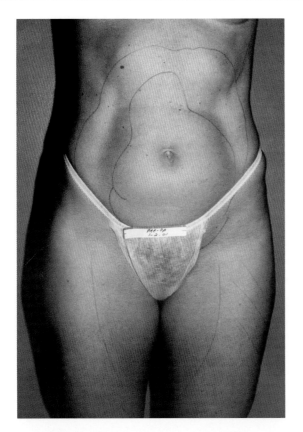
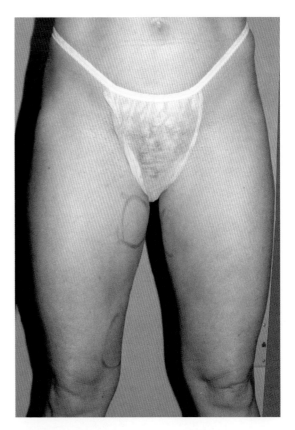

Figures 6-23 and 6-24   In the final analysis, the right side was not over-resected, and it was corrected using "spot" liposuction.

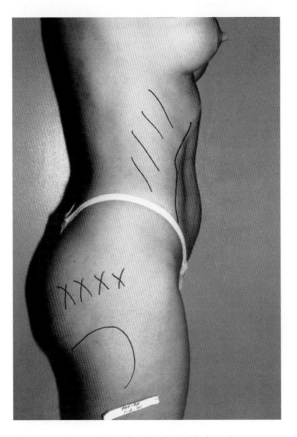
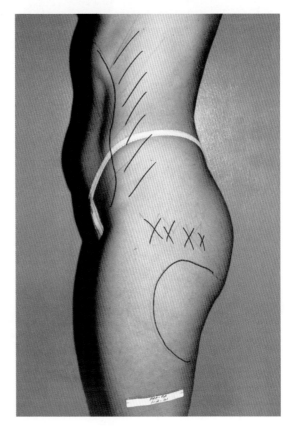

Figures 6-25 and 6-26   Folding of abdominal skin is no longer a contraindication. With taut abdominal musculature and the shrinkage factor of XUAL, these patients can expect a satisfactory result without the necessity of skin undermining and removal.

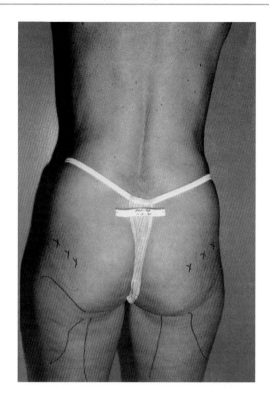
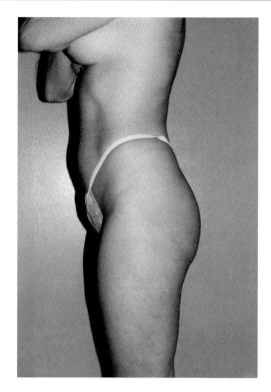

Figures 6-27 & 6-28   *Surprisingly, secondary "touchup" XUAL was not required in the abdomen (XUAL), the flank and back (XU only), or the inner aspect of the thigh (XUAL).*

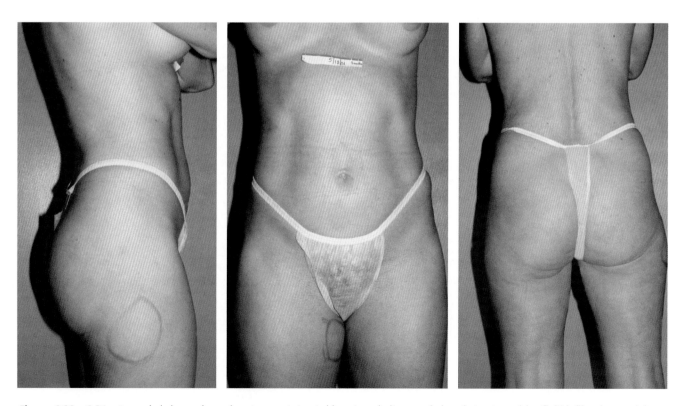

Figures 6-29 – 6-31   *Areas circled are minor edematous spots treated by external ultrasound alone but not requiring fluid infiltration.ermining and removal.*

The Versatile Flat-Bladed Cannula

In certain areas, the use of flat dissection to free up additional subcutaneous tissue is an advantage. One such area is the knee, which because of the contouring, is more difficult to liposuction evenly. With the use of a flat-bladed cannula (see Fig. 6-32), a sufficient subcutaneous level can be cleanly dissected to maintain contouring. Many surgeons believe that knee fat is softer and more easily damaged. It is certainly true that the transition between the knee and the inner part of the thigh is frequently bridged by an area with very little fat, often leading to over-resection. It is this anatomy and the distribution of fat that are more important than the ease of suctioning. The flat blade is also useful in abdominoplasty for thinning the superficial fat beyond the "French line" incision (see Fig. 6-33).

A second important area for liposuction with the flat-bladed cannula is the "banana roll," especially in patients undergoing secondary liposuction. In this instance, the flat blade is *pointed upward* toward the skin rather than the reverse (see Fig. 6-34). Because skin retraction is essential in this area, a wide area on either side of the buttock fold is suctioned with this flat blade, and then compression garments complete the contracture and reshaping of the curve of the lined gluteus muscles.

In the preoperative evaluation it is important to identify patients who have a *low gluteal attachment,* described in the vernacular as "low slung." These people will not achieve the rounded contour that you see in these pages.

LIPOSUCTION OF THE CALF AND ANKLE

In the early years of liposuction, few surgeons were bold enough to operate on calves or ankles. Anecdotal reports of sloughing and hematomas led innovators to establish a universal approach championed by Buck Teimourian, Gerald Pitman, Robert Ersek, and Richard Mladick. By 1989, surgeons were reporting large numbers of cases with good results. Certain foreign surgeons reported a low level of satisfaction, which led to further improvement of the techniques used today.

Once considered too risky for consideration, liposuction of the calves and ankles has a place in the armamentarium of the aesthetic surgeon. Dr. Richard Mladick (plastic surgeon, Virginia Beach) has offered advice from his extensive experience in this area so that other surgeons may achieve similar results.

In any individual the requirements may be different for the left and right sides. Multiple incisions are needed for thorough cross-tunneling. In correspondence from Dr. Mladick, he stated the following: "The incisions illustrated (see Figs. 6-35 and 6-36) allow access for the

> **CLINICAL PEARL**
> It is suggested that surgeons have considerable experience in body liposuction before attempting to correct fatty deposits in the calf and ankle. The following suggestions from Dr. Mladick are of importance:
> - Do not overestimate the improvement that you will achieve on initial consultation with a candidate.
> - Be sure that enough fat (a minimum pinch test) is present to warrant the procedure.
> - Inject the super wet fluid so that the tissues are tense, usually 600 to 1000 cc per leg.
> - Cross-tunneling should be at a very superficial level.
> - Compression is important postoperatively for at least 2 months.
> - The Byron Medical curved cannulas for calf liposuction shown in Figures 6-5 and 6-6 are helpful in addressing patients with circumferential fat versus localized fat (see Fig. 6-7).

best conforming, using both concave and convex small cannulas."

There is a transition zone that must be defined by horizontal and oblique suctioning. It may be medial and sometimes lateral and should be addressed to give the leg a more attractive shape. Entry points allow liposuctioning around the curves horizontally or obliquely (see Figs. 6-37 and 6-38). Convex cannulas are used more for vertical suctioning on the medial and lateral sides of the leg (see Fig. 6-39).

> **CLINICAL PEARL**
> After injecting the "super wet" solution, calves are corrected first from above downward. Then the ankle is suctioned upward to above the mid-leg with overlapping of the superior suctioning. The cannulas shown (see Figs. 6-37 and 6-38) were designed specifically for calf and ankle liposuction (Mladick System by Byron Medical).

> **CLINICAL PEARL**
> Patients must be examined while both standing and sitting. The most reliable test is the "pinch test." Marking must be circumferential, with the superior marks made just below the knee and the inferior marks just below the malleoli. To aid in orientation, Dr. Mladick suggests midline anterior and posterior marking, as well as outlining the transitional zone on the medial lane where the calf narrows into the Achilles tendon. Note that the frog position is preferable for addressing the medial aspect of the leg but that the lateral decubitus position with the leg turned slightly and pulled toward the surgeon allows better access laterally.

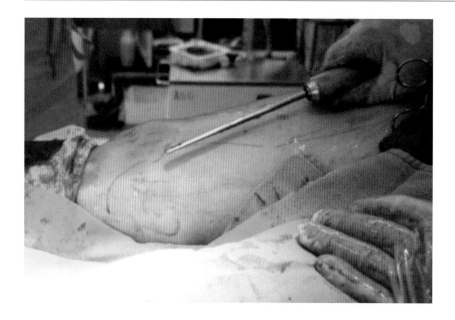

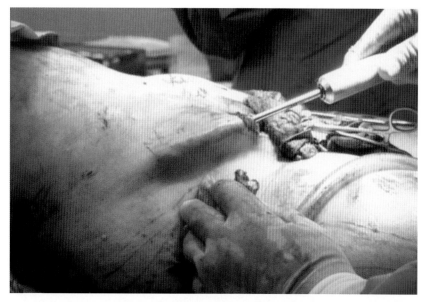

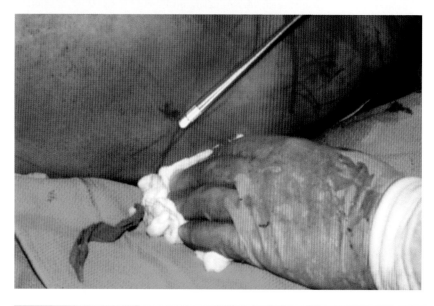

Figures 6-32 – 6-34 The versatile flat-bladed cannula, ideal for the "champagne groove," knee, and "dog-ear."

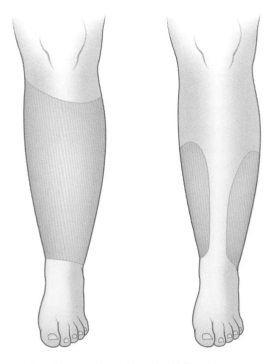

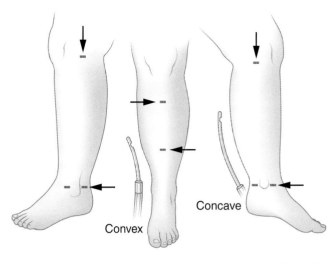

Figure 6-36 *Bidirectional approach to the lateral aspect of the calf with curved cannulas.*

Figure 6-35 *Planning the ankle and calf liposculpture.*

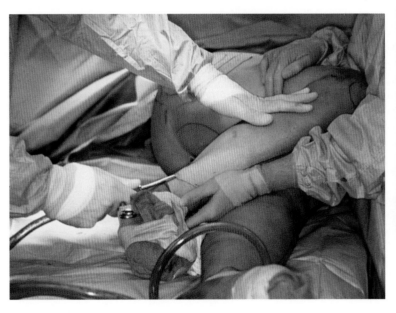

Figure 6-37 *Tip position controlled by hand pressure feedback.*

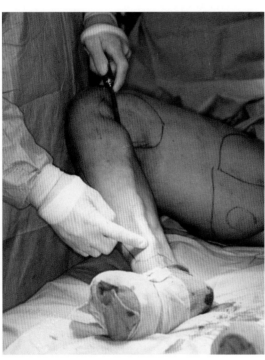

Figure 6-38 *Assessing the degree of correction (see text).*

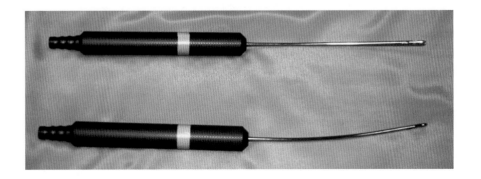

Figure 6-39 *Cannulas preferred for the calf and ankle (Dr. Mladick).*

A word of warning is in order: "Avoid the skin over the Achilles tendon when addressing the fatty deposits in the ankle." It is also important to determine whether these "bulges" are truly fat or simply thickening of the joint capsules. Incisions are made on each side of the malleolus to remove fat in the pre-marked areas (see Figs. 6-40 and 6-41).

CLINICAL PEARL

For calf and ankle suctioning, Dr. Richard Mladick suggests that the surgeon wrap the completed first leg tightly with an elastic bandage to prevent excess edema and bruising. After completing the second liposuction, the first side is unwrapped so that incisions can be closed. He prefers tight surgical stockings and then $1/2$-inch foam rubber held in place by an elastic bandage. The leg is covered from the foot to the ankle. Sequential compression machines are used in the recovery room and are suggested for postoperative care at home.

Although patients may walk immediately after surgery, it is ill advised to stand in one place without moving, and the leg should be elevated as much as is possible. Even more so than in the trunk, accurate marking of *areas of varying thickness and lesser fat deposits is essential* in ankle and calf rejuvenation. Patients operated on by Dr. Mladick show that a thorough preoperative evaluation and "game plan" can achieve excellent results in patients with both thick and thin, long and short legs and calves (see Figs. 6-42 to 6-49).

CLINICAL PEARL

Readers are aware that caution is advisable when liposuctioning a fatty calf and that evaluation of the contribution of muscle and fascia is as important as execution of the procedure. Not a good idea: Endoscopic resection of the gastrocnemius muscles as described in the recent literature.

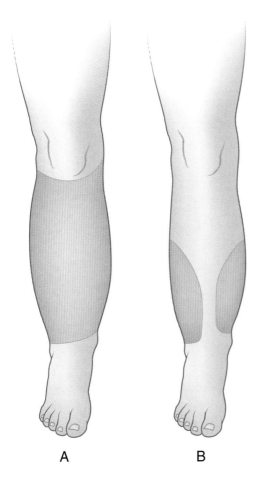

A   B

Figure 6-40   *Typical fatty distribution in advanced calf and ankle deformity.*

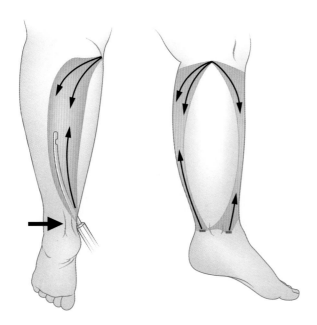

Figure 6-41   *Curvilinear approach to the lateral aspect of the calf.*

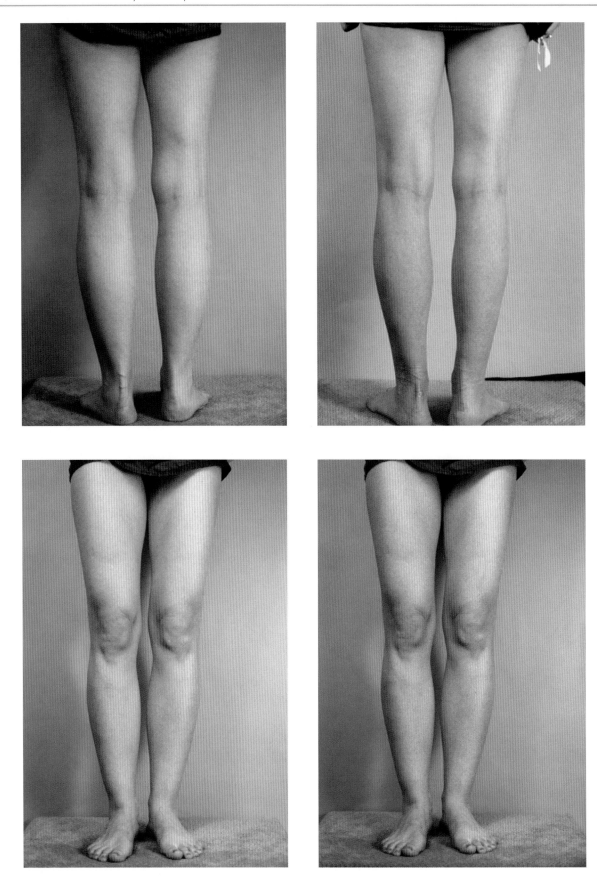

Figures 6-42 – 6-45 *Minimal fatty deposit category and results of liposculpture (Dr. Mladick).*

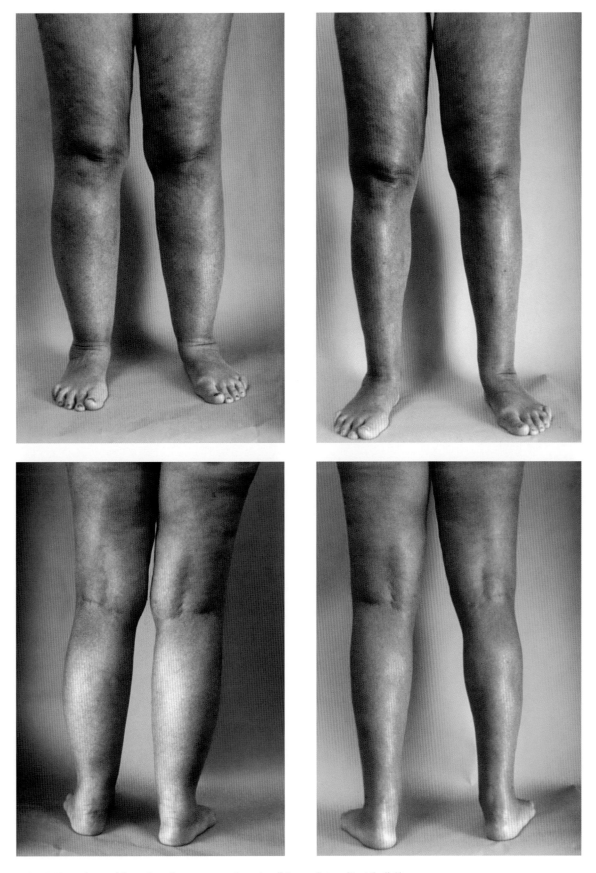

Figures 6-46 – 6-49 *Advanced fatty deposit category and results of liposculpture (Dr. Mladick).*

LIPOSUCTION OF THE ARMS

Liposuction of the arm for minor deformities did not completely correct the skin laxity because there was no method to induce skin contracture other than compression and postoperative massage. As shown in Figures 6-50 and 6-51, removal of fat left an acceptable reduction in arm thickness, but the loose hanging skin mars the result. This patient rejected skin resection. With the advent of liposuction with ultrasonic assistance, skin retraction is universal, and in patients such as this, a smooth contour would have been obtained with either UAL or XUAL. In the initial studies of ultrasound, we compared our results with those in patients such as this and found to our delight that skin retraction improved the operative results tremendously; accordingly, skin resection has rarely been required since initiating the program.

XUAL of the Arms

In patients with moderate fat deposits and age-related skin laxity, UAL and XUAL with circumferential application of ultrasound in the operative and postoperative periods will induce skin contracture (see Figs. 6-52 and 6-53). The *fatty deposits are limited to the lower fold of the arms* and are approached through a pinhole opening in the antecubital fascia and the shoulder. Without the skin contracture afforded by XUAL, the resultant hanging skin had made this procedure unacceptable. Postoperative application of ultrasound, massage, and compression aided in skin retraction. The final contour (see Figs. 6-54 and 6-55) is comparable to the results once obtained by standard excision with removal of the skin scar. After our initial experience in arm reduction with XUAL, we have not treated a single patient with skin excision for arm deformities (except in the extreme weight loss/gastric bypass group).

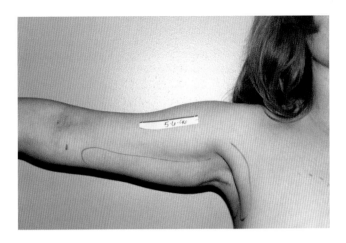 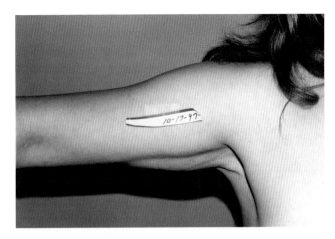

Figures 6-50 & 6-51 *Satisfactory arm reduction with XUAL with no skin excision/scar. Skin contracture to this degree did not occur in similar cases treated by SAL.*

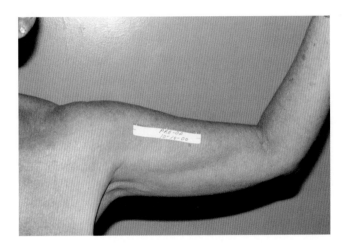 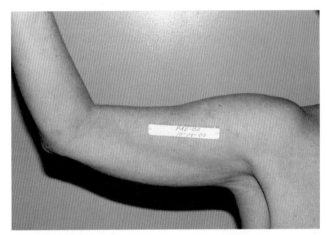

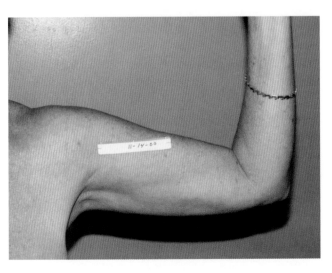 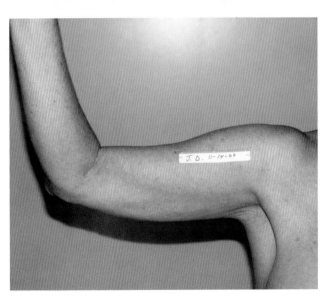

Figures 6-52 – 6-55 *In an older patient even more wary of scars, satisfactory reduction is accomplished by XUAL. The entire circumference is treated to aid in contraction, but only the lower midline treated fat is extracted.*

Case in point—Arm reduction with liposuction alone

This patient presented a number of challenges, and with the priorities of facial surgery and abdominal and extremity liposuction, the addition of abdominal repair and surgical excision of skin in the arms would have resulted in greater risk than was acceptable. The patient is shown with the preoperative markings in October 1997, at the initiation of the XU study. Without making promises, it was hoped that the addition of XU would reduce the redundancy of the mid-abdomen and allow retraction of the arms without surgical incision (see Figs. 6-56 to 6-59).

Surprisingly, there was excellent regression of the high hip rolls, the mid-abdomen, and the inner aspect of the thighs in 30 days (see Figs. 6-60 and 6-61), but the uncorrected underlying abdominal musculature left a curved contour (see Fig. 6-62). Compression and massage of the upper arm region was continued for 6 weeks after the initial XUAL procedure. The photographs taken 21 months after these procedures showed regression of the arm tissues, with no rippling or "flapping" as would have been expected. This contouring of a difficult arm problem was accomplished with two entry points and XUAL. *Before our experience with XUAL, this patient would have undergone a skin excision of the classic arm reduction type, with subsequent scarring and limitation of clothing so that she would have been required to cover the scars.* She would have worn long sleeves the rest of her life. Such was not the case. At 3 years, the position of the arms and contour are maintained (see Figs. 6-63 to 6-66). At this point, she was agreeable to a "Victoria's Secret" small-incision limited abdominoplasty with secondary liposuction.

Case in point

This woman is a typical middle-aged individual who should respond to only arm reduction of the classic type with an incision from the axilla to the elbow (see Figs. 6-67 and 6-68). With our experience in skin shrinkage in response to XUAL, patients in this category are now offered XUAL so that we can evaluate whether removal of the weight as in standard liposuction and the additional skin shrinkage with XUAL could possibly allow these individuals to benefit from the lesser procedure. XUAL was used after infiltration of the upper part of the arms in this individual with the "bat wing" deformity. A single liposuction procedure was performed and compression dressings applied. In the initial series, no additional XU treatments were given, but this practice has become a standard in aftercare. Because skin shrinkage in the arms had never occurred with other modalities, these individuals were advised to wear compressive garments for 3 months. As noted in the subsequent photographs (see Figs. 6-69 and 6-70), the skin shrinkage that was evident at 2 weeks continued to improve past 3 months. Despite weight gain, this woman has not regained fatty tissue in her arms, and the skin shrinkage has persisted in the 3-year follow-up evaluations.

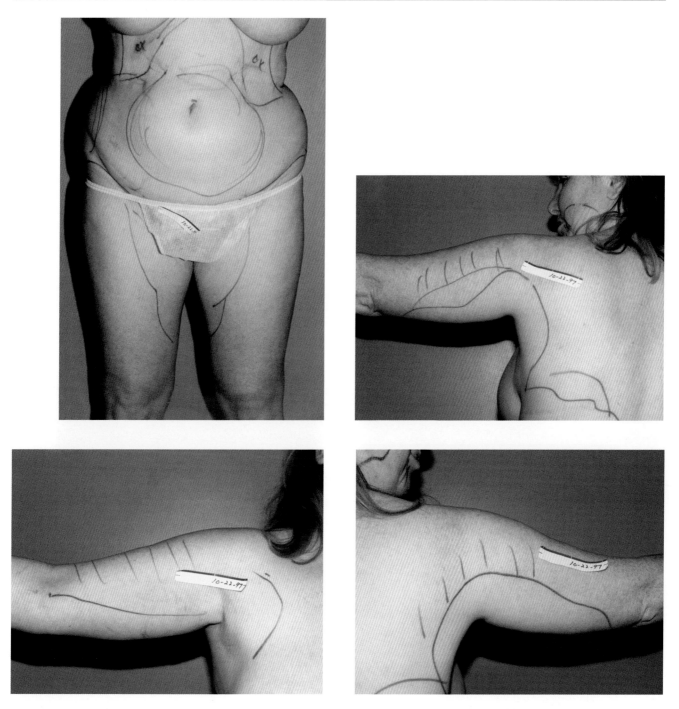

Figures 6-56 – 6-59 *Avoiding skin excision. In the 1997 evaluation group, patients in this category who would have benefitted from an abdominoplasty and standard arm reduction volunteered to have these areas, including other areas, treated by XUAL alone.*

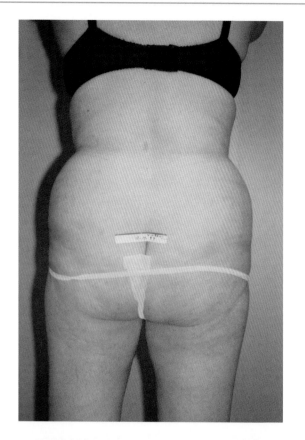

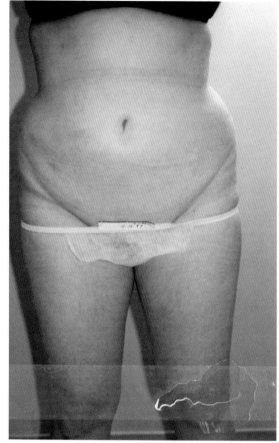

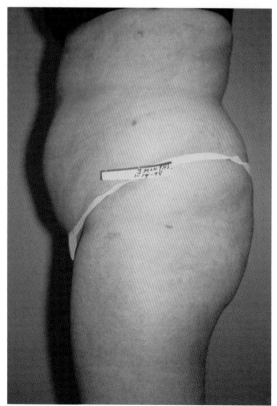

Figures 6-60 – 6-62 *Without muscle/fascia plication, the abdomen is not flat, but there is no skin fold at 3 months. Body contouring includes fat grafts to the buttocks and smooth contouring of the thighs.*

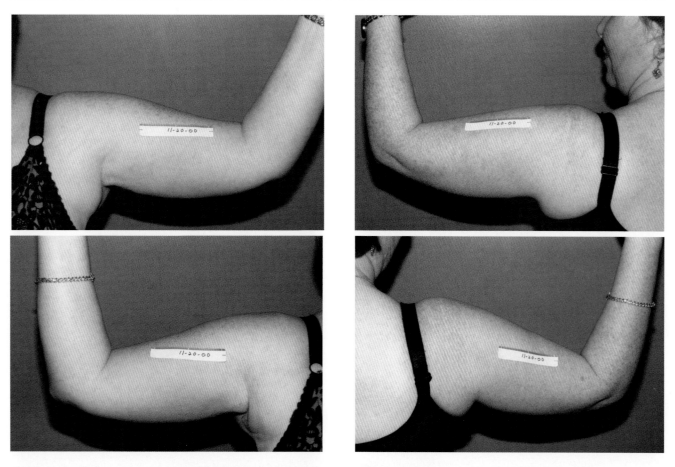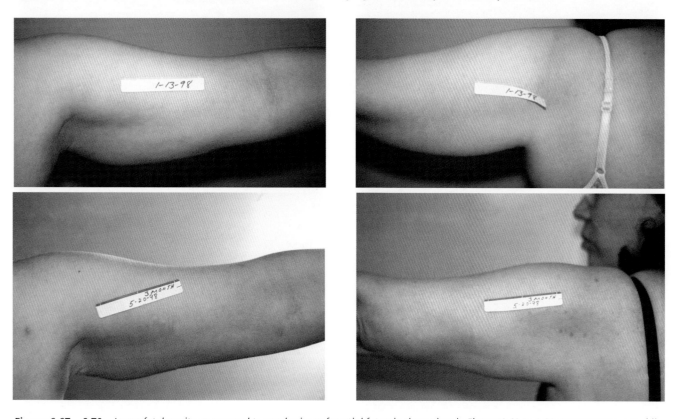

Figures 6-63 – 6-66 Arm contour restoration has been stable despite weight gain as shown by the 1- and 3-year results.

Figures 6-67 – 6-70 Lower fat deposits, as opposed to nearly circumferential fat as in the patient in Figures 6-63 to 6-66, recontour more rapidly.

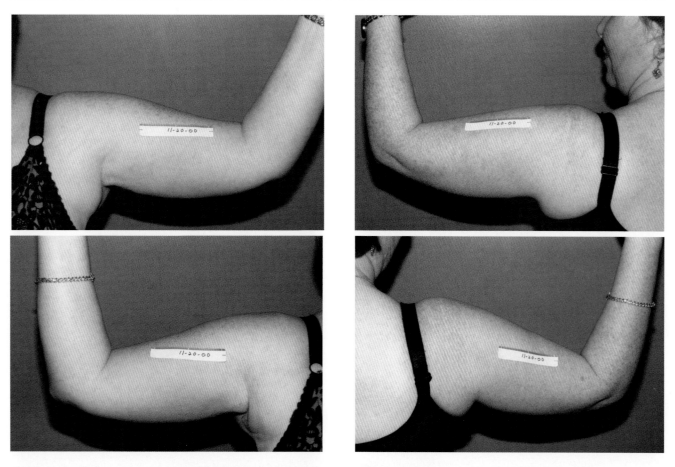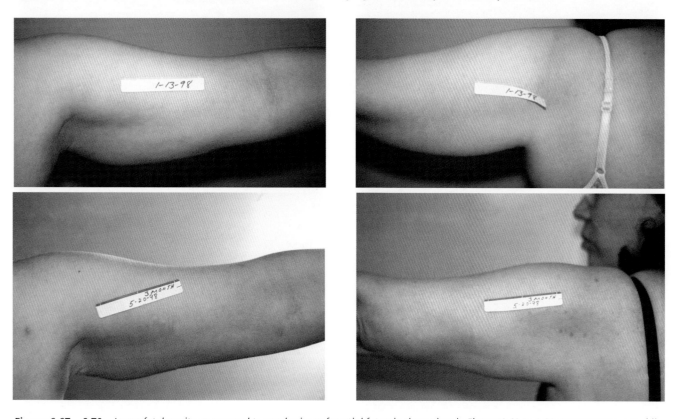

Liposuction of a Minimally Deformed Arm

This patient has only a moderate amount of arm fat but a greater degree of skin laxity (see Figs. 6-71 to 6-74). Before the advent of XU, liposuction would have been ill advised. Using XUAL to assist in skin contracture, a modest amount of fat was liposuctioned through two entry points, which resulted in the rapid shrinkage noted in the 2-month photographs (see Figs. 6-75 to 6-78). Ultrasound was applied in the postoperative period at 24-hour intervals for 3 days. Continuous compression was maintained for 4 weeks, an empirical rule based solely on previous experience with liposuctioning of arms that indicated little if any inclination of this tissue to retract or shrink. With XUAL, this patient was spared a skin excision procedure that would have resulted in a linear scar on the inner aspect of the arm, totally unacceptable for her lifestyle.

In the posterior arm view photograph, the liposuction extends well beyond the arm itself to include the posterior axillary fold. In many patients, only the anterior axillary fold shows a fat deposit, but in this case the opposite was true. Three-year photographs (see Figs. 6-79 to 6-82) show that the retraction has been maintained despite fluctuations in weight.

Reference

1. Cárdenas-Camarena L, Tobar-Losada A, Lacouture AM: Large-volume circumferential liposuction with tumescent technique: A sure and viable procedure. *Plastic and Reconstructive Surgery*, 1999;104:1887-1899.

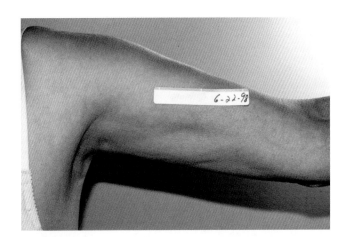
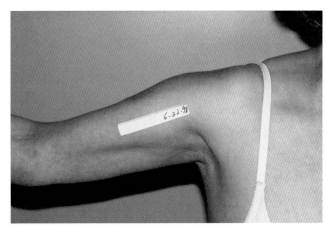
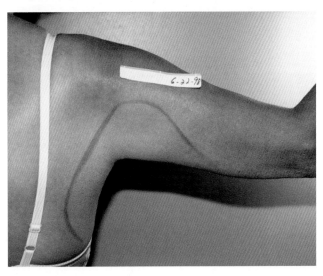
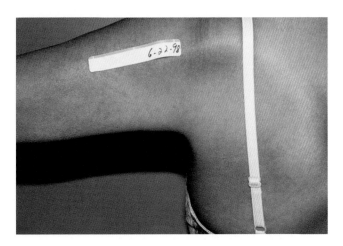

Figures 6-71 – 6-74 *Continuation of arm contour improvement. Initially seeking revision of a previous abdominoplasty with a high incision and wishing to avoid other scars, this lady's arm deformities were considered for XUAL reduction with other procedures.*

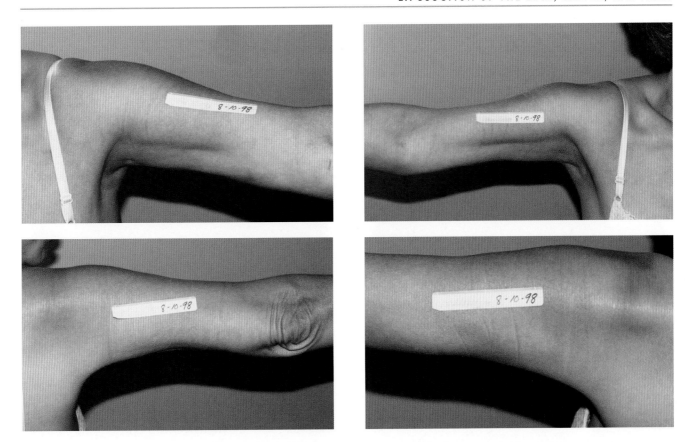

Figures 6-75 – 6-78   *In 1998, 2 months after circumferential XU and XUAL of the marked areas, good regression and reshaping are apparent.*

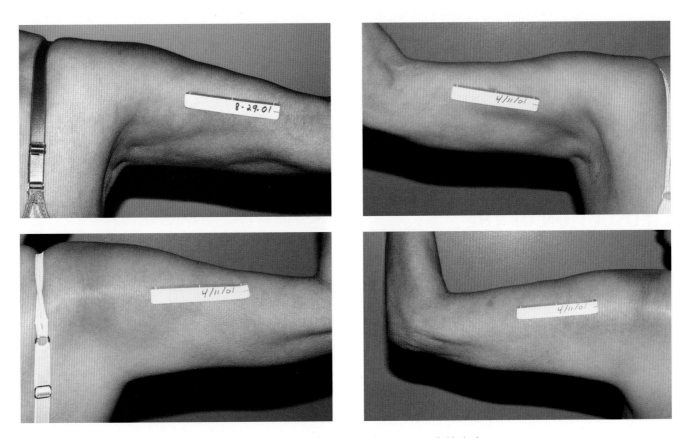

Figures 6-79 – 6-82   *Re-evaluation after 30 months shows good fat contour, but a degree of skin laxity.*

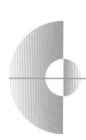

CHAPTER SEVEN

Breast Liposuction

Breast liposuction was prohibited because of legitimate fears that interpretation of mammograms would be impaired. As has been pointed out by Courtiss and subsequent authors, calcification may occur but is easily distinguished from the calcification of malignancy. Liposuction is generally used with breast reduction surgery to balance the sides, reduce certain areas that are thicker at the end of the procedure, and of course, reduce the lateral extension of the breast and the superior axillary fat pad.

Although "liposuction breast reduction" without incisions is a popular topic, anecdotal reports of patient dissatisfaction are discouraging. The general consensus is that liposuction alone may be used to marginally reduce a fatty breast or in patients who are not candidates for major procedures and care little about the aesthetic result of their breast reductions. Mastopexy of the various types will not usually require liposuction because partial reduction may be carried out on one side or the other for balancing; yet the use of liposuction in these procedures can be important not only in the lateral area as described but in the axillary fat pad as well.

LIPOSUCTION OF THE MALE AND FEMALE BREAST

Liposuction has played a role in gynecomastia since its first development and initially allowed plastic surgeons to reduce the length of the incisional lines, thus reducing scarring and the incidence of hypesthesia. Liposuction has been used as an adjunct in female breast reduction for balancing and removal of the anterior and axillary folds and the posterior "tail of Spence" area. The extensive use of liposuction in the lateral areas allowed surgeons to abandon the long "anchor" scar for breast reduction.

To avoid the complications of surface scarring, surgeons have used liposuction as a *primary* means of breast reduction and find it appropriate for a subgroup of patients in whom breast shape is unimportant, usually the elderly. The advantage is the simplicity of the procedure, but obvious irregularities occur even with experienced surgeons. The procedure is used in a certain subgroup of individuals who prefer the simpler procedure because of age, health, or fear.

Traditional breast reduction involves an incision in the shape of an inverted T, with complications of sensory loss, scar breakdown, and nipple necrosis primarily related to the size and length of the breast, the patient's age, and reduced blood flow resulting from the incision line. To avoid these problems, the "lollipop" procedure, in which the horizontal line is eliminated completely, and circumareolar reduction were developed. Despite a number of technical improvements to reduce the skin gathering in the lollipop "LeJour" breast reduction, the emerging trend is improved circumareolar reduction, in which liposuction plays a role.

Reporting on a 10-year experience with a circumareolar procedure for mastopexy repair and reduction in 1985, I was on a panel with Luiz Toledo, Adrien Aiache, and Louis Benelli at the Beverly Hills Review of Aesthetic Plastic Surgery (RAPS). The Benelli infolding procedure, called "round block," de-epithelialization for suture security with areolar reduction, and the use of liposuction were introduced to the American plastic surgery group at that time. Their results were better than I personally had achieved.

Other surgeons in South American and Europe plus the American surgeons Aiache, Schlesinger, Dinner, and others have contributed to the development of this procedure in which the breast is coned subcutaneously and measures are taken to reduce areolar spread and vascular embarrassment. Liposuction is used as a major part of the reduction, but each reduction and mastopexy procedure involved resetting the areolar position.

Quite surprisingly, the issue of fat regrafting in the breast resurfaces at regular intervals despite the obvious fact that this procedure is clearly "below the standard of care." The breast is the only area in which fat grafting will be subjected to x-ray analysis: the mammogram. Fat grafts are not only in contact with the resident bacteria within the breast but also calcify and permanently obscure the development of breast carcinoma. Despite this knowledge, basic to any trained surgeon, some individual will periodically promote depositing fat obtained in liposuction for breast enhancement. This practice is to be condemned, not only for the obvious complications of fat necrosis, infection, and distortion but also for the virtual death sentence incurred by eliminating any value that could be obtained from mammography. The only exception is the use of superficial fat and dermis grafts in a badly damaged breast. If these procedures are performed, it must be with the patient's clear understanding that this *superficial* corrected area will be visible on mammograms but will not obscure the breast parenchyma. Subcutaneous grafting with synthetic materials, dermis fat, or for small defects, fat or fat dermis grafts, will then be acceptable and will avoid the aforementioned hazards.

PATIENT SELECTION

Among male gynecomastia patients, the ideal candidate for liposuction removal is one with primarily fatty tissues. In most male patients beyond the teenage years, there is an extra component of thick breast tissue that must be resected. If this thick tissue is not extensive, liposuction aided by sharp cutting cannulas is the preferred choice. If a male breast is truly pendulous, a secondary procedure would be contemplated because shrinkage may not give a smooth contour. An elliptical incision may be planned for skin reduction both above

and below the areola in these unusual cases (see Figs. 7-1 to 7-6).

Among female breast reduction patients, those with bulky breasts who are not candidates for general anesthesia are considered for bulk reduction by liposuction. Unfortunately, most patients do not have fatty tissues sufficient to reduce the bulk of the breasts to their satisfaction, and this issue must be discussed. The use of ultrasound-assisted liposuction (UAL) to melt the fibrotic portion has been advocated, but complications, including reduced blood supply and fat necrosis, make this consideration less likely. As several authors have pointed out in large series, many patients do not wish to undergo an extensive procedure and are not concerned whether a nipple position is altered or the breast contour is smooth and acceptable in ordinary clothing. For these individuals, one may offer liposuction reduction as a first or second choice. Liposuction also plays a role in equalizing breasts, particularly in the operating room. Even though planning has taken into account differences in the left and right side, liposuction may be used for final shaping. It is also advisable to use liposuction to remove the axillary tail area, thus avoiding an incision in that area and reducing any overhangs in the upper axillary fold from abnormal fat deposits.

CLINICAL PEARL

Dr. Adrien Aiache (plastic surgeon, Beverly Hills) has been involved in breast liposuction from the very beginning and was the first author to perform this type of surgery and report it in the first lipoplasty book. This technique is extremely limited because the breast is often only a combination of breast tissue and some interspersed fat, and only in older patients who have a larger amount of fat is liposuction useful. In younger women with breasts composed of essentially glandular tissue, liposuction is impossible and useless. As a consequence, the only situations in which liposuction is useful are as follows:

- When it is associated with mammary reduction or is performed as a stand-alone procedure consisting of suction of the fat surrounding the breast tissue in the chest wall
- In older patients if some of the fat can be observed at the superficial layers of the breast tissue itself so that suctioning is possible

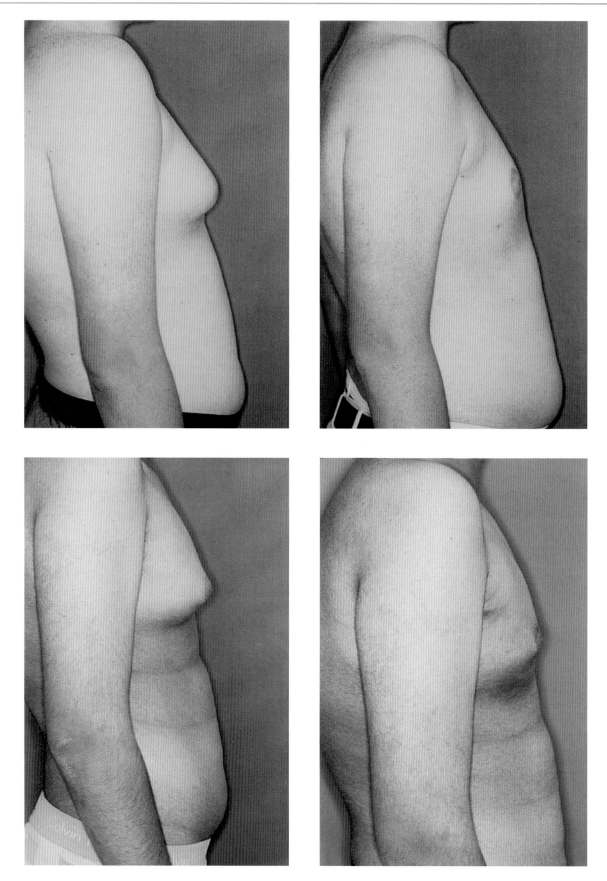

FIGURES 7-1 – 7-6   *Gynecomastia correction with liposculpture. Note the excellent contour of the realigned skin cover (Dr. Hamas).*

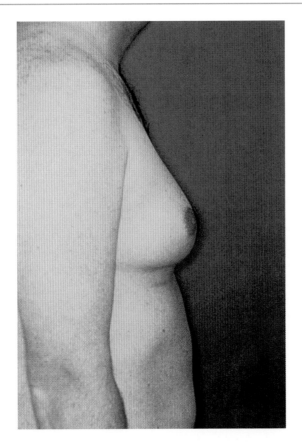 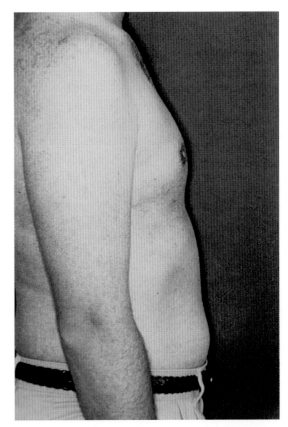

FIGURES 7-1 – 7-6   *Continued*

LIPOSUCTION FOR GYNECOMASTIA

Male patients are counseled regarding the standard request for reduction of mid-abdominal fat and "love handles" and whether gynecomastia should be addressed. In many patients older than 20 years, gynecomastia is a major concern. Problems with gynecomastia include the fibrotic nature of the central breast tissue and the necessity for pathologic examination of breast tissue that is removed under even the most benign of circumstances. Open excision is rejected by most male patients if an alternative is offered. Liposuction variants for gynecomastia were proposed by Dr. Hilton Becker (plastic surgeon, Boca Raton) and Dr. Gary Rosenberg (plastic surgeon, Delray Beach). New cannulas tapered to penetrate this fibrous tissue were effective and soon replaced "open" excision in most cases. However, removal was time consuming. Sharper pointed cannulas are now in general use. UAL was suggested as the better alternative, but mammographic studies after removal by UAL showed that only limited fibrous tissue was gone. The larger incisions, costlier equipment, and greater time requirement for UAL, as well as the risk of seroma and skin burns, have led Dr. Robert Hamas (plastic surgeon, Dallas) to design a liposuction cannula with a sharp pointed tip and sharpened openings. These cannulas cut strips of fibrous tissue and breast parenchyma (Gram's Medical). Fibrous tissue, breast tissue, and fat are removed simultaneously.

When cutting edge cannulas are used, surgeons reported less complicated removal of breast tissue. Pathologic study confirmed the presence of breast and fibrous tissue in the aspirates. Liposuction with these cannulas corrected gynecomastia to Dr. Hamas' satisfaction in 57 of 88 cases. In earlier cases, liposuction was performed twice to achieve the desired result. It is predicted that with greater experience, the practice of following liposuction with open excision will be abandoned in all but the most pendulous male breasts.

Regardless of whether removal is performed with the syringe technique or with liposuction machines, tissue removed from the male breast should be submitted for pathologic examination. Patients must be aware that although carcinoma of the male breast is a rare occurrence, such examination protects both the patient and the surgeon.

Case in Point—XUAL for Gynecomastia

In Figure 7-7, the areas for release of the submammary fold are marked and the areas for external ultrasound-assisted liposuction (XUAL) circled, including the anterior axillary fold and areas above the breast where XU will be applied without liposuction. In addition, this patient exhibits the usual male pattern of fat deposits and transition zones (see Figs. 7-8 to 7-10). Gynecomastia may be approached with UAL, cutting suction-assisted lipectomy (SAL), cannulas such as the "Brazil needle," or a combination. In this instance, use of the cutting cannulas was preceded by an application of XUAL, which softened the fibrotic part of the breast as well as the surrounding fat. The single entry point for liposuction is the red dot in Figures 7-9 and 7-10. Resolution is virtually complete at 1 month (see Figs. 7-11 to 7-14). Compression is used for only 7 days, but with additional massage in our spa program. Male patients will not wear girdles and are uncomfortable with the jacket-type compression devices. We abandoned the use of these jackets in favor of 6-inch elastic bandage wraps, which can be removed more easily for showering and after exercise and of course are less expensive. This patient was shown how to apply the compression so that the upper chest folds and axillary line areas are included. Various abdominal binders are provided and used continuously in the first 7 days. Most male patients show such rapid regression after ultrasound pretreatment that they can change to spandex exercise shorts that cover the upper part of the abdomen after this time. At 4 months, correction of the gynecomastia is illustrated (see Figs. 7-15 and 7-16), as well as better shrinkage of the love handle areas than we could achieve without UAL.

The procedure was further facilitated by the design of the Rosenberg breast dissector, which was easily inserted through a 3-mm incision. The dissector made it a simple matter to elevate the inframammary crease from the underlying chest attachments.

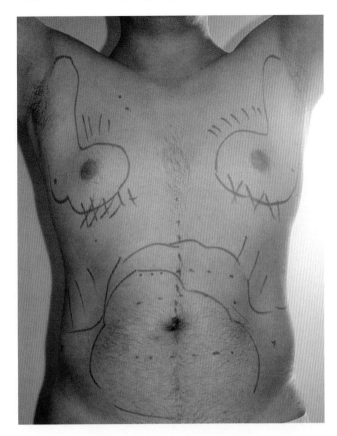

FIGURE 7-7 *Typical planning for simultaneous liposculpture of the male breast, abdomen, and flank (circles). XX lines indicate areas in which skin and subcutaneous tissue will be elevated with flat dissectors. Vertical lines indicate "transition zones" where external ultrasound will reduce fat thickness.*

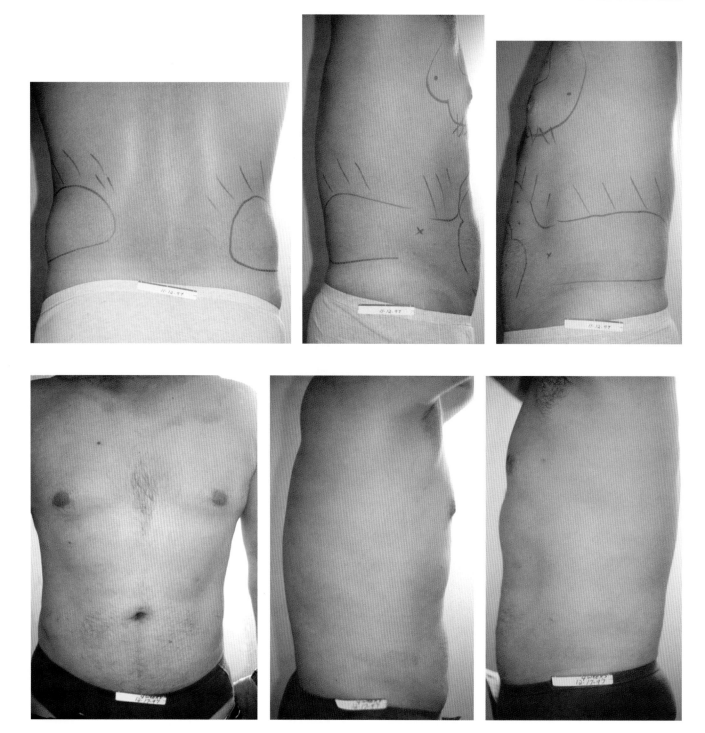

FIGURES 7-8 – 7-16 *Preoperative markings with washable ink at first consultation contrasted with the final result of liposculpture with XUAL.*

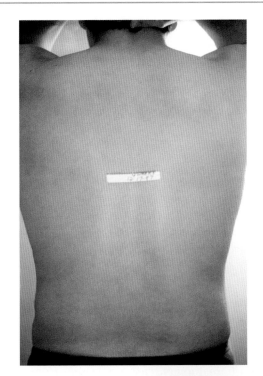
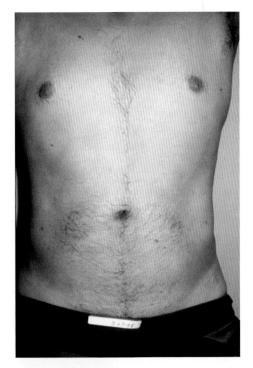

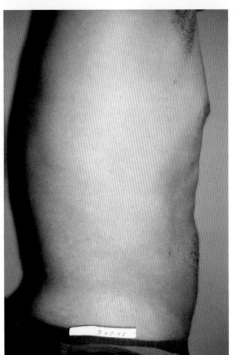

FIGURES 7-8 – 7-16   Continued

How I Do It—
Dr. Gary Rosenberg (Plastic Surgeon, Delray Beach)

Over the past 2 decades that I have been performing gynecomastia surgery I have confined my technique to suction lipectomy only. The technique has changed little since I first described suction lipectomy alone for gynecomastia in 1984.

At first, my colleagues were not able to repeat my results and quipped at the audacious notion of being able to suction the parenchymal and glandular tissue of gynecomastia. It was not until I first described thin cannulas 2.3 mm in diameter that others were able to reproduce the results.

In the first paper, I described hydrostatic dissection for the first time, which later took on the name of tumescent liposuction. This technique facilitated suction removal of the subareolar glandular and parenchymal tissue. The Rosenberg gynecomastia cannula has remained unchanged at 2.3 mm in diameter and 5 cm in length.

Once the Ultrasound Task Force finally released its secretive information, those of us who could have helped many more patients with earlier release of this information were able to expand the applications. The use of internal ultrasound, in conjunction with suctioning for removal of gynecomastia tissue, facilitated the procedure. However, increased deformity resulted because of the large incisions. The risks were also increased multifold as a result of the nature of the internal ultrasound apparatus.

In 1994 I was introduced to the concepts of XUAL by Barry Silberg, M.D., of Santa Rosa, California. He appreciated the obvious application of this technique, which avoids the pitfalls of internal ultrasound. In addition to the increased efficiency of fat removal, I have found that skin shrinkage was facilitated.

The XUAL technique facilitates removal of glandular and parenchymal tissue, as well as fatty tissue. The improved skin shrinkage that is immediately apparent after using XUAL versus other techniques also improves the results. Today's patient is a highly motivated individual who does not want to have much downtime. Return to full activities the day after surgery and the superior results of this technique make this procedure highly popular in my practice.

Technique

I personally prefer to perform the procedure with the patient under general anesthesia. Once the patient is asleep, each breast is infiltrated with the super wetting solution (1 L of lactated Ringer's solution, 500 mg lidocaine [Xylocaine], 1 mg of epinephrine). External ultrasound alone (XU) is applied with the Silberg EUA apparatus set at 3.0 W/cm with the 10-cm² head. Ultrasound is applied for 5 to 7 minutes, depending on the size of the breasts and the density of the parenchymal tissue. A 3-mm incision is made at the 12-o'clock position on the areola. Next, the Rosenberg 2.3-mm cannula is used to remove the subareolar and periareolar dense glandular and parenchymal tissue. A 3.5-mm cannula is then used for circumferential subcutaneous suctioning from the clavicle to the mid-axillary line to the sternum to 10 cm below the inframammary crease. A second incision at the anterior axillary fold is used for cross-suctioning. Finally, through the 12-o'clock incision, the Rosenberg 3.5-mm breast dissector is inserted and the inframammary crease released from the underlying attachments to the pectoralis fascia, serratus anterior fascia, and rectus abdominis fascia.

The incisions are closed with 4-0 Prolene suture. Reston foam is used for 5 days and a compressive garment for 2 weeks. Patients are allowed to return to full activities the day after surgery without exception.

Case in Point—Combining Solid Silicone Pectoralis Implants with Lateral Liposuction

In the case illustration, Dr. Adrien Aiache (plastic surgeon, Beverly Hills) combines subpectoral silicone implants with liposuction. Several companies manufacture implants in a number of shapes. Planning and placement of these solid implants depend entirely on patient requirements and the physical dimensions of the area. Softer solid materials have replaced the cigar-shaped hard silicone implants originally used. Liposuction plays a role in these patients as shown. Liposuction has reduced the fatty tissues located in the anterior axillary line so that placement of the implants will give the desired forward projection without loss of definition (see Figs. 7-17 to 7-20).

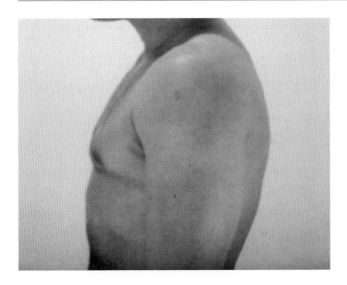
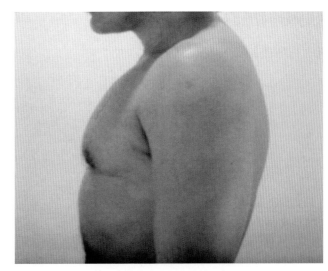

FIGURES 7-17 & 7-18 *Patient for simultaneous breast liposculpture reduction and augmentation with a pectoral silicone prosthesis (Dr. Aiache).*

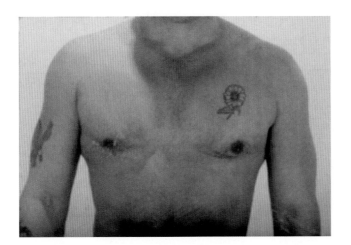
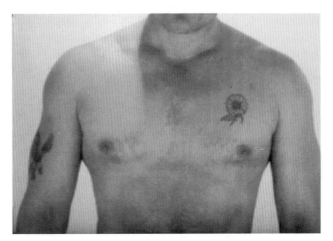

FIGURES 7-19 & 7-20 *Liposculpture plays an important role in these cases as shown.*

LIPOSUCTION OF THE FEMALE BREAST

Although the Food and Drug Administration has not endorsed ultrasonic liposuction for breast reduction, more surgeons are using it as a primary procedure in selected patients. The results are definitely not what one would consider attractive, but in certain high-risk individuals or elderly patients with poor medical status, breast reduction by liposuction is the choice. Peter Fodor (Los Angeles) uses power-assisted liposuction (PAL), which is particularly effective in dense breast tissue. Preoperative radiographs frequently help by showing the areas that can be liposuctioned and those that would resist. Peter has these patients wear a bra for 3 months to aid in the remodeling process.

Lawrence Gray (Portsmouth) has analyzed 500 cases of breast reduction by liposuction. In his view, problem patients rarely ask for repositioning of the nipple. They always complain of the bulk of the breasts. This may not be true in the practice of other surgeons, but in the group in which the breast is 60% to 70% fat and shape and appearance are less important, liposuction is a good alternative to traditional surgery.

How I Do It—Dr. Woodrow Baxt (Plastic Surgeon, Paramus)

Liposuction as the sole means of breast reduction has been reported in our literature for over 10 years but has not achieved the universal acclaim that it should. A large audience of women would love to be one, two, or even three cup sizes smaller if they had just not seen it shown on television. The idea of extensive scars and the substantial recuperation required have turned them away from the idea of surgery. They are not necessarily looking for the "perfect breast," but they would like to be a little smaller.

CLINICAL PEARL

Liposuction and Breast Reduction

The major limitation is the inability to predict the exact size or position the nipple at the exact appropriate location. This shortcoming is said to be readily accepted by the large majority who have already rejected traditional operations because of fear of pain, scarring, and prolonged healing. The asymmetry that I see in reports of this technique would be unacceptable to most aesthetic surgery patients. The problem of scarring has already been addressed in great detail by the prevalent use of the circle technique, or internal breast reduction-mastoplasty.

With the "scarless" reduction, we have a procedure to match their expectation. Breast reduction via liposuction has the following virtues:

- Outpatient procedure
- Intravenous sedation
- One half to 1 hour of surgery required
- Back to work and play in a few days
- Almost painless
- Can be offered at significantly less cost than the traditional breast reduction

Figures 7-21 to 7-26 offer illustration of these attributes.

We have developed several refinements in the last few years. I do not use any form of ultrasound for potential medicolegal reasons only (I use external ultrasound on all other liposuction cases). I instill twice the amount of fluid as I plan to remove in actual breast tissue. Most surgeons who have performed enough traditional reductions can quite accurately estimate the amount that they expect to remove. I then remove the amount that I have instilled. If I am expecting to remove 500 g of tissue, I will instill 1000 cc and remove 1000 cc. All of this assumes good surgical judgment and symmetrical breasts. Asymmetry is obviously trickier, but the same basic rule applies. I will use implant sizes preoperatively to estimate the amount of difference and then follow the guidelines just given. Regarding cannulas, I use an aggressive three-hole cannula in the 3- and 4-mm range, and it works well. I work actively under the skin over the entire breast first because it is easier than after the bulk of the fat is removed. Having tried the power-assisted device and found no appreciable difference, I keep it simple and use all muscle power. I make one or two incisions in the inframammary fold and often crisscross from an incision in the axillary fold. Our pathologist is always notified in advance to expect this specimen, which is sent in a separate container. We have occasionally been able to obtain some insurance coverage. I like ice postoperatively and firm taping with Microfoam, but it has been too uncomfortable.

Patients are told to resume an activity that they are comfortable with because there is nothing the patient can do to ruin the operation. Massage begins as soon as possible. The patient should be prepared to feel hard, lumpy, and bruised for a few months. All breasts have been soft by the time of the 3-month follow-up visit. As with other liposuction procedures, they will improve for up to a year. Skin shrinkage has been remarkable, with a 2- to 5-cm elevation of the nipple.

Liposuction has opened up a huge new audience of women who have rejected breast reduction for all of the obvious reasons. We are all fond of saying that our

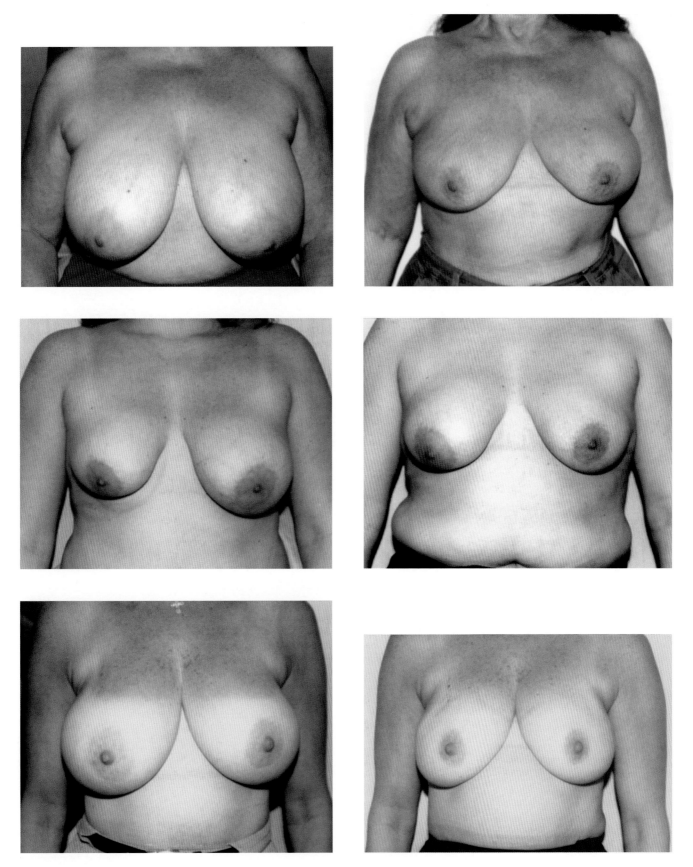

FIGURES 7-21 – 7-26   *In carefully selected and counseled patients, a reduction in bulk is a less invasive procedure. The results obtained are acceptable in these individuals (Dr. Baxt).*

happiest patients are those who have undergone breast reduction, but now the happiest of my breast reduction patients are the "scarless" ones.

> **CLINICAL PEARL**
>
> If you didn't know what "medial syndesmosis" is, don't feel dumb. It's the presternal fat in large-breasted women, and it responds to suctioning.

Partial Breast Reduction

The 20-year-old patient in Figures 7-27 to 7-29 underwent partial breast reduction by Dr. Robert Hamas (plastic surgeon, Dallas). A total of 440 cc was removed after a 250-cc infiltrate. Note that nipples measuring 25 cm preoperatively measured 23 cm at her 2-year postoperative examination. She has not gained weight and has definitely been reduced from a 34D to a 34C. The Gram cutting cannulas shown in Figure 7-29 are particularly useful for removing thick breast tissue in male gynecomastia procedures.

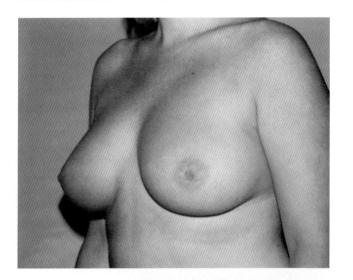
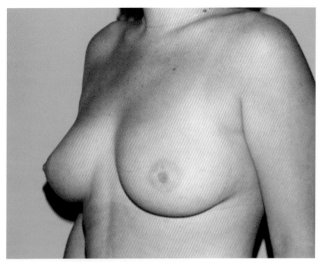

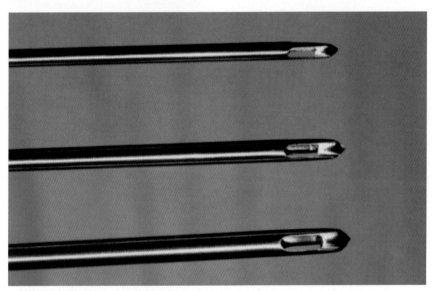

FIGURES 7-27 – 7-29 *This 20-year-old patient had a partial breast reduction by Dr. Robert Hamas (plastic surgeon, Dallas). A total of 440 cc was removed after a 250-cc infiltrate. Note that the nipples measuring 25 cm preoperatively measured 23 cm at her 2-year postoperative examination. She has not gained weight and has definitely been reduced from a 34D to a 34C. The Gram cutting cannulas shown in the accompanying illustration are particularly useful for removing thick breast tissue in male gynecomastia procedures.*

Liposuction of the Breast Aided by "Super Wet" Infusion

Use of the "super wet" solution has simplified the planning of multiple procedures such as illustrated in this patient, in whom liposuction will be performed in multiple areas with regrafting of fat in the hips and a circle procedure breast-lift performed. Details of the circle procedure include the use of super wet pump solution to separate the skin and subcutaneous tissue of the lower two thirds of the breast, elevation of the nipple to a new position, and internal creation of a mound. Final adjustment is performed with liposuction.[1]

Case in point

Liposuction plays a role beyond reduction of the breast's shape. In this patient, without creation of a mound, there would be elevation, and resetting the breast would be incomplete. However, liposuction is used in the posterior axillary line (see Figs. 7-30 to 7-36), as well as in the interior axillary fold. If there is asymmetry, as shown in Figures 7-34 to 7-36, liposuction is used in a preliminary fashion to reduce the bulk of the larger breast. Although the results of the breast-lift show good symmetry and position, resection of the back folds must be repeated (see Figs. 7-37 to 7-42). The lateral views (see Figs. 7-41 and 7-42) show excellent resolution of the anterior axillary and posterior axillary fat deposits, as well as breast position and symmetry. The mid-flank folds have been reduced but not eliminated (see Figs. 7-38 to 7-42). Successes include reshaping of the buttocks with fat grafting (see Fig. 7-38), shaping of the high hip and banana roll (see Figs. 7-39 and 7-40), and shrinkage of the excess skin after full abdominal liposuction (see Fig. 7-37).

With use of the "super wet" solution and external ultrasound to distribute the epinephrine to all of her tissues, there was no necessity for blood transfusion and the procedure moved forward rapidly, with completion in less than 3 hours. It is interesting to note that the transition areas of the mid-back resolved whereas liposuction of the major folds was incomplete. We recommend that these patients be offered a secondary procedure at no cost or a minor facility cost. Local anesthetics will suffice. If resolution is not complete in 3 months, as in this case, one should proceed without further delay. Resolution of body liposuction is continuous over a period of 3 months, and further improvement is not to be expected.

Prevention of a "Tomato Breast" Appearance in Mammaplasty— Ulrich T. Hinderer, M.D., Ph.D. (Plastic Surgeon, Madrid)

In 1992, at the IPRS International Congress in Madrid, I presented a paper on periareolar dermopexy with retromammary mastopexy, which is, as far as I know, the first donut-type technique. At the beginning I used the technique for breasts with minor ptosis, and thereafter I started to use it for both hypoplasia and tubular breasts, combined with implants. Lately, its use has been very much expanded as the "circumareolar dermoglandular plication procedure."

The procedure has proved safe and reliable in almost 200 patients and has the following advantages:

- No full-thickness skin incision or excisions are performed.
- Only the epidermis is incised or excised.

Except for patients with hypertrophy, the skin is not dissected from the gland, nor the gland from the pectoralis fascia, which increases vascular safety. The dermoglandular unit of the breast through Cooper's ligaments is stabilized by a single or multiple plications. The scar is only circumareolar, which reduces psychological stress and discomfort and achieves early recovery.

The disadvantages are twofold:

- Widening and irregularities of the periareolar suture line may occur and often require postoperative scar revision at 6 months, which by the way is also frequently necessary in conventional breast reduction techniques for correction of the scar and possible "dog-ears."
- For circumareolar plication and all techniques that do not achieve satisfactory forward projection of the central breast mound, flattening of the NAC with periareolar bulging can occur, appropriately termed a "tomato breast" appearance by Basset.

The circumareolar bulging is corrected by means of *liposuction of the corresponding area and downward.* However, liposuction is never performed in the area of the central breast cone, which would further reduce its projection. Liposuction can also be used in other mammaplasty techniques when there is insufficient forward projection of the frontal breast mound. If insufficient, several vertical glandular plications beneath

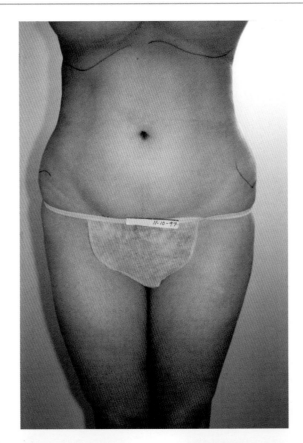
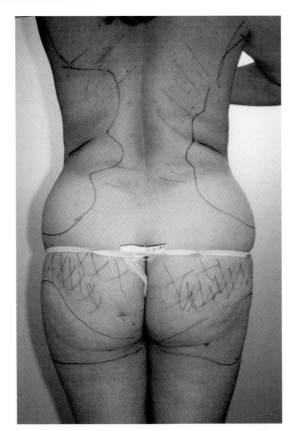
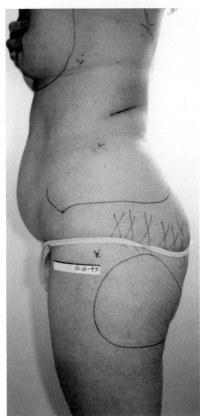
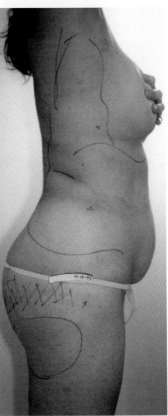
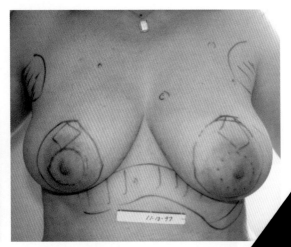

FIGURES 7-30 – 7-34   *The role of lipoextraction in breast asymmetry. This patient is marked for hip, abdomen, flank and thigh XUAL with regrafting to the mid-buttock. These "bloodless" procedures may be safely combined with a "minimal blood loss" circumareolar mastop wet" fluid is injected into all areas. Note the breast asymmetry and prominent axillary pads and "tail of Spence."*

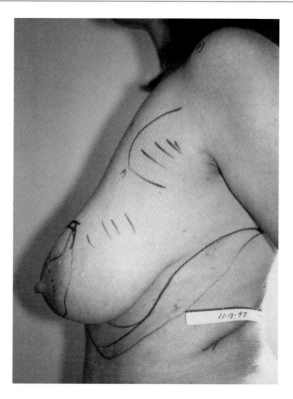
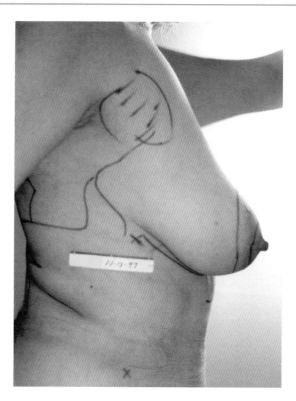

FIGURES 7-35 & 7-36   *The extent of circumareolar de-epithelialization, asymmetric supra-areolar wedge excision, and balancing liposuction.*

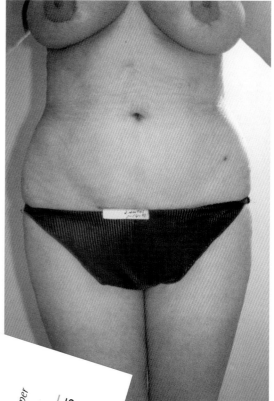
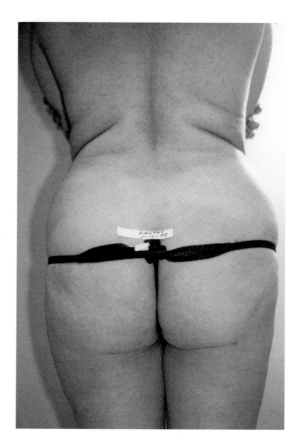

liposuction in asymmetric breasts includes several areas of planned and intraoperative fat removal to obtain

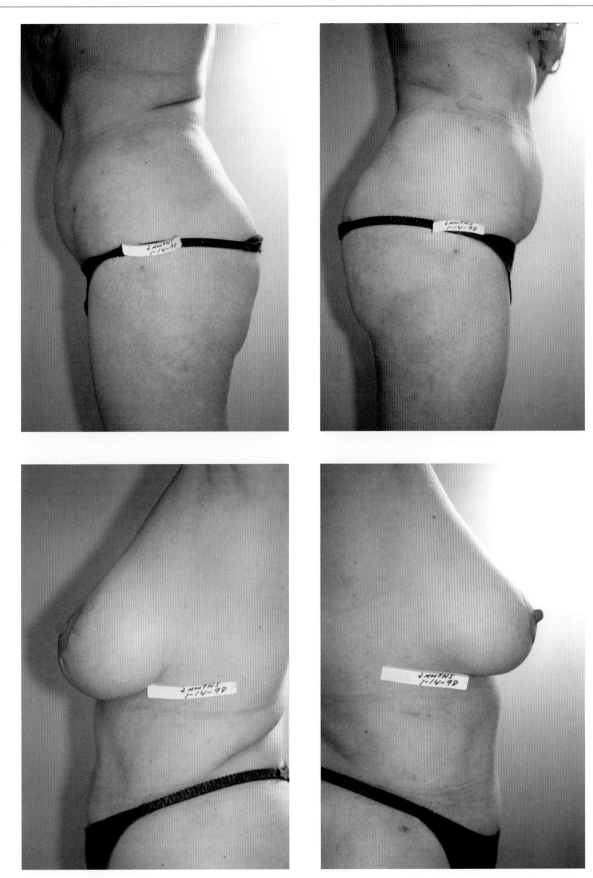

FIGURES 7-37 – 7-42   *Continued*

the subdermal network, which has to remain with the deep dermis to guarantee circumareolar plication without vascular complications, may be performed additionally. Erol and Spira used a similar technique at the base of the breast—rotation-invagination—to improve forward projection of the breast mound.

Editor's Note: Dr. Hinderer was one of the innovators who made an impression in my early career, both with malar and facial surgery and with circumareolar breast surgery. It had become apparent that a greater degree of invagination and reshaping was required than described by Erol and Spira. The concept of complete internal shaping was presented in 1985 at a RAPS meeting in Los Angeles. Dr. Louis Benelli, Dr. Luiz Toledo, Dr. Adrien Aiache, and I gave presentations and compared techniques and results. Dr. Toledo added an additional refinement, liposuction, when liposuction was considered to be a dangerous procedure in breast surgery. Dr. Benelli discussed the "round block" with a de-epithelialized ring. This circular suture largely prevented distortion of the nipple complex. I advocated a double suture and methods of building a conical breast mound beneath the skin. The double suture prevented areolar stretch and, with the "Texas diamond" excision, stabilized the nipple-areolar complex in the preferred position.

Our textbook *Circumareolar Techniques in Breast Surgery*[1] combined our experience with the procedures. Like Dr. Hinderer, we have eliminated the "tomato breast" by performing a greater degree of plication, as well as incorporating the liposuction that he describes.

FAT GRAFTING OF THE BREAST

Although fat grafting of the breast is inherently undesirable because fat grafts calcify in the same manner as early malignancy and the bacteria living in breast tissue can lead to early infection and disappointment, in some instances, dermis fat or fat grafting may play a role.

Case in Point

In the patient pictured, a silicone implant from the early 1980s had ruptured with migration into soft tissue. After removal of the capsular tissue and the implant aided by "super wet pump dissection," a deficit in soft tissue in the upper inner quadrant of the right breast still remained after her breast reconstruction. With time, after adjustment of the breast contour to the textured gel prosthesis and internal repair, the following procedure was initiated to supply the soft tissue in the area. The usual pectoralis major and minor rotation flaps were not an option because of destruction of these tissues from migration of the silicone.

A "crescent" excision was planned above each areola of the reconstructed breast. This tissue has de-epithelialized and was prepared as a dermis-fat graft. The center of the breast is noted in the preoperative markings (see Fig. 7-43). Because of the limited tissue and the lack of soft tissue on either side of the defect, fat grafts obtained with the syringe technique are prepared for placement directly into the subcutaneous tissue medial to the dermis-fat graft repair (see Fig. 7-44). The patient was warned repeatedly that this area must be identified on subsequent mammograms.

The two dermis-fat grafts obtained from the upper portion of each breast are sutured together as a unit and will be placed in the defect with a "pull-through" suture or fixation. After placement of the grafts, fat and dermis, closure is initiated as shown to reposition both areolas at a higher spot by suture to subcutaneous tissue in the preferred position and subsequent multilayered closure of the defect.

If the patient is carefully counseled that local spot augmentation of a deficit with fat grafts will result in an abnormal mammogram of that specific area, fat grafts can be beneficial in complex breast repairs and

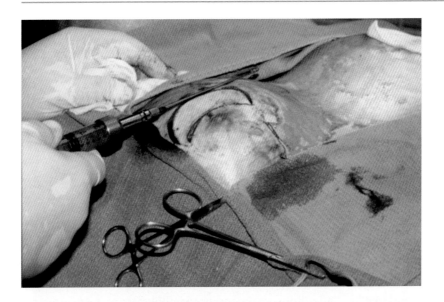

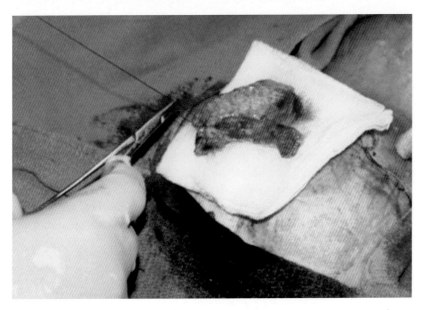

FIGURES 7-43 & 7-44 *Smaller subsurface defects in breast repair are addressed by multilayer subdermal fat grafts. Larger defects are corrected with dermis-fat grafts, shown here and obtained from the periareolar area.*

reconstructions. Radiologists are advised in advance that this procedure was performed for surface elevation.

Reference

1. Wilkinson TS, Toledo LS, Aiache AE: *Circumareolar Techniques in Breast Surgery.* New York, Springer-Verlag, 1995.

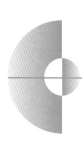

CHAPTER EIGHT

Liposuction of the Face and Neck

Once greeted with enthusiasm as a method of reducing fatty cheeks and jowls, liposuction of the head and neck soon fell into disfavor. Experienced surgeons found that irregularities in the face were magnified by even the most concise application of this technique. Reduction of nasolabial fold fullness by liposuction is still advantageous, as well as larger lateral fat pads of the jowl and neck. Other surgeons prefer to reduce these areas under direct vision and approach them through a "submental tuck" incision, which allows for reduction of the overhanging "witches chin" deformity. External ultrasound techniques will further dissolve superficial fat pads in the subcommissural, nasolabial, malar pad, and jowl areas.

In the typical older patient, fat accumulates in these visible spots while "melting" of circumoral tissues occurs. Fat regrafting plays a role not only in lip enhancement but also in filling subcommissural depressions and elevating and filling the chin and nasolabial depressions. These safe procedures are designed to create a more natural effect without the extremely taut face that occurs after an ill-advised attempt to stretch out the nasolabial folds. I have found that the use of external ultrasound postoperatively not only reduces bruising and edema but also seems to induce further contracture of facial tissues, which is a process that continues over many months and enhances the result of the mid-face– or "complete" face-lift.

In no other area of the body have there been such extreme pendulum swings. Liposuction was initially embraced as a means of removing neck fat in the submental triangle, as well as in the jowl areas and cheeks, often with disastrous complications. It soon became apparent that furrowing, skin damage, contracture, and deep scarring accompanied these attempts at facial rejuvenation. When the "super wet" techniques were introduced, surgeons were still dismayed to find that a percentage of patients exhibited worsening of the facial contour when liposuction was used outside the "safe zones" of the jowl edge. Reports of facial paralysis after liposuction and irreparable scarring from attempts to curet or laser burn the undersurface of the neck skin in an ill-advised effort to induce skin contracture in conjunction with liposuction emphasize that planning based on sound surgical principles is of extreme importance in this unforgiving area. Liposuction may be used in the neck as an isolated procedure in younger adults who do not have bowing of the platysma. A bidirectional approach to removing superficial fatty tissues in the neck results in a degree of skin retraction and a pleasing restoration of contouring in young adults. Until the advent of ultrasound-assisted liposuction (UAL) and external ultrasound-assisted liposuction (XUAL), retraction in these areas rarely occurred in older adults, and the wrinkling excess skin could be corrected only by classic face-lift procedures.

PATIENT SELECTION

A current misconception is that any form of liposuction will correct descent of the mid-face musculoaponeurotic system, which is routinely repaired and repositioned in modern face-lift procedures. The same misconception applies to the submental triangle, in which fat removal should accompany treatment of lax skin and platysmal bands. Direct excision plus plication of the platysma and low neck division of the bands, in conjunction with removal of superficial and deep fat, is the procedure of choice. For each individual, the degree of skin laxity must be judged so that one may avoid misleading patients about the efficacy of procedures that are simpler than rhytidectomy with submental platysmal repair.

On the other hand, certain young adults have fatty faces that respond well to classic liposuction. In others, removal of the Bichat pad is a better procedure, in combination with some degree of liposuction of the jowl areas. The patients to be presented in this chapter demonstrate the usefulness of liposuction in the classic face-lift, the fatty-faced young adult, and the classic submental bowing of the platysma with prominent superficial and deep fat pads. Restoration of facial contours with fat grafting is an integral part of restoration in these categories of patients. More recently, the skin shrinkage afforded by UAL and XUAL have also changed our perception of the role of liposuction. Skin retraction from the jowl area downward accompanies careful fat removal by UAL. This technique produces a more natural "clean" jowl line. With XUAL, patients who do not accept a more complex procedure, even rejecting the so-called mid-face–lift, can be helped considerably with lesser procedures in combination with XUAL shrinkage of the cheek, jowl, and neck.

"En bloc" fat resection of the neck was presented as early as 1920 and 1932. In the American Society for Aesthetic Plastic Surgery teaching course of Dr. Lawrence Robbins, the success of scissors dissection in the submental triangle is demonstrated as being considerably better than liposuction alone. Long-term induration and inadvertent removal of superficial subcutaneous fat often mar the results of closed liposuction. "En bloc" resection under direct visualization results in thorough clearing, whereas liposuction often requires "cleanup." In addition, one has easy access to the platysma during direct neck fat excision.

LIPOSUCTION OF THE FACE

Before the development of XUAL, liposuction of the face was a commonly performed procedure. Even with small cannulas and meticulous attention to detail, "furrowing" and skin irregularities occurred. In young individuals such as the one illustrated in Figures 8-1 and 8-2, the combination of Bichat pad removal from within and "wet" superficial liposuction with small cannulas was the only alternative at the time of this 1983 surgery. The

shaping of his face is a reflection of his age and skin quality (see Figs. 8-3 and 8-4). Further evolution of the edematous areas is noted in the later photograph, which shows good highlighting of his natural malar eminences and resolution of the original rounded, jowly cheeks (see Fig. 8-5).

Mid-cheek liposuction and liposuction beyond the "safe zones" of the jowl and submental fat pads are less

> **CLINICAL PEARL**
>
> "Superficial liposculpture of the face" refers to multilevel suctioning starting with the 3-mm, 15-cm-long cannula and performed with a syringe suction technique. It is especially recommended for contouring the submental triangle. A 1.5-mm, 15-cm-long flat-tipped cannula is used for superficial suctioning in the jowls and the area beyond the nasolabial fold. The holes do not face the skin surface, and the cannula is inserted beneath a pad of subcutaneous fat that is preserved. With this technique, experienced surgeons are approaching the mid-face and linking this dissection of the face to the neck to avoid the furrowing appearance that has always discouraged surgeons from liposuctioning in this area. Others, however, believe that there are better ways, safer and more efficient, such as XUAL for shrinkage or careful UAL.

likely to be problematic today. Additional infusion ("super wet") provides a few millimeters of cheek fat expansion for safety in preventing over-resection of subcutaneous fat.

> **CLINICAL PEARL**
>
> To illustrate how pioneers in technique may lead us astray, the use of large volumes of fluid infiltrate (tumescent technique) in face-lifts certainly did not prove to be advantageous. Not only is it more difficult to gauge the amount of fat that is left on the skin flap (and fat is a precious commodity in the face), but the additional stretching of the skin from the overabundance of infiltrate also proved to be a drawback. This is not to say that infiltrate fluid does not give the surgeon an extra margin of safety. Moderation is the answer.

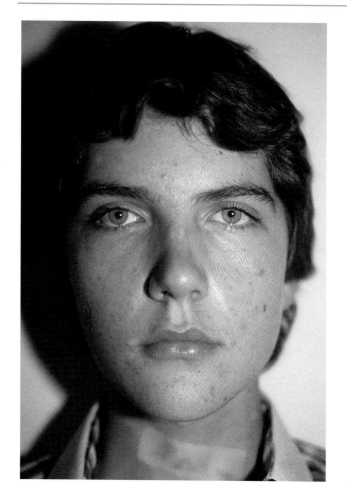
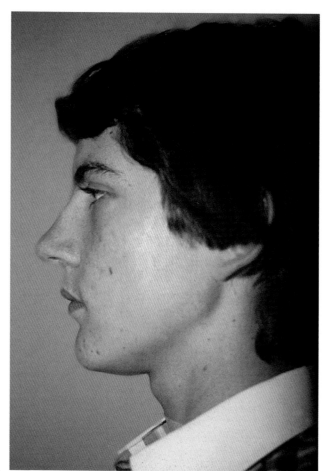

FIGURES 8-1 & 8-2   *Careful liposculpture in selected "jowly" younger patients was our only option in the 1980s.*

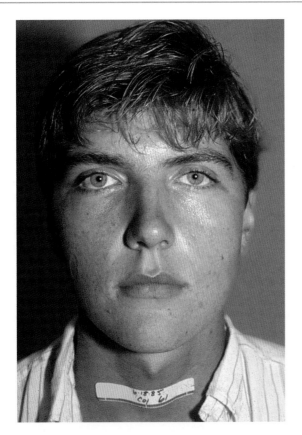
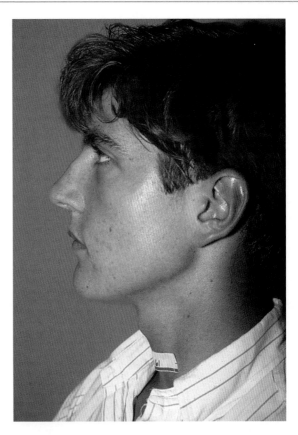

FIGURES 8-3 & 8-4   *Bichat pad removal was once too exotic and was never discussed, but facial improvement was achieved.*

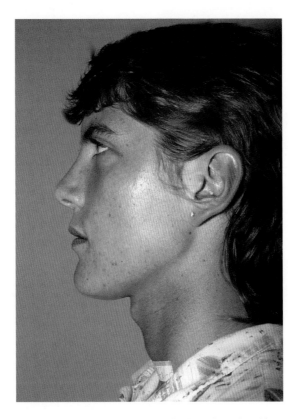

FIGURE 8-5   *Five-year photographs show the sculpted jaw line from suction-assisted lipectomy.*

HOW I DO IT—Liposuction and Face-Lifts—David Foerster, M.D. (Plastic Surgeon, Oklahoma City)

By liposuctioning the submental area, working from either side, I have been able to obtain excellent results during a face-lift procedure without the need for open lipectomy. In fact, it has probably been 15 or 16 years since I have had to perform an open lipectomy. The liposuctioning technique thoroughly cleans out the area that open lipectomy doesn't quite complete, plus avoids the incision. Furthermore, it appears to take less time to heal and soften when compared with the open approach. While marking the patient preoperatively, I mark the incisions and skin flaps that I plan to use, as well as a separate superficial musculoaponeurotic system (SMAS) and separate skin flaps and the submental area to be suctioned, with extension as far down as the sternal notch, if needed. In most cases, it is necessary to go only halfway down the neck.

During the face-lift procedure, when the flaps are elevated, I remove the fatty deposits in the sub-mandibular triangle between the sternal mastoid and the jaw line at the edge of my dissection. I use a small cannula and begin liposuctioning with the flap down so that I can see the areas that I am treating. I usually go beyond the midline so that when I treat the other side, I have a bit less to do and can be sure that the midline areas are well done. Because there is virtually no platysma muscle in that submental region, depth is determined by how much fat is present. I nearly always do quite a bit of superficial liposuctioning, as well as remove the bulk of the fat in that area, which allows a much deeper and sharper cervical mandibular angle and gives a much cleaner neck appearance (Figs. 8-6 to 8-9). Once the liposuction is completed, it is necessary to lift the flap up and clip the little residual bands between the deeper portion of the skin and the soft tissues of the neck. Otherwise, they will act as tethers or checkreins, which is undesirable. Thus, when I tighten my SMAS and neck flaps, I am able to achieve excellent contour of the anterior of the neck, and the need for a secondary procedure is almost zero.

Author's Technique

Since 1997, in patients whose facial deformity can be corrected by liposuction alone, the use of XUAL softens the mid-cheek, jowl, and submental fat, tightens the skin, and produces fat atrophy in the "transitional area" beyond the safe area for liposuction. In Figure 8-10, a single entry point with a small stab wound in the submental line allows access to the mid-cheek. A second aspiration is performed from the earlobe area, with special care taken to avoid passing the cannula into the subplatysmal area, which might damage the seventh nerve. Addition of the "super wet" infusion adds a safety factor and facilitates liposuction.

CLINICAL PEARL

Better to Be Experienced than Overconfident
Only a few experienced surgeons will use a small UAL cannula in the face. They believe that the contour is smoother if the fat is melted. Other surgeons report disastrous facial burns and irregularities.

Remember that the safe zones are thicker jowls and the upper part of the neck, not the cheeks and certainly not the lateral portion of the neck. Liposuction of any form in these areas has caused more grief for plastic surgeons than any procedure in recent memory. Another advantage of XUAL is that these peripheral areas, the so-called transition zones, will show a degree of fat dissolution without the risk of furrowing.

CLINICAL PEARL

Yukio Shirakabe (Tokyo) began performing face-lift operations in combination with open and closed liposuction of the neck in the early 1980s; he used a crisscross approach to avoid waves or rippling. Many surgeons have followed this innovation with a variety of open liposuction techniques when cervical fat is exposed on the grounds that more concise suctioning would be obtained under direct vision than with the closed technique.

CLINICAL PEARL

Steve Block (Oak Park) also finds that XUAL will help face-lift patients achieve the result that we desire. He uses XUAL before making the incision and finds that the skin contracture is "remarkable." He adds one other factor, "cooking the SMAS." After subcutaneous dissection, Steve uses a Valley Lab Bovie "spray" and passes this over the SMAS. There is at least a 25% contracture, which appears to be permanent. The results were corroborated by Dr. Barry Silberg (Santa Rosa), who is also a proponent of nonsurgical shrinkage of the face with XUAL.

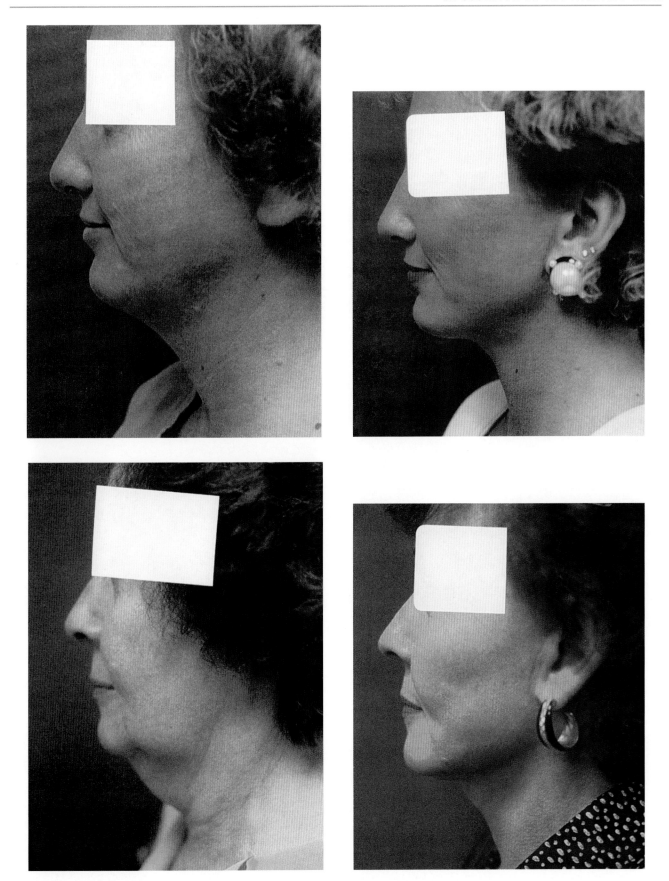

FIGURES 8-6 – 8-9 *Skin retraction and probable platysma trauma as a result of neck liposculpture from a lateral face-lift incision can result in good contour without platysmal plication (Dr. Foerster).*

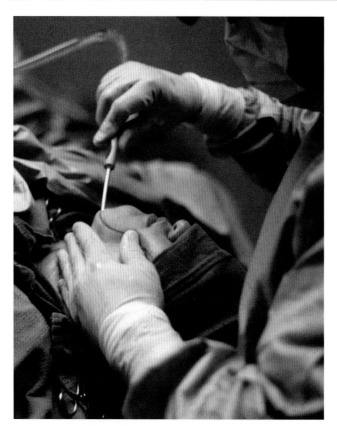

FIGURE 8-10 *Liposuction of the "safe zone" above the platysma is less likely to over-resect facial fat if the opposite hand acts as a guide to position the cannula.*

SUBMENTAL TUCK

Restoring a useful flat under-jaw area and a clean mandibular line is one of the goals of aesthetic surgery. Liposuction plays a role, of course, but it is now confined primarily to the jowls and nasolabial fold. At one time everyone jumped on the bandwagon, and the neck was liposuctioned merrily. Too often, we saw these patients with prominent bands and without the clean line that we wanted, simply because we had neglected the platysma. I began performing platysma surgery some 20 years ago, but we could not assure patients that it would be long lasting. We used this technique only in those with very fatty necks and prominent bands. We should have performed platysmorrhaphy in almost 100%! Like bad pennies, those patients are coming back now with stretched skin and prominent neck muscle bands. Those fortunate ones who had the platysma resectioned with plication and removal of the deep and superficial fat pads still have their jaw lines 30 years later.

The following important points should be considered when correcting this important zone:

1. Keep the incision short and high in the submental fold. Good surgeons advise you to make the incision lower down, but it shows and it's your scar.
2. Do your superficial liposuction as soon as the skin is opened, but don't be brave enough to try to suction the subplatysmal fat. It's easier to remove it under direct vision.
3. Clear only one side at a time. It's easier to control the bleeding through a small incision.
4. Pull the platysma toward the midline and use flat-bladed scissors to trim off the remaining fat. You will be surprised by how much you left behind.
5. Divide the platysma as low as possible in the neck. You will start your plication of the divided muscle just at the hyoid.
6. While it's fashionable to talk about a new "full-neck corset" repair, that's what we performed in 1971

and it's still a good idea. If you divide too high and repair too high, you will have a "Dick Tracy" cutoff.

7. Always leave a little fat at the base of the dissection to make the transition zone more natural.

8. It's almost always indicated, so go ahead and resect part of the platysma. That gives you good access to the submental fat and good muscle to sew together.

9. Use figure-of-eight sutures. I prefer "nonabsorbable" rather than "absorbable." Mersilene will last longer, but all the braided sutures, such as Neurolon, have a disturbing tendency to become untied. That's not true of Dexon and Vicryl.

10. After you have completed the midline plication, take another look and you may find fat that hasn't been trimmed. Put your finger on the edge of the mandible and push downward. You may see a bulge that could easily cause a visible blip postoperatively.

11. Always drain this area.

12. At the end of the procedure, reblock the regional nerves with bupivacaine (Marcaine).

Ultrasound Sculpturing of the Cheeks in Combination with Bichat Pad Removal, Submental Repair, and Chin Augmentation

The addition of ultrasound to correct a jowly face (see Figs. 8-11 and 8-12) is complementary to the other restorative procedures. Rapid resolution of mid-facial edema with protraction and smoothing of the nasolabial folds is evident at 2 weeks (see Fig. 8-13) and at 6 months (see Fig. 8-14). In our experience, males undergoing this combination procedure previously did not lose the facial edema this rapidly. The remodeling of the face shown in the frontal view (see Fig. 8-15) was 90% complete within 3 weeks of the original surgery. The effect of Bichat pad removal is to accent the highlights of the cheek, and ultrasound provided smoothing of the jaw line contour, as well as retraction of the cheek skin.

Case in Point—"First, Do No Harm"

This patient is a newly retired executive who "does not have the time" for a face-lift. After a long discussion of the advantages of face-lifting with posterior repositioning of the platysma, he agreed to undergo a lesser procedure. The results have been to his expectations. The procedure chosen was a "submental tuck" with application of external ultrasound alone (XU) to the cheeks and neck and direct removal of fat from the single incision in the submental fold.

For these individuals, especially those with thicker skin, the only question is the degree of shrinkage that will be afforded by undermining and the addition of XU. Because no guarantees are made that the neck will be as smooth as in a face-lift patient, the use of these techniques gives an alternative to certain individuals who have time or financial constraints.

> **CLINICAL PEARL**
>
> Alan Matarasso (Plastic Surgeon, New York)
>
> Patients must recognize that they have to "give" something—whether it be accepting scars, allowing for adequate downtime, or quitting smoking—to get the results that they desire. Plastic surgery may be a glorious blend of art and a science, but it is still surgery—not magic.

Technique

The procedure begins with infiltration of a 0.125% lidocaine (Xylocaine) "super wet" formula from the malar eminence to the clavicle. External ultrasound is then administered after a 5-minute wait. After 6 to 8 minutes the skin begins to show a heat reaction. At this point the jowl fat is beginning to break up and will disintegrate and spread with pressure. No direct removal of the jowl pad is necessary. This is an advantage in that liposuction around the rim of the mandible has been associated with seventh nerve palsies. After elevating the subcutaneous tissue from the underlying fat of the anterior neck under direct vision, the platysma is grasped and brought toward the center so that defatting can be performed with flat-bladed scissors. Our preference is the blunt-tipped Wilkinson face-lift scissors (Snowden-Pencer, Padgett). Using the blunt tips for dissection and for spreading in the area of the edge of the sternomastoid avoids nerve injury. The central fat pad is then grasped, elevated, and removed as a unit by a simple maneuver. Pressing downward with the scissors spread wide facilitates removal of muscle and fat above the deep fat pad. This maneuver affords excellent visualization. When bleeding has been controlled from the cut platysma edges, the remaining deep fat pad can be trimmed as necessary. With the platysma once again stretched, a cutting cautery is used at the level of the hyoid to divide the platysma. It is important that this division be carried back at least 3 or 4 cm to destroy visible banding.

The platysma is plicated in the midline with figure-of-eight absorbable sutures. My preference is 2-0 Vicryl. The anterior neck contour is now re-established. Once the platysma has been sutured, small amounts of fat along the rim of the mandible can be easily removed

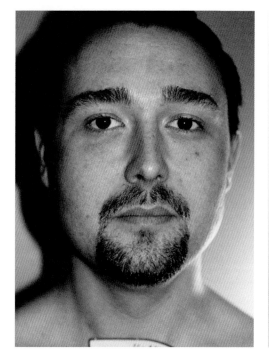
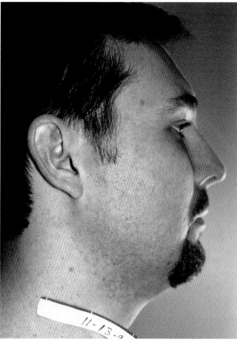

FIGURES 8-11 & 8-12
Ultrasound pretreatment for facial contouring. This young man with a receding chin, concealed by a goatee, also asked for correction of the cervical angle and fatty neck as a first volunteer for sculpture by external ultrasound alone.

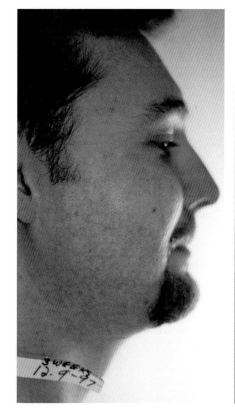
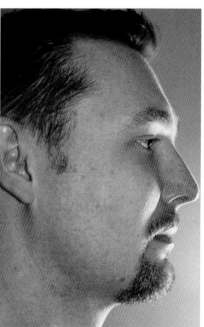
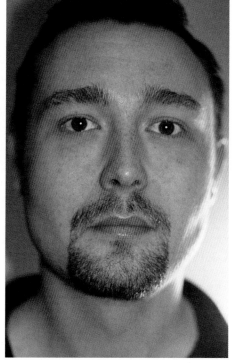

FIGURE 8-13 *Three weeks after a "submental tuck" and cheek ultrasound with a silicone chin prosthesis. Note the early cheek and neck contraction.*

FIGURES 8-14 & 8-15 *At 1 year, there has been further beneficial cheek and neck remodeling with no further treatment or weight loss.*

under direct vision. A helpful maneuver is to place a finger above the mandible and press downward so that the fat bulges away from the underlying musculature and vessels.

It is always necessary to drain this area. A small butterfly apparatus with a suction tube is sufficient. Closure of the small incision proceeds in a lateral-to-medial direction and ends with a subcuticular suture. Compression is applied to this area, as well as the jowls and cheek. In these individuals (see Figs. 8-16 to 8-18), wider undermining of the skin is helpful, although contracture will occur more from ultrasound than undermining.

As noted in postoperative photographs (see Figs. 8-19 to 8-21), at this early stage there is good contouring of the skin in the jowl and neck area. This contouring continues for months with further resorption of XU-treated fat in the jowls and mid-cheek. The nasolabial folds are addressed during the initial XU treatment. Dissolution of fat in the nasolabial fold along with concomitant shrinkage of the mid-cheek gives the youthful appearance noted and is further improved with postoperative ultrasound (see Fig. 8-22). Liposuction of the fold may be indicated in certain instances.

It is important to realize that no harm has been done. There has been no attempt to cauterize the undersurface of the skin by either electric cautery or laser, and the known complications of scarring and distortion are avoided.

Case in Point—Transient Paralysis of the Face after Liposuction

Technical Forum had surveyed a number of plastic surgeons about this phenomenon and reported that transient paresis was indeed rare but was reported clandestinely until the February 1989 issue. It was not limited to any cannula, any anesthetic technique, or any entry spot. Paresis occurred after open suctioning and closed suctioning. In most cases surveyed, nerve function returned after 3 to 4 months. When asked for an opinion of the etiology, I speculated that nerve injury occurred at the ear when the cannula entered the face or at the crossing point of the mandible near the oral commissure. The latter would be more suspect because the mandibular branch of the facial nerve may be more superficial in these two spots and would probably be more easily damaged. Gerald Pitman (New York) believes that inadvertent deep entry played a role in the cases he reviewed.

Advice would include avoidance of vigorous cross-suction in the "no man's land" between the edge of the commissure and the appearance of true jowl fat. Use slow penetration rather than a tearing motion. Be certain that the cannula is superficial if liposuction is performed in this area near the lips outside the fatty jowl (and with the advent of XUAL, it is not usually necessary to suction). Finally, be aware that it is conceivable that muscle hypertrophy was misinterpreted as being fat.

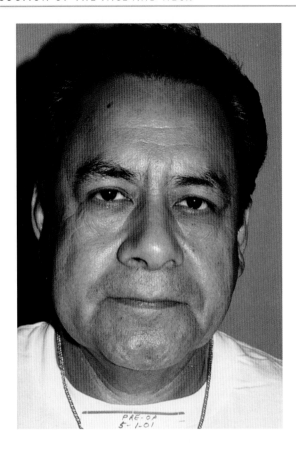

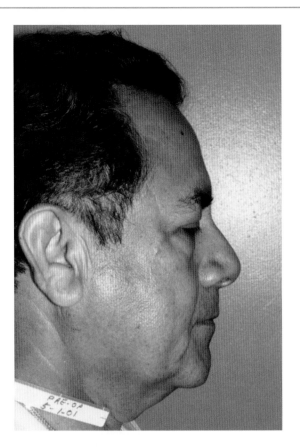

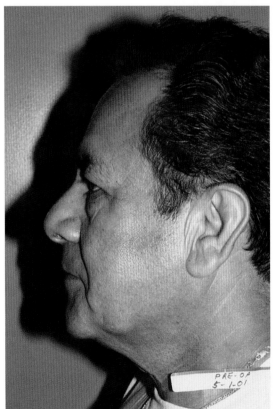

FIGURES 8-16 – 8-18 *The difficult male face. Thicker skin, prominent cheek musculature, and larger jowl and Bichat fat often require secondary facial skin tucks.*

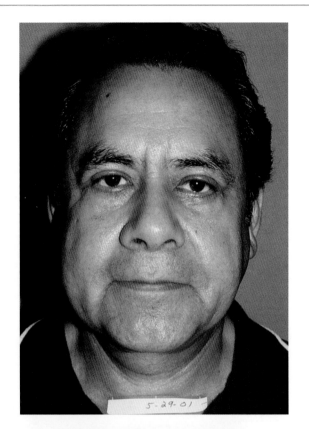
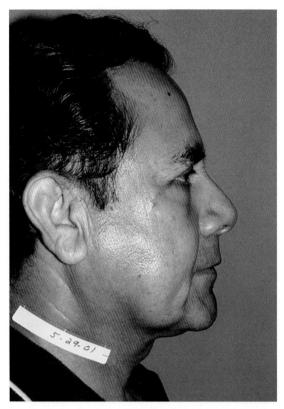
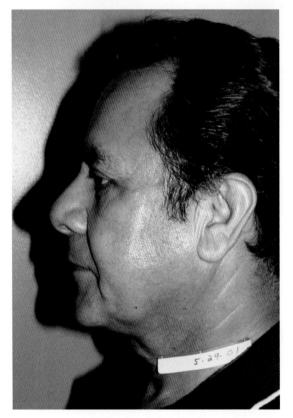
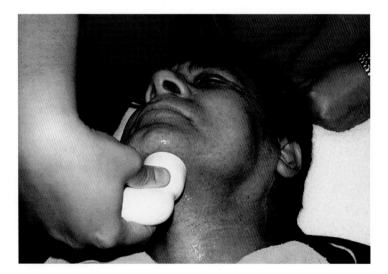

FIGURES 8-19 — 8-22 *Residual jowl fat and cheek redundancy are first addressed by postoperative injection and XU.*

Case in Point—Correction of the Bichat Pad Contribution to Cheek Fullness

This patient in Figures 8-23 to 8-25 exhibited primarily thickening and bowing of the submental musculature with a deep fat pad. In addition, she wanted to thin her face in the midsection but did not have a large subcutaneous fat pad. Removal of the Bichat pad from an intraoral approach is the procedure of choice. Failure to diagnose the role of this intramuscular fat pad and plan for removal would have been an error.

With a small incision at the submental fold, the superficial and deep fat pads were removed manually, the platysma was divided low in the neck and resected medially, and then the usual plication with the multilayered suture technique was performed. In the 3-week photograph, there is still edema in this area. Today, this is treated aggressively with postsurgical XU. Postoperative XU was not used in similar individuals in the original 1997 study, so we could gauge the effect of a single treatment.

Even at 3 weeks one can see that the cheeks are beginning to show flattening after resection of the rounding in the jowl area (see Figs. 8-26 to 8-28). This process continues for 60 to 90 days postoperatively.

The same patient shows very rapid resolution of edema in her 3-week photographs after XUAL of the high hip, inner thigh, banana roll, lateral hip, and abdominal areas along with regrafting of fat into the valley in the mid-buttock zone (see Figs. 8-29 to 8-36).

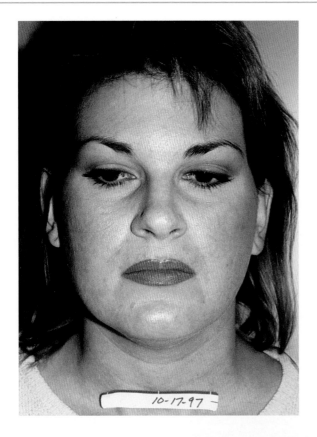
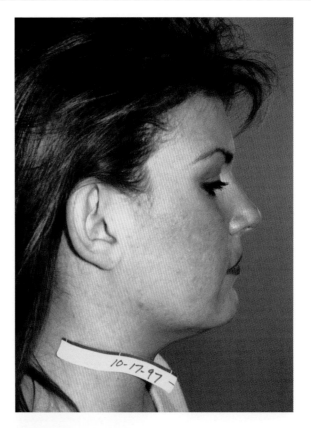
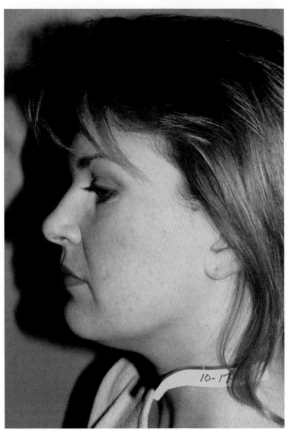

FIGURES 8-23 – 8-25 *Early improvement in facial shaping by intraoperative XU. Prominent platysmal bands and moderate jowl fat will be corrected by platysma plication and XU.*

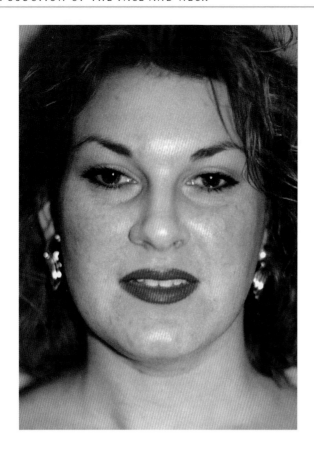
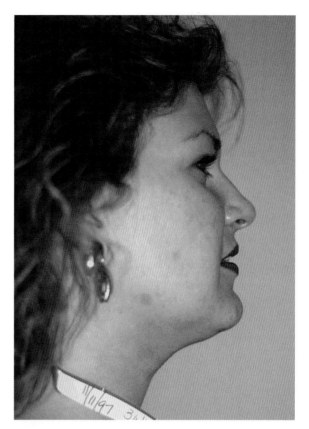
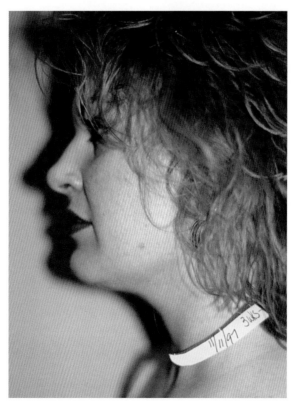

FIGURES 8-26 – 8-28   *Contouring nearly complete at 30 days.*

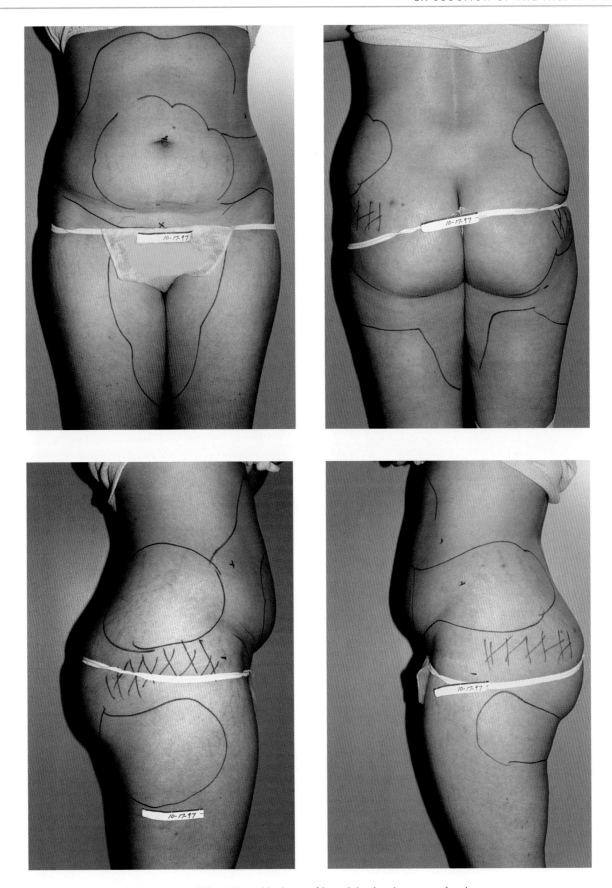

FIGURES 8-29 – 8-32 *The major procedure will be XUAL and body regrafting. Abdominoplasty was refused.*

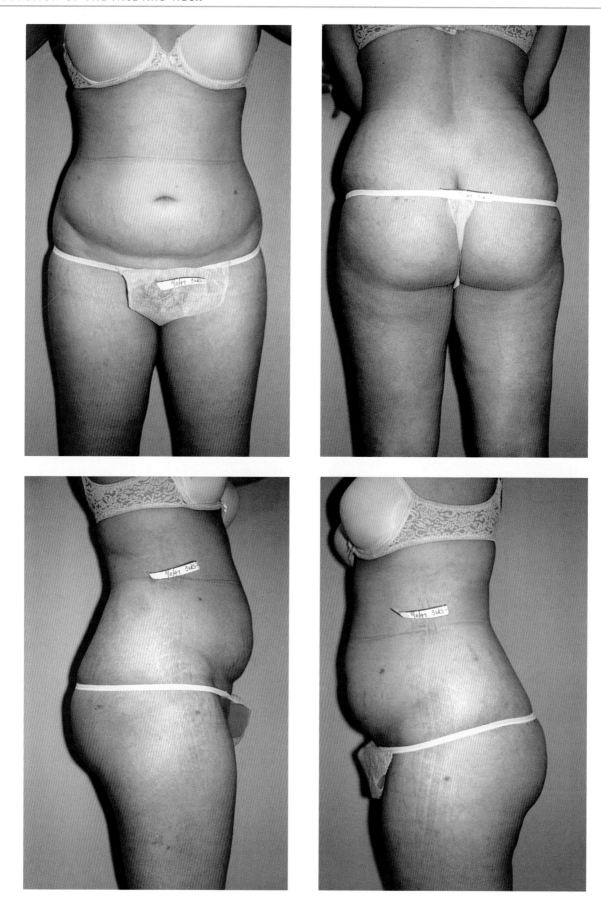

FIGURES 8-33 – 8-36   *Rapid reshaping of XUAL body sculpture at 30 days.*

FACIAL RESHAPING WITHOUT SURGERY

In the initial evaluation of XU, reports of facial recontouring with the prototype machines in the hands of Dr. Steven Hoefflin prompted a search for volunteers. In the patient illustrated in Figure 8-37, the correct choice for her would have been submental lipectomy with muscle plication and at least a mid-face–lift. Because other procedures were contemplated, she agreed to a trial of a single application of XU for 6 minutes to the face and neck after "super wet" infiltration. Preoperative photographs show the typical mid-face descent with jowls, prominent nasolabial folds, and a prominent platysma with subplatysmal and superplatysmal fat, best seen in Figure 8-38, in which the patient holds her preoperative photograph 1 month after the application of ultrasound. Even at this early point it is obvious that there is skin retraction with flattening of the nasolabial folds and resolution of the jowl and superficial submental fat pads. At the time of this application, the degree of retraction of the nasolabial folds was not appreciated. In subsequent patients, additional application time over the nasolabial fold was planned to improve the results that in this patient were surprisingly acceptable. At 4 months, without weight gain or loss, there has been further regression in the jowl, mid-cheek, and even the nasolabial fold, plus regression of the deep fat pad as well (see Figs. 8-39 and 8-40).

The patient was generous in allowing us to use XU primarily as a means of convincing not only our observers but also other physicians of the efficacy of XU application. She also underwent complete abdominal repair, which was complicated by tissue necrosis after a fall 3 days postoperatively. Taking care of this complication was unpleasant, but it was mitigated by her delight in the facial improvement. This is an additional advantage of a minimal cost procedure that may be offered to patients. When a patient is happy with one area, there is a tendency to tolerate the inevitable prolonged recovery if a complication occurs elsewhere!

CLINICAL PEARL

Direct fat excision from the nasolabial fold has been supplanted by suction-assisted lipectomy (SAL) of the nasolabial fat and undermining during face-lifts.[1] The supplemental use of XU-induced skin contracture is an addition to direct attack of the nasolabial fold.

The first choice for many patients is small-cannula liposuction of prominent nasolabial folds from an intranasal approach. Liposuction cannulas are inserted to reduce the bulge of the nasolabial fold; then the area beyond the fold itself is undermined. The fat removed or fat from a different donor site is placed in tunnels medially when the nasolabial groove has been elevated. Regrafted fat is placed in three different levels beneath the fold. XU to induce contracture of the cheek completes the procedure.

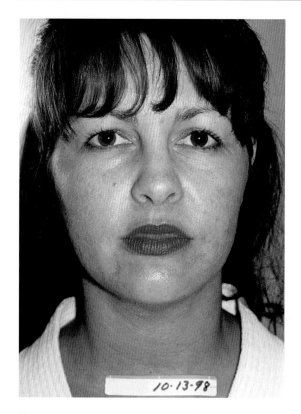

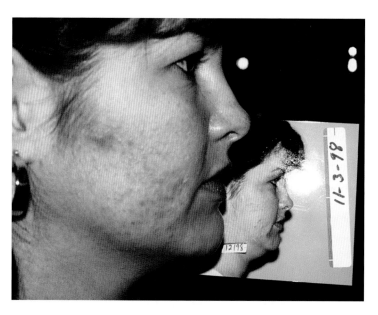

FIGURES 8-37 & 8-38 *Contrast to patients who refuse platysmal repair and are treated by XU alone. Patients undergoing major plastic surgery procedures may choose the lesser alternative of XU alone to improve neck and jowl contour.*

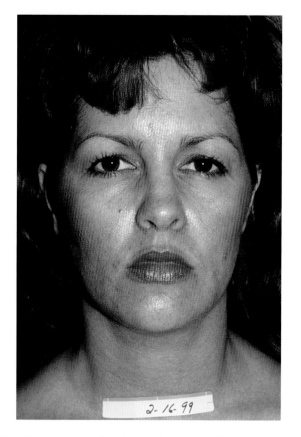

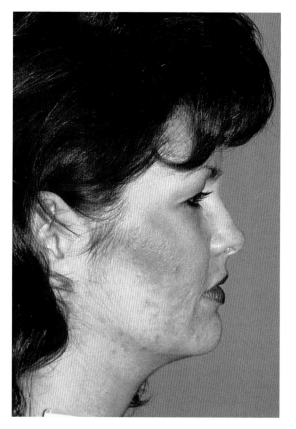

FIGURES 8-39 & 8-40 *Continued reshaping at 4 months versus the 1-month contour in Figure 8-38.*

Facial Sculpturing with Ultrasound

While undergoing reconstructive surgery, the patient in Figures 8-41 to 8-43 volunteered to have XU with infiltration applied during the operation to improve the appearance of her face. Without weight gain or loss, reshaping is evident in these areas after a single application of ultrasound (no liposuction): a cleaner jowl line, less prominent nasolabial folds, and retraction of the platysma from dissolution of the superficial and deep fat pads (see Figs. 8-44 to 8-46).

Offering External Ultrasound When a Patient Refuses Surgery

In the initial evaluation of XU for facial recontouring without surgery, the patient in Figure 8-47 refused our recommendation of internal repair of the submental triangle or face-lifting. External ultrasound was applied after local infiltration for 6 minutes.

At 1 month, skin retraction and fat redistribution became evident (see Fig. 8-48). The deep fat pad and nasolabial folds were attacked vigorously with XU.

At 60 days, further contracture is evident, thus illustrating that the effect of the XU process is ongoing (see Fig. 8-49). Subsequently, these patients report continuing remolding of the face for up to 12 months after XU.

Case in point—XU with aggressive skin care

Although it was our impression that some improvement in skin quality occurred after the application of XU without surgical intervention, there was also a question of whether an aggressive skin care program would have provided the reversal of facial descent illustrated by the patient in Figures 8-50 to 8-52. Our clinic provides complete spa facilities, which in addition to post-operative body care, offers skin rejuvenation with various techniques, including microabrasion, the Duke University vitamin C topical program, and in certain patients, the addition of a graduated tretinoin (Retin-A) program.

Our staff was not prepared for the changes evident in this patient 2 months after a single application of XU, 5 days of compression, and our standard skin care program. As noted in the postoperative photographs (see Figs. 8-53 to 8-55), there has been rounding of the lower part of the face with resolution of the nasolabial folds and jowls, retraction of the skin of the neck and cheek, but little effect on the deep subplatysmal fat pad. Her recent evaluation in 2003 showed further regression of the jowl area. It is suggested that patients who are willing to undertake skin rejuvenation also be offered the additional improvement afforded by XU without surgical intervention.

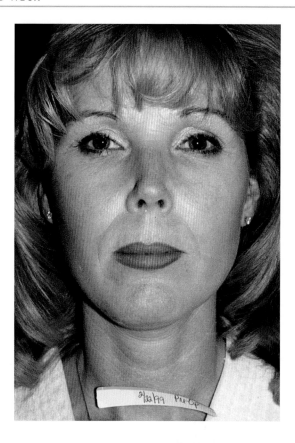

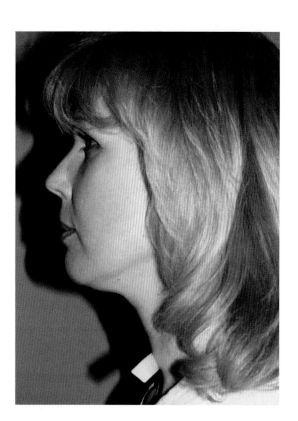

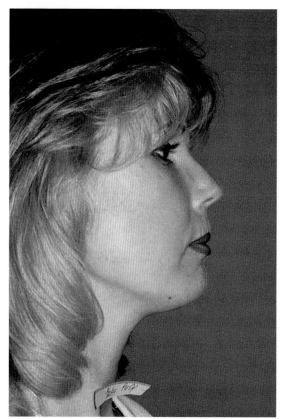

FIGURES 8-41 – 8-43 *Patients with minor corrections are often the most appreciative. Minor degrees of facial fat accumulation rarely warrant surgical intervention.*

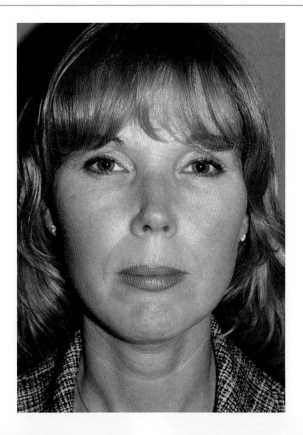

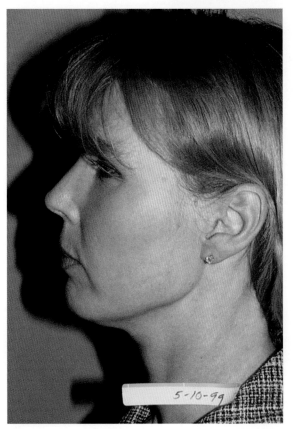
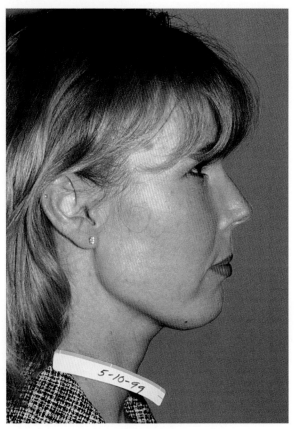

FIGURES 8-44 – 8-46   *Infiltration followed by immediate and daily XU results in visible "improvement" without surgery.*

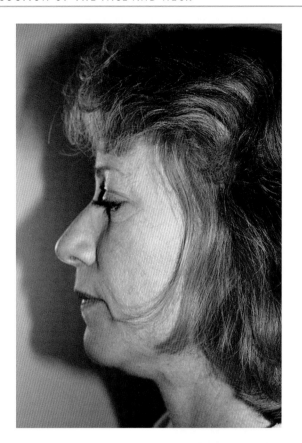
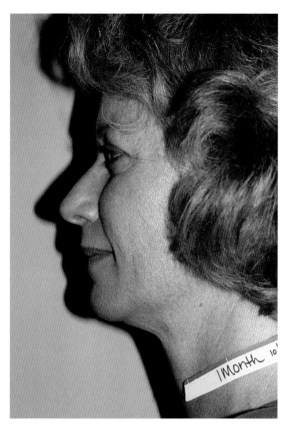
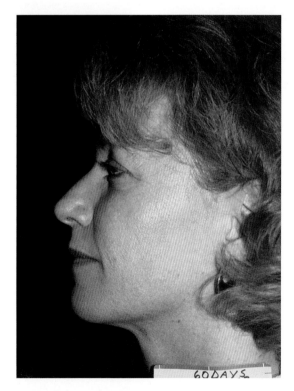

FIGURES 8-47 – 8-49 *Remodeling after even a single XU treatment is an ongoing process in the first 2 months.*

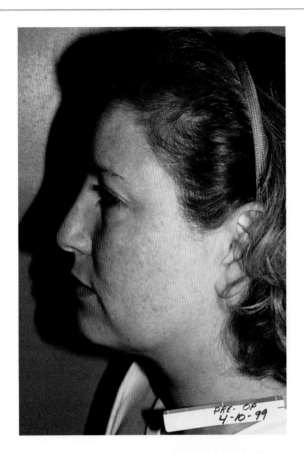
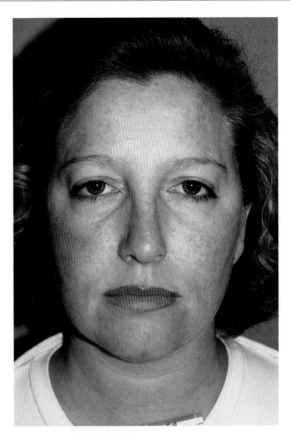
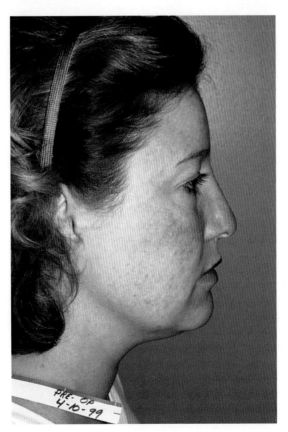

FIGURES 8-50 – 8-52 *Facial contour improvement with XU and a skin care program. A "tired" appearance is worsened by neglected skin quality. A series of three XU treatments is planned.*

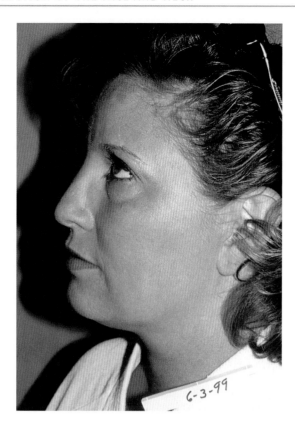
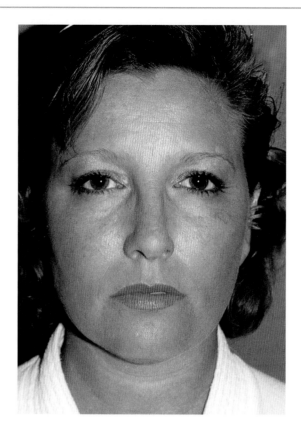
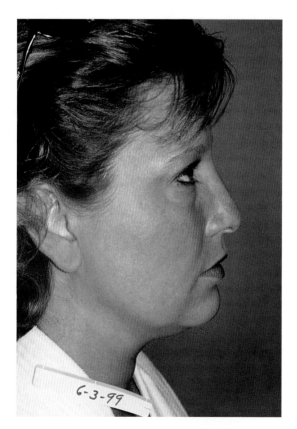

FIGURES 8-53 – 8-55   *At 2 months, contour shows "improvement" with good skin quality and appearance. Microabrasion, topical medication, and vitamin C programs are credited.*

ULTRASOUND AS AN ADJUNCT TO MINIMALLY INVASIVE SURGERY

Malar Pad Removal with XU

After a consultation that included a recommendation for submental repair with liposuction and chin augmentation, this patient chose to undergo only XU of the face and neck and lower lid blepharoplasty. The malar pad has always been a problem, even when it is elevated and anchored. Often, soft tissue fullness was obtrusive. Steroid injections, liposuction, and other modalities have been used to reduce this prominence, but overcorrection was common and required secondary fat replacement. The patient in Figures 8-56 to 8-58 has large C-shaped pads extending from the pupil area laterally. Five weeks after blepharoplasty and XU applied during surgery and for 2 consecutive days, the fat pads are beginning to resolve (see Figs. 8-59 to 8-61). There is also shrinkage of the submental fat, which left the platysma exposed, and early resolution of the jowl pads. At 3 months, the malar pads are flattened, the patient's face is less rounded in the jaw line area, the palpable fat above and below the platysma has disappeared, and only the visible platysma bands are left for future plication (see Figs. 8-62 to 8-64).

CLINICAL PEARL
A consultation is often as much about what surgery won't achieve as what it will.

Advantages and Disadvantages of Facial XU

There is a downside to XU of the face. In the patient shown, descent of the mid-face was only one of the problems that should have been corrected. She agreed to undergo blepharoplasty and submental repair of the platysma along with XU from the malar area to the mid-neck. In the second photograph 1 month after these procedures, her jowl pads have receded, the mid-cheek has tightened, and there is no redundancy of the upper part of the neck (see Fig. 8-65). The decision to have a face-lift, made before her choice of the lesser procedure, will be deferred. For the patient this is a good choice because rejuvenation is less expensive and less complex. For the surgeon, however, it is a "lost face-lift!"

ULTRASOUND AS AN ADJUNCT TO FACE-LIFT PROCEDURES

XU in older individuals with poor skin tone who are undergoing face-lifts is definitely helpful. In these individuals the internal repair is far more important than the redraping and contouring of the skin. The area of jowl fat adjacent to the mouth was considered to be a "no man's land" (see Fig. 8-66). Liposuction in this area endangered branches of the facial nerve, and the branches that crossed the mandible inferiorly were vulnerable to UAL as well as standard dissection techniques. This mid-60s woman participated in the early evaluation of XU and face-lifting. Her poor skin tone, prolonged exposure, and unique resistance to aftercare are commonly encountered in "ranch women." Contouring of the face continued to improve postoperatively rather than deteriorate after a single application of XU. Liposuction was avoided, and defatting was carried out only under direct vision in the submental triangle. The visible jowl and submental fat was removed with the flat-bladed Wilkinson face-lift scissors used to dissect solid tissue.

Although many individuals recover rapidly from face-lift surgery with little bruising, it was unusual to see that older patients in this category responded as well as younger patients with the assistance of XU treatment during surgery and in the early postoperative phase (see Fig. 8-67).

With "super wet" infiltration and general anesthesia, abdominoplasty with XUAL, including revision of her vertical midline scar, proceeded rapidly and safely without complications (see Figs. 8-68 and 8-69). The total operating time was 3 hours, an additional safety factor. "Power pump" super wet infiltration for dissection and to provide comfort for early active mobilization also reduces operative time and morbidity.

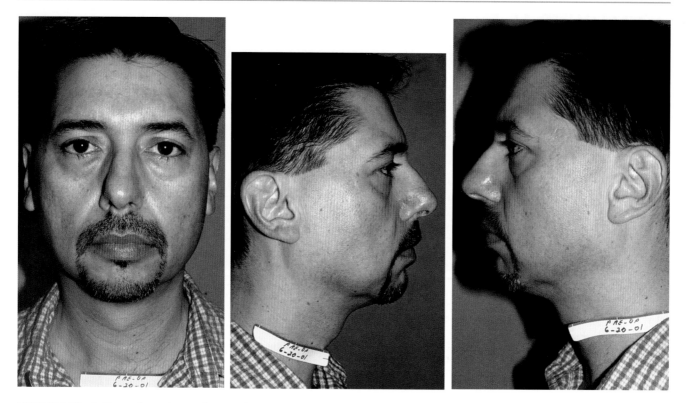

FIGURES 8-56 – 8-58 *Malar pad regression. Despite counseling, this gentleman chooses only blepharoplasty and facial XU because of cost and recovery time.*

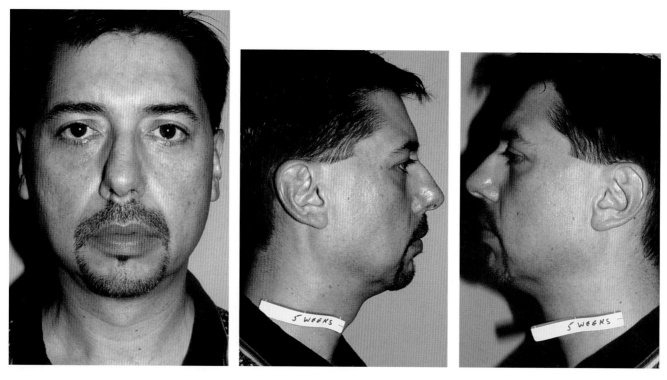

FIGURES 8-59 – 8-61 *At 5 weeks, the blepharoplasty incisions are still visible, but the jowl and malar pads are regressing.*

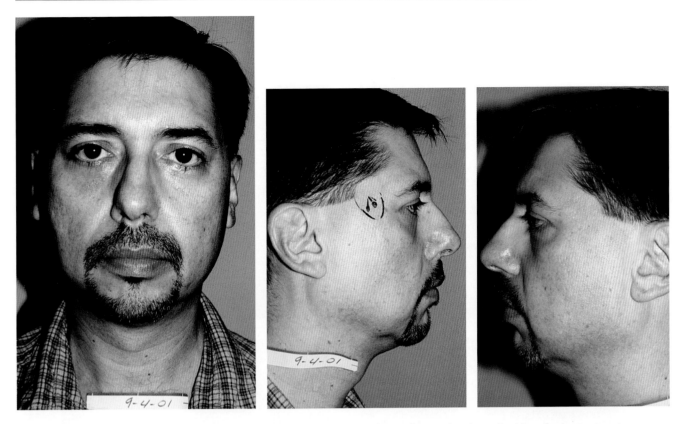

FIGURES 8-62 – 8-64   *Continued remodeling and obliteration of the cheeks, submental fat, and malar pads with no further treatment.*

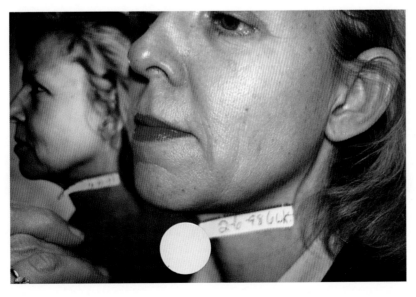

FIGURE 8-65   *Older patients rarely defer face-lifting as this lady did. Blepharoplasty, a submental tuck, and XU were not the recommended combination and should have left her with facial folds and hanging neck skin, but the improvement was so satisfactory that she has not returned for the face-lift!*

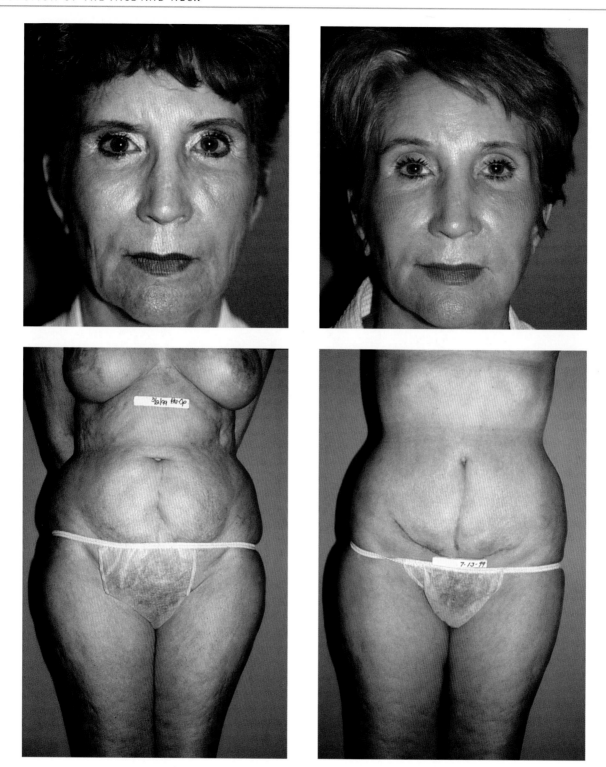

FIGURES 8-66 – 8-69 *Ultrasound as an adjunct to face-lift and abdominoplasty. By limiting blood loss and facilitating quick recovery, an abdominoplasty with flank XU and XUAL was selected, as well as XU face-lifting and XUAL-derived fat grafts to obtain the improvement illustrated.*

PERSISTENCE OF FAT GRAFTS ENHANCED WITH SKIN CARE PROGRAMS

The patient in Figures 8-70 and 8-71 is shown in 1986 in a preoperative black and white photograph while planning for a face-lift, rhinoplasty, blepharoplasty, and fat grafting of the perioral area and, to a limited degree, the vermilion of the lips (see Figs. 8-70 and 8-71). The 1-year postoperative photographs show smoothing of the soft tissues aided by an aggressive skin care program on an outpatient basis (see Figs. 8-72 and 8-73). These fat grafts, which were placed in the vertical ridges of the upper lip, above the white roll margin of the upper and lower lip, in the vermilion, and in the entire perioral area, were intact. A light chemical peel from 1986 was helpful as well.

Subsequently, additional fat grafts were placed in 1991, and she continued to follow an aggressive home skin care program. The program has not changed her normal skin color but is helping to prolong the surgical corrections.

Fifteen years after the initial procedure (see Figs. 8-74 and 8-75), the decision was made to perform a "mini" skin excision in front of her ears and to fill in new atrophy-related depressions in the commissure areas. It will be noted that her skin color has remained normal and that the original fat grafts from 15 years before are also still in place in the upper lip, the white roll area, and the vermilion of the upper and lower lips.

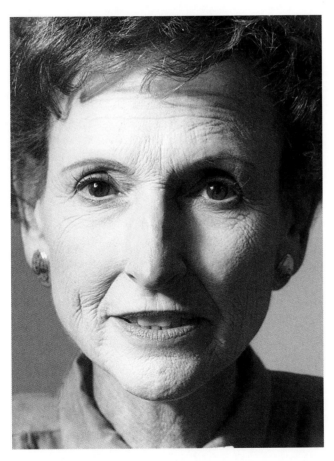
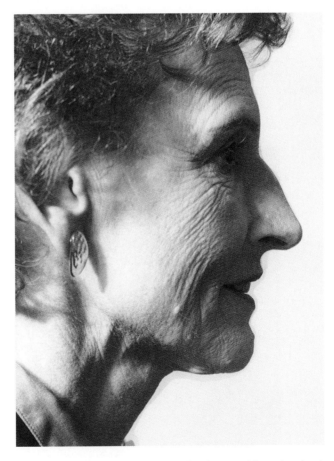

FIGURES 8-70 & 8-71   *Long-term fat grafts. The 1986 surgery plans included rhytidectomy, a submental "tuck," rhinoplasty, and lip and perioral fat grafts with a "light" chemical skin peel.*

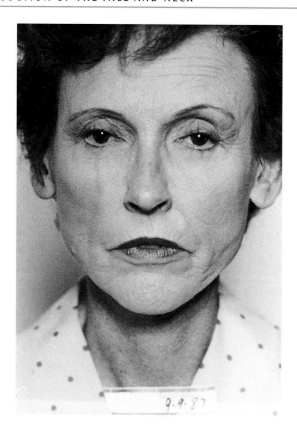
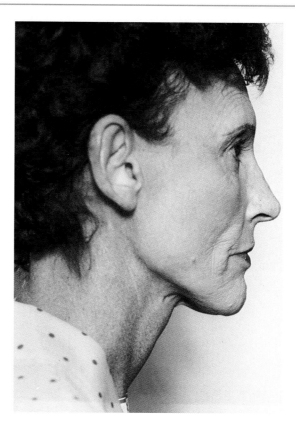

FIGURES 8-72 & 8-73   *Result of this combination at 1 year before an extensive skin care program.*

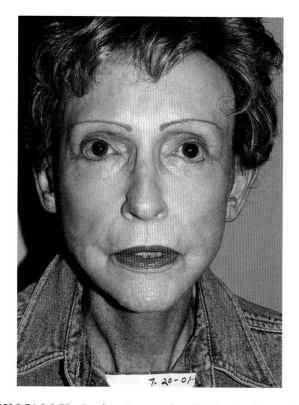
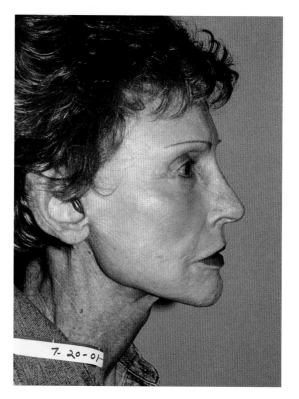

FIGURES 8-74 & 8-75   *Result at 15 years. The original perioral fat grafts were augmented at intervals. The lip correction is from 1986 grafts.*

FAT GRAFTING AS AN ADJUNCT TO FACIAL REJUVENATION

This woman had a multitude of problems, and many resulted from previous surgery. Malar implants have been placed, but positioned above the orbital rim (see Fig. 8-76). The residuals of Bell's palsy (see Fig. 8-77) further accentuated the asymmetry of her face. She had wide atrophic scars of a mid-face–lift with descent of her untouched neck and jowl (see Fig. 8-78), which were compounded by extremely poor skin quality. Beginning in 1991, this patient was placed on an intensive skin care program, and surgery was scheduled. The small malar implants were replaced with mid-cheek Terino malar shells, and the preauricular scars were revised (see Figs. 8-79 and 8-80), but only minimal tightening of the facial skin resulted. A complete repair was scheduled for the future. She chose instead to have fat grafting of the nasolabial fold, the commissure, and the upper and lower lip and requested a very full lip contour. The operative photograph shows the effect of multilevel fat grafting (see Fig. 8-81).

Four years after the surgery the lip enhancement shown in Figure 8-82 was acceptable to her surgeon but not to the patient! Figure 8-82 shows the effect of the fat grafting in the cheek and perioral deficits and equalization of the effect of her Bell's palsy. In addition, the quality of her skin was considerably improved. She has chosen to use skin-lightening formulas in addition to the standard procedures of fruit acid peels and topicals, and her face has changed from being corrugated and darkly pigmented to one more suitable to the blonde that she ultimately chose for her hair color. An additional fat graft was performed for a minor lip volume increase. Five years after this fat graft and 9 years after the original fat graft, an unrelated surgery was scheduled. She requested a further increase in lip volume, which resulted in the recontouring shown in Figures 8-83 and 8-84. This degree of lip enhancement is unusual, but it matched the photographs she presented at each of her consultations. Surprisingly, she asked for more fullness in certain areas of the lips, which was accomplished under local anesthesia (see Figs. 8-85 and 8-86).

This case illustrates the permanence of facial fat grafting in the lower part of the face, the nasolabial area, and the lip. Even though she has chosen a very large lip enhancement, her lips remain soft and pliable and pass the "kiss test" with flying colors.

CLINICAL PEARL

Lip Enhancement Is Not Rocket Science, but It Is a Minefield
If the patient has no vermilion to speak of, you're wasting your time using fat grafts. An alternative is a very firm insert, but such inserts will not be acceptable because they are visible and palpable and frequently extrude. "Lip roll" vermilion repositioning is the best choice.

All non-autologous grafts are temporary. Fat grafts, if properly performed, are permanent. Pre-tunneling withdrawal deposits and all the technical details that were worked out in the past are essential. One must also caution patients that the lips often shrink with age and a successful lip enhancement in 1986 will require a touchup fat graft in 2003.

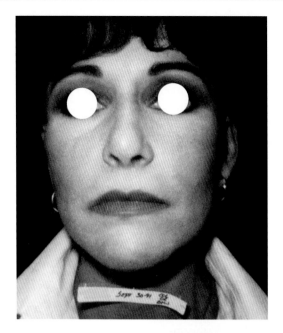
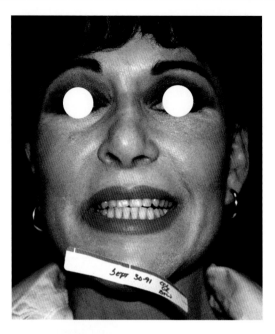
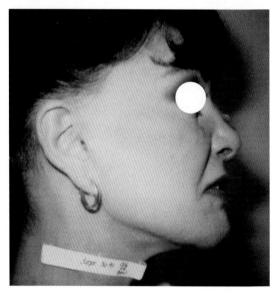

FIGURES 8-76 – 8-78 *Facial revision enhanced by strategic fat grafts, skin rejuvenation, and progressive volumetric lip enhancement in a brunette with oily skin and a thin lip phase after surgery and Bell's palsy. Correction included facial grafts, replacement of the malar implants, and scar revision.*

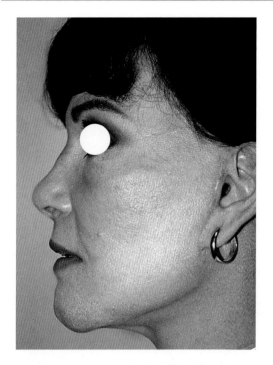 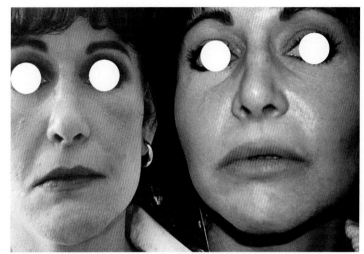

FIGURES 8-79 & 8-80   *Result of multilevel lip grafts.*

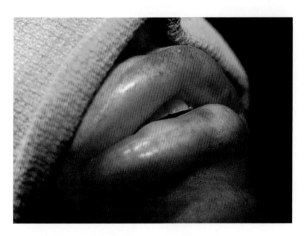

FIGURE 8-81   *When full lips are desired, overcorrection as shown has little risk of disappointing the patient.*

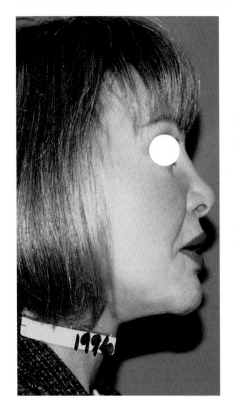
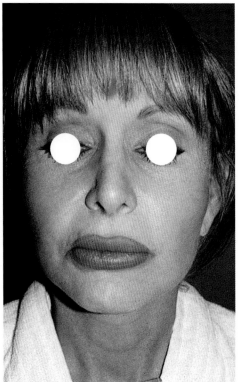
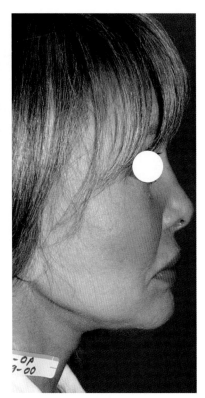

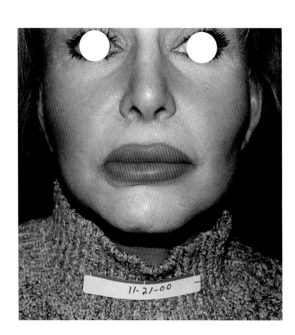
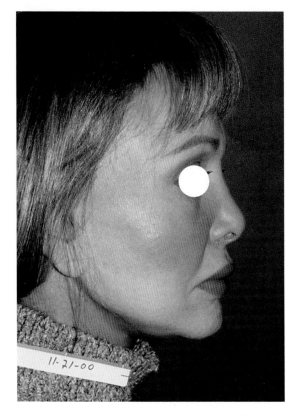

FIGURES 8-82 – 8-86 *Woman with smooth skin and a full lip phase. Revision of a mid-face–lift and a carefully discussed further lip enhancement with fat grafts achieved this strongly desired result.*

USEFUL CANNULAS IN FACIAL SCULPTURING

The tip design shown in Figure 8-87 is on 2-mm cannulas available with a Luer-Lock configuration or with attachments to fit into a syringe liposculpture device. At the top of the illustration is the "micro" removal cannula designed by Luiz Toledo. This small cannula can be used for removal as well as for very small regrafting techniques. The middle cannula facilitates harvesting of fat. The strips of fat that are suctioned are just wide enough to be placed in the prepared tunnels during fat grafting. The lower cannula, which is one of my designs, incorporates a dissection tip with a rough end to elevate depressions such as acne scars and an opening to serve as a delivery system. This variation of the "Toledo pickle fork" is useful for transnasal elevation of isolated depressions, which can be grafted immediately after soft tissue dissection. In general, however, it is preferable to perform a separate dissection with the Wilkinson rhytidissector (Byron Medical). The handle of this dissection device facilitates more precise maneuvering of the tip to create subdermal tunnels, release scars, and free the nasolabial fold and beyond.

NECK DEFORMITY FROM LIPOSUCTION

Aggressive liposuction can produce the neck deformity shown in Figure 8-88, even without curettage or cautery of the undersurface. Although liposuction alone may suffice in a younger individual with a fatty neck and minimal subplatysmal fat, in an older patient, such over-resection is a risk. Visible platysmal bands are complicated by contracture and scarring of the overlying skin. As has been often stated, "facial fat is a precious commodity," and the deformity would have been less obtrusive if a sufficient layer of subcutaneous fat been retained. The procedure of choice for these individuals would have been an open platysmal resection and re-anastomosis in the midline, followed by "en bloc" fat resection assisted by liposuction.

Correction in these individuals is extremely difficult, especially if some form of laser or cautery has been used and deep scar contracture has occurred. Fat regrafting, redraping of the skin, re-anastomosis of the platysma at the low division, and even dermal grafts may be required to restore an acceptable appearance to these individuals. To a self-proclaimed "liposuction specialist" who lacks surgical expertise and appreciation for the anatomy, contouring of all structures in the neck may seem unimportant, as well as beyond a person's capability, but they are important! Liposuction alone only addresses one part of the problem.

CLINICAL PEARL

Staying out of Trouble in the Face
"Facial fat is a precious commodity." Anyone who has worked with liposuction in conjunction with face-lift would certainly agree. Those of us who have seen overly resected patients such as those pictured in this chapter realize that to the surgeon, the liposuction may seem to have been performed well, but these resulting deformities were not from something as dangerous as laser treatment of the undersurface of the skin or sharp curettage, but from simple over-resection.

The marginal mandibular nerve crosses the mandible in a superficial position to innervate the lips, thus making it vulnerable to UAL. Dr. James Grotting (Birmingham) palpates the facial artery and marks it so that his UAL cannula, 1.5 to 2.0 mm, stays far away from this area.

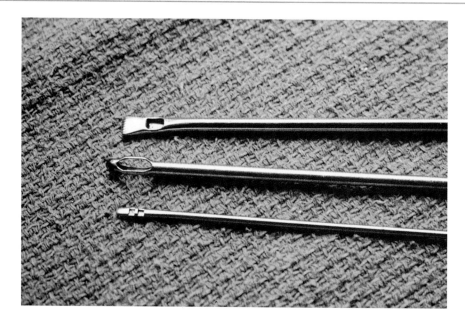

FIGURE 8-87 *Ultrafine cannulas for facial sculpture and fat grafting (see text).*

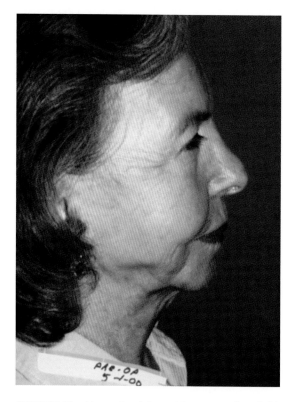

FIGURE 8-88 *Liposuction injury without correction of skin laxity, platysmal banding, or facial descent is more difficult to correct and requires longer recovery than a properly planned and executed primary procedure does.*

SCULPTURING THE ANTERIOR NECK

Before XU, patients such as the 40-year-old man in Figures 8-89 and 8-90 would have been rejected for neck contouring, but he has thicker and elastic skin. Accordingly, he was offered a procedure of direct plication of the divided and resected platysma with direct-vision en bloc fat removal plus liposuction along the jowl edge and above. Although recovery was prolonged, the results of this local approach were acceptable. In contrast to XUAL patients, whose recovery is very rapid, with skin shrinkage occurring in even less than ideal candidates, a 6-month photograph with the degree of contouring shown was considered unusual in 1989 (see Figs. 8-90 and 8-91).

Note in the lateral postoperative view (see Fig. 8-91) that jowl reduction has been accomplished by fat removal without excision of the Bichat pad. The frontal postoperative view (see Fig. 8-92) shows good resolution of the jowl fat, which was removed with liposuction as well as skin contracture. Liposuction in the cheek is performed from two entry points. The first is from within the nostril to initially reduce the nasolabial fold and then fan out with cross-suctioning in the upper part of the jowl. The second point is behind the ear with entry in a superficial plane. These liposuction areas then overlap with the neck elevation of soft tissues, which is accomplished through the small incision in the submental fold. Wide undermining in patients with good skin tone resulted in uniform skin contracture. There was no attempt to cauterize, scrape, or otherwise damage the dermal tissue to induce this degree of shrinkage.[2]

> **CLINICAL PEARL**
>
> Fat removal in face-lifting may vary significantly from person to person. It is certainly wise to avoid fat removal outside of prominent jowl pads. The "closed technique" of liposuction is recommended to initiate the procedure, even if one removes up to 25 cc. Subplatysmal fat should be removed during open exploration because of variable motor nerve positions. Open liposuction may be performed above the platysma for a "cleanup," or one may choose scissors excision while the platysma is stretched, according to the experience of the surgeon.

> **CLINICAL PEARL**
>
> Dr. Eugene Courtiss (Boston) reminded us in 1986 that liposuction is *not the answer for the majority of patients with fatty necks*. This is still true. One must plicate the platysma and redrape the skin. For all except younger patients with good skin retraction and a flat platysma, this advice is still relevant today. However, the addition of XUAL intraoperatively has broadened the patient base of those who benefit from a "tuck" without face-lift.

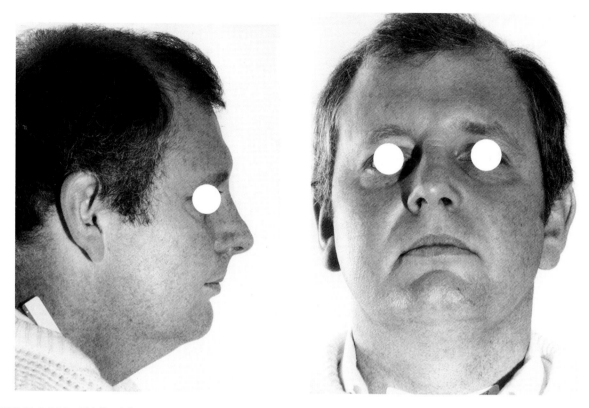

FIGURES 8-89 & 8-90   *This "jowly" man may obtain a satisfactory correction with a liposuction-assisted submental "tuck" because of natural unassisted skin draping and contraction.*

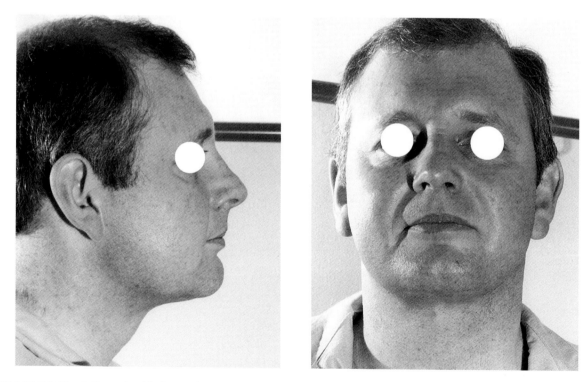

FIGURES 8-91 & 8-92   *At 5 months, this degree of edema was to be expected.*

ROLE OF LIPOSUCTION IN SECONDARY FACE-LIFTS

In 1993, this patient had a face-lift with upper blepharoplasty, a submental "tuck," and fat grafting in the nasolabial folds, commissures, and glabella. Her deep-set upper eyelids are natural, and she has never requested fatty augmentation to fill the upper eyelid.

Seven years later, she exhibits minimal descent of the skin but not the SMAS of the face, with reaccumulation of fat in the submental triangle and lower part of the neck (see Figs. 8-93 to 8-95). Surgery confirmed that the internal platysma repair was still taut, as was the mid-cheek SMAS lift. Her primary concern was skin stretching on the lower part of the face. External ultrasound was used before a surgical retightening procedure that included spot liposuction of jowl fat from an anterior and posterior approach. Note that her hairline is in good position above the ear and the incision is inside the tragus.*

One year after this procedure, she requested adjustment of a small amount of laxity in the upper jowl line and a new fatty accumulation above the clavicle, perhaps influenced by the old thyroidectomy scar (see Figs. 8-96 and 8-97). Approaching this problem is relatively uncomplicated. External ultrasound and local anesthesia were used; the cheek and neck were infiltrated with local anesthetic, and shrinkage of the skin and new fatty tissue and further contouring of the jowl area will result.

CLINICAL PEARL

Advances in plastic surgery anesthesia have vastly enhanced what we can achieve in surgery and have improved operative time and facilitated more rapid recovery.

---

*Use of an advancement suture of the skin to the base of the tragus in front of the ear creates the natural shadow shown in the photographs.

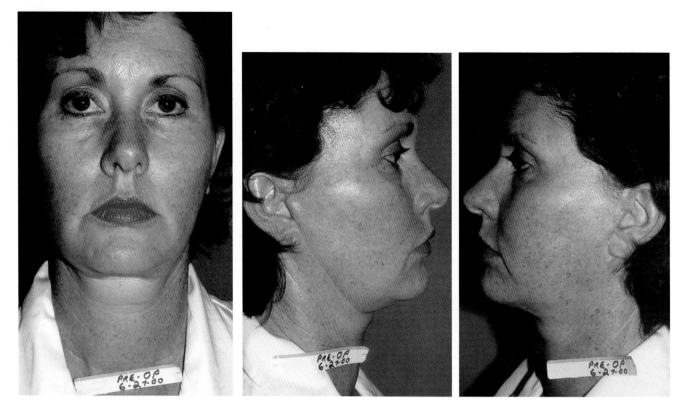

FIGURES 8-93 – 8-95   *Minor adjustment in secondary surgery facilitated by ultrasound treatment. After complete SMAS and platysmal repair, this common problem was confined to the relaxing facial skin, plus a new fat deposit in the sternal notch.*

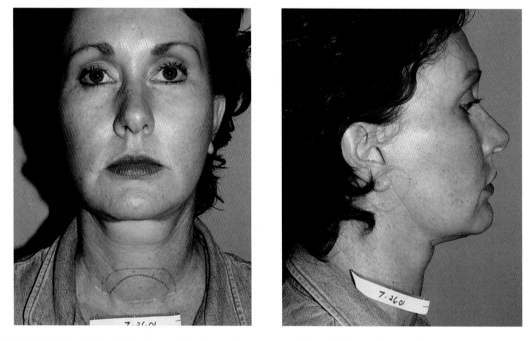

FIGURES 8-96 & 8-97   *Minor "skin tucks" and XU of the face and upper part of the neck plus aspiration of the sternal fat restored the lost contour.*

Case in Point—When a Lesser Procedure Is Preferred

Analysis of the preoperative photographs in Figures 8-98 to 8-100 would call for a recommendation of a face-lift, submental "tuck" repair, fat grafting, and some form of skin rejuvenation surgery. After discussion, this patient declined the major procedures and agreed to proceed with lesser repairs, with the possibility of future surgery for the interior of the cheek and face. With the advent of XUAL, fat grafting in the perioral area and internal repair in the neck were selected, and the patient agreed to a vigorous postsurgical skin care program primarily involving a home care regimen.

Conceding that we had little expectation that the excess skin in the neck would conform to the newly repaired platysma and that the fat grafting with XU would reduce the nasolabial fold only a minor degree without internal facial repair, it was a pleasant surprise to watch and document the continuing improvement in this patient's facial contours.

Contracture of the cheeks and dissolution of the jowls were apparent within 3 weeks of surgery. At 8 weeks, her frontal appearance had improved greatly (see Fig. 8-101), and there was continuing contracture of the neck skin that

had not been apparent 30 days before (see Figs. 8-102 to 8-104). The improvement in skin quality and appearance is also apparent.

CLINICAL PEARL
The elastic ability of the skin to contract is the "rate-limiting" factor in many plastic surgery operations. Even with skin excision procedures, surgery won't restore skin quality or tone.

Contracture of the skin after the initial series of XU applications seems to be an ongoing process. Although the changes are subtle, there is definitely an improvement in the appearance of her face and neck in photographs taken 4 months after the procedures (see Figs. 8-105 to 8-107).

This patient illustrates the wisdom of agreeing to perform lesser procedures in patients who for financial or time constraints cannot comply with the recommendations for full facial repair. Although the aging process appears to be reversed, eventually the mid-facial deep tissue descent will convince this category of patient to proceed with a mid-face or full-face repair.

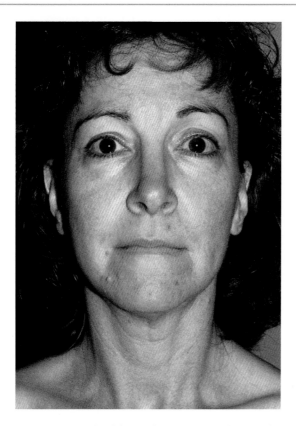
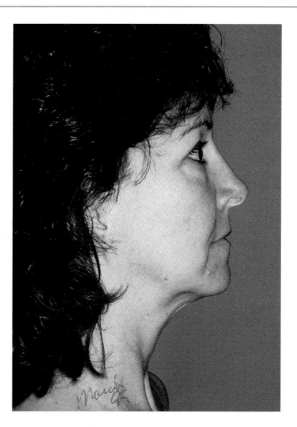

FIGURES 8-98 & 8-99 *Maintaining patient loyalty. Despite extensive counseling, certain patients will choose a less reliable course and ignore recommendations—in this case, choosing a "tuck" without a complete face-lift.*

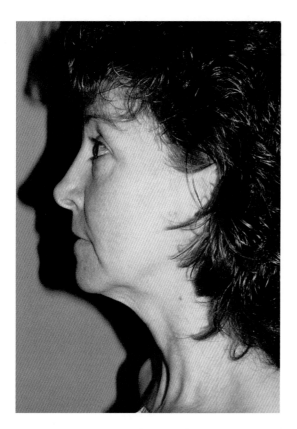
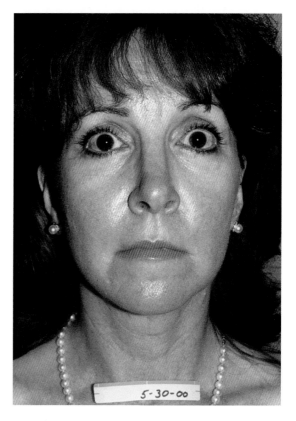

FIGURES 8-100 & 8-101 *As expected, lax skin folds conceal the taut internal anterior platysma repair. A course of monthly XU treatments was proposed and accepted.*

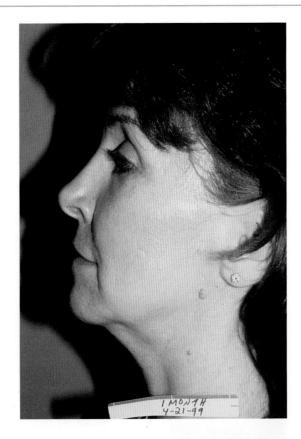
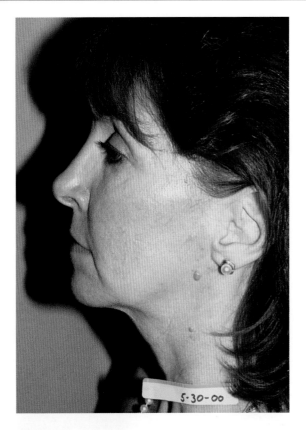
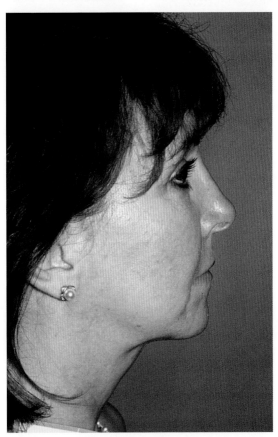

FIGURES 8-102 – 8-104   *Progressive skin contouring from the application of XU.*

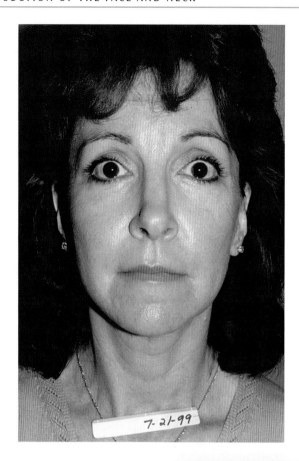
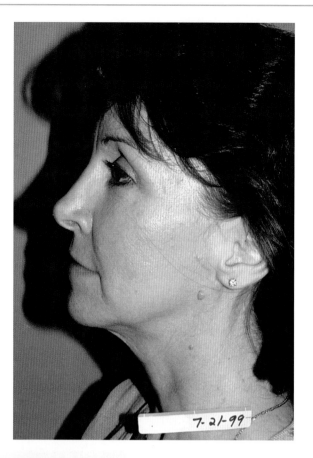
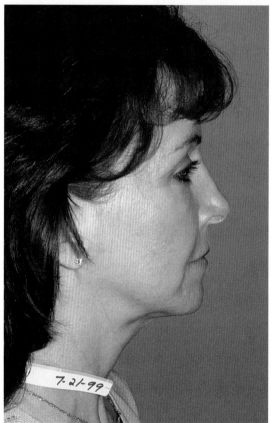

FIGURES 8-105 – 8-107 *Acceptable regression after 4 months of XU treatment.*

Case in Point—"Facial Fat Is a Precious Commodity"

Over-resection of facial fat as illustrated in Figure 8-108 is almost impossible to correct. The use of dermis fat grafts as well as multilevel free fat grafting is helpful. In patients with damage to the overlying dermis from ill-advised cautery or laser application, scarring and contracture of the neck skin will prevent expansion to a more natural appearance.

Lesser degrees of over-resection lead to the "Dick Tracy" appearance in which a prominent laryngeal cartilage is revealed and is unsightly. Direct excision of the superior laryngeal cartilage is an acceptable aesthetic procedure and is particularly useful in transsexuals who wish to lose the prominent cartilage that indicates masculinity.

Case in Point—SAL versus XUAL in Facial Rejuvenation

Small cannulas have traditionally been the choice for reduction of nasolabial folds, jowl pads, and mandibular fat deposits during facial rejuvenation. The patient shown in Figures 8-109 and 8-110 underwent liposuction with a mid-face–lift in 1995, which produced acceptable correction. Anterior and posterior repositioning of the platysma gave a clean jaw line. After 6 years, however,

there were signs of continued aging (see Figs. 8-111 to 8-113), with stretch of the skin but maintenance of the jaw line repair. The fat grafting used for lip enhancement, the blepharoplasty, and the skin care program had been helpful. The counseling session discussed additional fat grafting, a "skin tuck," and the use of XU for shaping of the face. The procedure was performed with ketamine-diazepam (Valium) intravenous sedation and "super wet" local anesthesia. Much more rapid recovery was reported than occurred in 1995.

Secondary fat grafting was applied to the nasolabial area, the subcommissure, and at her request, the upper and lower lip for further enhancement. In addition, she began the vitamin C SkinCeuticals skin rejuvenation program with microabrasion. The resulting improvement in skin quality complements the improvement in facial contour (see Figs. 8-114 to 8-116).

It is not unusual for patients who have enjoyed lip enhancement to request additional enhancement after a period of years, and it is also common for individuals in high-stress environments to show continuation of perioral atrophy. This patient illustrates the permanence of submental repair, the impermanence of perioral rejuvenation with fat grafting because of natural aging factors, and the soft natural result of lip fat grafting. An additional benefit is resolution of the jowl fat and further tightening of the lower cheek laxity in the postoperative period.

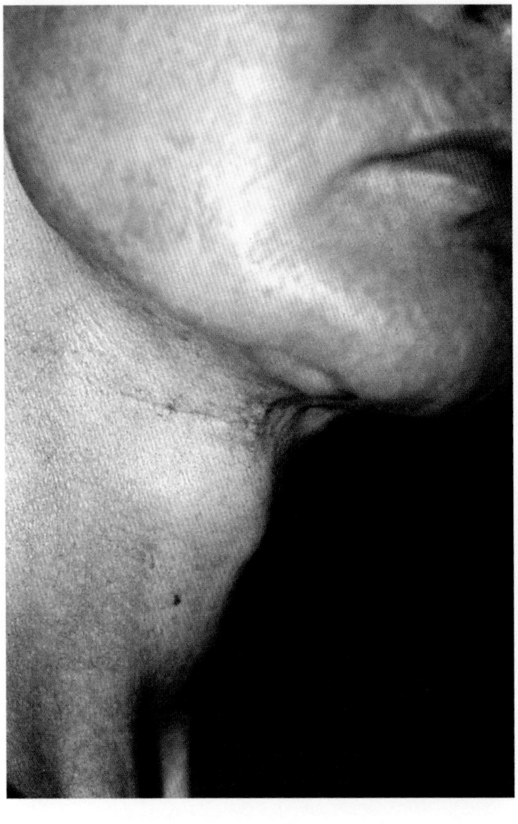

FIGURE 8-108 *Over-resection of facial fat is almost impossible to correct, as shown in this figure.*

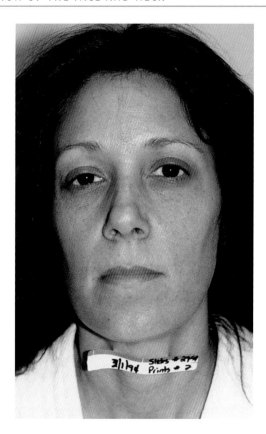
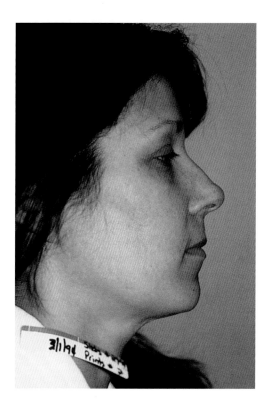

FIGURES 8-109 & 8-110 *Facial enhancement with ultrasound and fat graft assistance. The patient is depicted before a submental tuck in 1994 and lip grafts.*

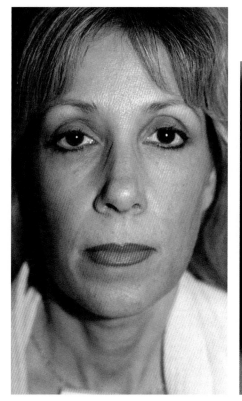
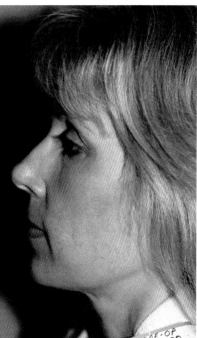
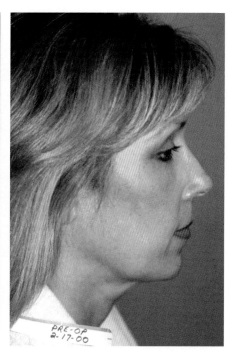

FIGURES 8-111 – 8-113 *Correction planned at 6 years includes ultrasound, mid-face–lift, an aggressive skin care program, and planned secondary lip fat grafting.*

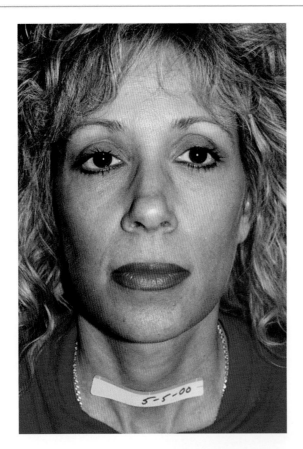
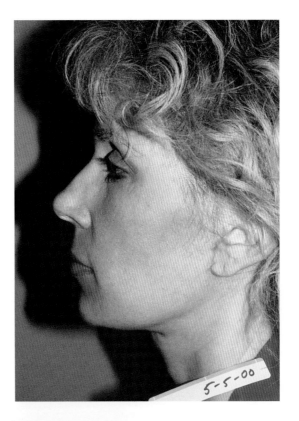
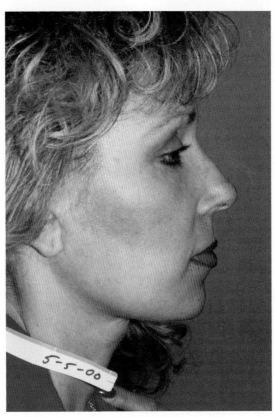

FIGURES 8-114 – 8-116 *All the elements of facial rejuvenation (surgical, topical, fat grafting, ultrasound) give this soft, natural, "not operated on" restoration.*

Case in Point—Submental "Tuck" with XU and Blepharoplasty as an Alternative to Face-Lifting, Improvement by Postoperative Steroid Injections

This patient was preparing for a complex breast reconstruction to repair deformities after failed breast reconstruction elsewhere and had asked whether facial rejuvenation could be accomplished with quick recovery. Although the best advice would include a face-lift, we agreed that liposuction, platysmal repair, blepharoplasty, and fat grafting in the perioral and nasolabial areas with XU for cheek shrinkage would be an acceptable alternative to correct the facial aging changes shown in Figures 8-117 to 8-119.

Before using XU, we would not expect contracture of facial skin in a patient of this age, and indeed, contracture was delayed by postoperative hemorrhage, which left the residual deformities shown in Figures 8-120 to 8-122. These thickened spots were corrected by a series of steroid injections (see Figs. 8-123 to 8-125). A final injection after these photographs eliminated the last traces of tissue edema.

Without XU for shaping of the jowl fat, slimming of the cheek, and retraction of the nasolabial folds, the results of the lesser procedures would have been unacceptable. Reduction of cheek fat by ultrasound, as well as contracture of the neck skin after surgical removal of fat and platysmal repair, makes this choice a consideration in individuals who prefer to delay face-lifting until the future.

References

1. Millard R: *Plastic and Reconstructive Surgery*, 1992;89:356-365.
2. Wilkinson TS: *Practical Procedures in Aesthetic Plastic Surgery*. New York, Springer-Verlag, 1994.

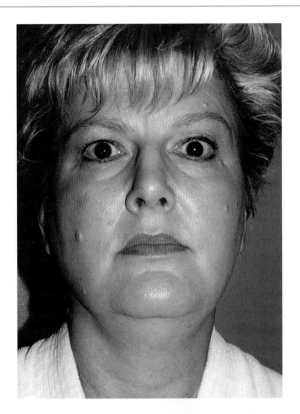
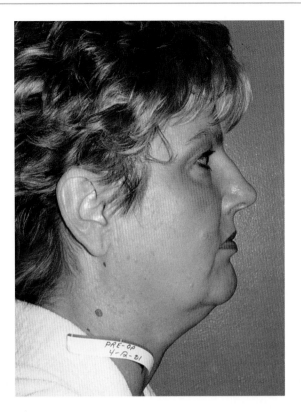
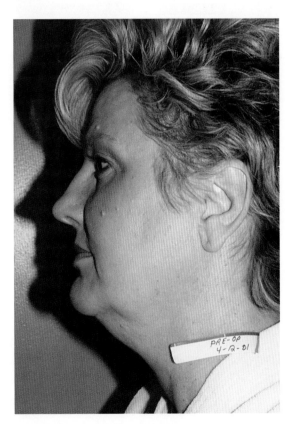

FIGURES 8-117 – 8-119   *As is often the case, a patient facing major body reconstruction will request "a little help" facially, but only agree to procedures associated with quick recovery. In this case, blepharoplasty and a submental "tuck" were chosen.*

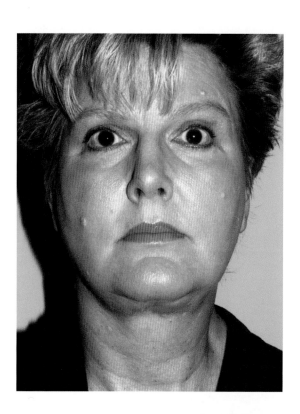

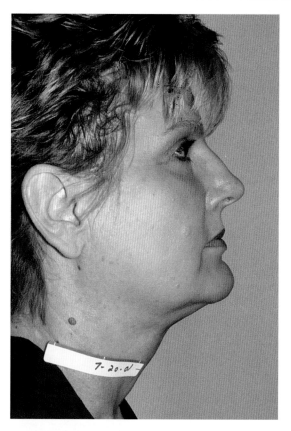

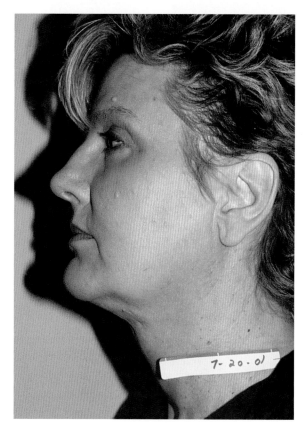

FIGURES 8-120 – 8-122   *Despite the use of ultrasound in surgery and complete cleansing of submental fat, irregularities remain.*

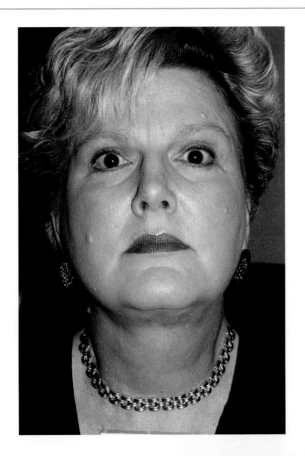

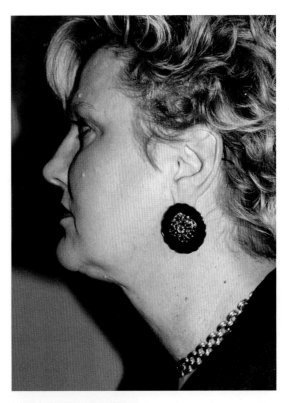

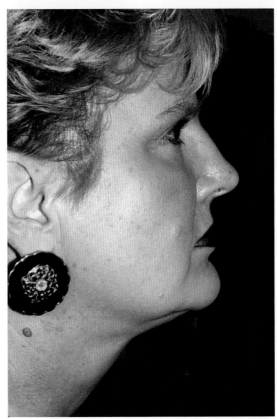

FIGURES 8-123 – 8-125   *Slow but progressive remodeling by XU treatment, augmented by steroid/lidocaine injections in specific areas.*

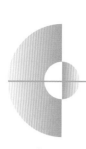

CHAPTER NINE

Fat Replacement

With the advent of liposuction came renewed interest in using fat as an autograft. Based on the French challenge, several American surgeons and I first evaluated and successfully performed fat grafting in 1984. Following the pressure injection technique of Dr. Fournier and others in 1982, fat grafting was so unsuccessful that it was almost abandoned. With the use of pre-tunneling and concentration techniques, surgical expertise in preparing areas for living grafts soon resulted in uniform success with a 70% to 80% rate of retention. Unfortunately, overcorrection is a greater problem for repair than undercorrection today.

Dr. Richard Ellenbogen (plastic surgeon, Los Angeles) began his trials of fat grafting in 1982. Articles describing his success and the necessity for technical maneuvers were rejected by our major journals. Ellenbogen initially used an insulin soak to increase fat survival. In retrospect, his 1987 experiences were important in that his meticulous technique allowed other surgeons to replicate his success, although the need to add insulin has been abandoned.

Materials used for augmentation in the nasolabial folds or lips included fascia, superficial musculoaponeurotic system (SMAS), dermis, and dermis-fat, but each had significant problems of thickness and palpability. Patients complained of feeling "a roll" beneath the surface. A few early reports in the plastic surgery literature showed that over 50% of transplanted fat remained stable. Dr. Yves-Gerard Illouz presented a patient whose post-liposuction "dent" was treated by fat grafting in 1984. Other surgeons quickly embraced the technique, but independently discovered that adipose cells are extremely fragile and must be placed in a prepared bed without tension or trauma.

Early clinical reports from South America from such respected authors as Chajchir, Zalas, and Loeb were often ignored, as were my publications in the North American literature. Dr. Paulo Matsudo (São Paulo)

noted variability in the absorption rate in 1988, but advocated fat grafting as the best choice for materials. Greater degrees of concentration, undermining, and multilevel placement of carefully harvested fat grafts have improved this soft tissue rejuvenation procedure. Matsudo's conclusions, however, are still appropriate; the most important advantage is that the procedure can be repeated with no artificial materials and the cost factor and surgical maneuvers are "very reasonable."

Syringe liposculpture was adopted because of the difficulty of filtering and obtaining fat for regrafting. I published articles evaluating a variety of fat traps, each of which was cumbersome, resulted in "suction trauma," and led to less than satisfactory harvesting. Many surgeons then expanded the use of syringe liposuction beyond the simple harvesting of fat to include precise facial sculpturing in the submental area and the nasolabial fold. By 1988, the liposuction machine was often abandoned in favor of body contouring with only the syringe technique! Incorporating the correction of superficial irregularities, or depressions and liposuction "dents," allowed surgeons to simultaneously remove fat and regraft in a single maneuver, thereby facilitating corrective procedures and reducing trauma to the cells to be transplanted.

Patients who complain that their faces look young but their hands look old should be offered a combination of three techniques. Miniature vein strippers can be made from small paper clips and the veins stripped through tiny incisions and direct threading. Lipografts placed into subcutaneous tissue are easily pressed into position and protected so that they will not be completely resorbed. It is important that manual labor be avoided for 3 weeks. Light chemical peels are usually applied from the fingers to the elbow. A subsequent skin care program involving various "fruit acid" peels, vitamin C products (SkinCeuticals), and tretinoin (Retin-A) complete the rejuvenation.

"Although we have long been envisioning the face in two dimensions, with the treatment of choice being to pull the skin out and essentially tightening the canvas of the tent, that perspective is changing. We now know that for more attractive results we need to pop things in by adding fat grafts."[1] Drs. Harold Clavin and Mark Burman (plastic surgeons, Santa Monica) have used fat grafting to recapture a youthful look for years. They state that "any doctor who concentrates on the procedure will rave about the results. Those who don't rave about it just don't know how to use it."[1]

Surprisingly, surgeons still tell patients that fat grafting "does not last." Today, many results are achieved in a single procedure, such as grafting for an atrophic lip. Patients certainly should be advised that grafts are permanent. Second or third procedures may be required, especially for those desiring larger lip enhancement or enhancement of atrophic areas in the face. Patients must be advised that facial fat atrophy is a natural and ongoing process and that subsequent touchup is therefore necessary.

HOW I DO IT—Fat Grafting—Richard Ellenbogen, M.D. (Plastic Surgeon, Los Angeles)

Since I introduced the first paper in the modern plastic surgical literature on fat grafting in 1982, my techniques and philosophy have changed drastically. I now believe that fat placed into the face will persist in various percentages in certain areas. Specifically, a high percentage of the fat placed at the cheekbones and zygomatic areas will persist. A lesser percentage will persist in the cheek area. Still less will persist in the nasolabial and chin area, and barely 10% of the fat will persist in the lips. However, the fat placed in the lips of some patients has remained photographically visible after only one procedure for many years afterward. The missing link with making 100% of the fat last is still missing. At this stage in my career, I use Coleman's instruments made by Byron, but I believe that the Lambros instruments made by Gram's Medical are equally as good. I do not inject the fat with needles.

Principles that I maintain are as follows:

1. Fat must be placed in toothpick-like strands to maximize persistence.
2. A minimal amount of adrenaline in the donor or recipient area increases "take."
3. Fat from the abdomen, inner aspect of the thigh, and upper part of the arm is identical as far as feel and lasting ability are concerned.
4. Refrigerated fat might as well be thrown out.
5. All areas of the face can be filled from the oral commissures without a visible incision.
6. I do not put fat in the forehead because even when the forehead receives botulinum (Botox) injections, the fat becomes lumpy and descends to the lower portion.
7. No more than 1 cc of fat can be placed under the eyelids, and it must be under the orbicularis muscle and done with great care. One hundred percent of fat in this position is retained. If not done properly, it becomes lumpy and cannot be corrected.
8. Faces age by two processes: sagging and deflation (loss of fat). For years, many of our procedures to correct sagging have yielded incomplete or unnatural results because the bulk lost in aging has not been replaced (see Fig. 9-1). Even in young women undergoing face-lifts, I use fat in the cheekbones, cheeks, lips, nasolabial folds, chin, and any other area that I feel demonstrates early fat loss (see Figs. 9-2 and 9-3).
9. Fat can be used for two purposes: to make something that never was (cheekbones, puffy lips, filled-out cheeks) or to replace fat that has been lost (atrophy of the labiomandibular region, nasolabial folds, etc.).

CLINICAL PEARL
There seems to be no difference in permanence of survivability with grafting of fat from any specific donor site. In 1990, the greatest experience with fat grafting was in individuals with facial atrophy, or Romberg's disease. Although it was interesting material to discuss preferences on a panel discussion, knee fat was no more or less effective than fat from any other donor site. Fat taken from the eyelid area does have a lower metabolic rate and can easily be used for bulk reinforcement, especially in deep facial creases. A multilevel technique of fat grafting is effective there as well.

Autologous Fat Reconstruction as an Office Procedure—Adrien Aiache, M.D. (Plastic Surgeon, Santa Monica)

Based on more than 2000 cases, Dr. Adrien Aiache has demonstrated how a simple technique can be useful as opposed to other products and surgeries that give only temporary improvement. Areas that can be improved include the frown lines, nasolabial folds, marionette lines, upper and lower lip lines, malar underdevelopment, postoperative fat defects, and the unsightly small depressions resulting from either surgical incisions or removal of deep lesions.

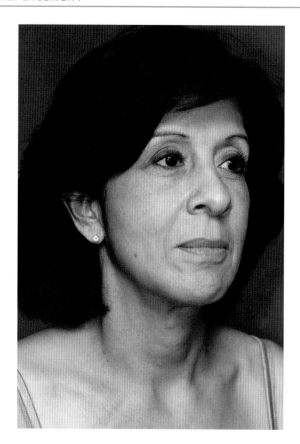
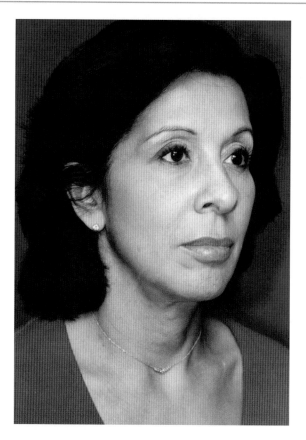
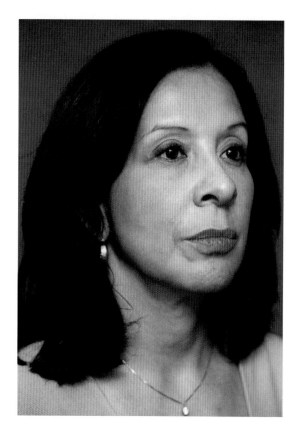

FIGURES 9-1 – 9-3   *Strategic fat grafting by Dr. Ellenbogen connected preoperative shadows. The connection is shown at 9 and 18 months after grafting of the chin, commissure, and nasolabial areas.*

CLINICAL PEARL

When presented with depressions in the skin after liposuction of any area, the usual method of correction is to liposuction the margins of the depression and fill the depression with autologous fat. It would be simpler, when using the wet technique, to apply ultrasound or a massager around the depression for 5 minutes and then liposhift the fat into the depression. The fat can also be loosened by breaking up the fat attachments with a cannula (without suction). Liposhifting consists of moving the loosened fat around the depression into the depressed area.[2] It is done by rolling a rod (old 8- to 10-mm straight liposuction cannula) firmly inward toward the depression from all angles.

Technique

The patient is supine with the head slightly raised. The material consists of a 10-cc syringe, a 22-gauge needle, a 14-gauge needle, and a 12-inch, 25-gauge needle. Local anesthesia is provided by 0.5% lidocaine (Xylocaine) with epinephrine 1:200,000.

Approximately 10 cc of the anesthesia fluid is drawn through the bottle cork into the syringe with a 22-gauge needle. The syringe is then connected to a 12-inch, 25-gauge needle. The anesthesia fluid is injected intraorally in the area of the infraorbital nerve and the mental nerve bilaterally.

If lip fat grafting is to be added to the procedure, the local anesthesia is then infiltrated along the upper and lower mucocutaneous junction of the lip and the vermilion border. The same syringe is filled with an additional 10 cc of anesthesia. Local infiltration of the iliac crest area or the inner part of the thigh is performed with the 25-gauge needle, and a wide area is infiltrated for fat extirpation. About three to four injections of the needle are made for this purpose. The 10-cc syringe is then connected to a 14-gauge needle, which is introduced into the same zone that has been anesthetized. The barrel of the syringe is pulled and kept open with the needle cap. Multiple back-and-forth motions are made in the donor zone to gradually retrieve fat mixed with blood. The syringe is set in an erect position or placed in a centrifuge. If centrifuging is performed, the syringe is obturated with a 22-gauge needle covered with its cap so that centrifugation will allow the blood to go down to the bottom of the syringe while the fat stays above. The blood is ejected, and pure fat is used for injection. The syringe is again capped with the same 14-gauge needle and the autologous fat injected.

If the nasolabial lines are to be corrected, the needle is introduced through the inner commissure of the lip, and approximately 8 to 10 tunnels are created with the 14-gauge needle subcutaneously under the nasolabial line, which has been marked with ink for proper identification. In some instances, fat is injected perpendicularly across this line, or sometimes fat is introduced by longitudinal parallel injections to add more material. The same technique is used for marionette lines, the upper and lower lip, and frown lines; however, the fat is injected along the line and not across it. About 1 to 2 cc of fat is injected into the nasolabial lines, 0.5 cc of fat along the frown lines, and 1 to 2 cc along the lip vermilion/skin junction line, as well as about 1 cc along the marionette lines themselves.

CLINICAL PEARL

To Centrifuge or Not to Centrifuge?
To some surgeons, preparing fat for regrafting is complex. Aspirated fat is washed first with lactated Ringer's solution, passed from one syringe to another, and then centrifuged at 1500 rpm for 1 minute. For others, simply placing the aspirated fat on a Telfa nonsticking absorbent pad is sufficient preparation. A minor degree of overcorrection is advocated by these physicians in comparison to those who use the centrifuge, but the end results are the same.

This process takes about 30 minutes and is performed as an office outpatient procedure without any premedication. Occasionally, the patient is allowed to take a tranquilizer, or with more squeamish patients, increments of midazolam (Versed) are injected intravenously as premedication. In short, this procedure has been found to

CLINICAL PEARL

Injectables
In the review article referenced earlier, discussion included platelet-rich plasma for "growth factors." Claims for growth factor enhancement of other injectables and tissue glues have no solid evidence that they are clinically effective.[1]

Dr. James Romano (San Francisco) states that certain patients, about 20% to 30% of his patient population, will not show improvement with fat grafts.[1] He abandoned further fat grafting, but this has not been the experience of others. Patient care factors as well as general health and other unknowns vary the result. Patients must not touch the grafted area! Secondary fat grafting, in my experience, is successful in the few patients who have had little improvement with an initial fat graft. As always, there are many technical factors that are either under the control of the surgeon or patient or are unknown at the present time. Each of the physicians who stated their experiences for *Plastic Surgery Products in 2001* agreed that fat grafting is "an artistic procedure" and is continuing to evolve. This view must be tempered by the experience of others who see patients with fat grafts from 1984 that still retain their shape, form, and restoration.

be extremely useful and has been performed by me for about 15 years without any serious problems. It is recommended as a superior technique for soft tissue augmentation as opposed to any other soft tissue injectable material on the market. In addition, it can be inexpensive because of all the characteristics mentioned here.

Filling Body "Divots and Depressions"

For deeper truncal anterior depressions, 50 to 60 cc of fat is placed in individual tunnels during withdrawal of the cannulas (see Fig. 9-4). The subcutaneous tissue is infiltrated, as well as the underlying gluteus musculature. There is some reason to believe that the fat survives to a greater degree in muscular tunnels than in subcutaneous ones. The end result is a contour that is acceptable with either technique, but better with multilevel grafting.

Autologous Fat Grafting in the Buttocks

Fat grafting of buttock dimples and mid-buttock depressions such as those illustrated should be a standard part of rehabilitation of body deformities with liposuction. Based on the Brazilian experience in 1984, undermining of the depressions and multilevel over-correction by fat grafting have been successful since that time. These patients were evaluated 16 years after fat grafting and showed only minimal regression. The natural tendency of certain women is atrophy in the mid-buttock area. The fat grafts are intact and seem to be a permanent addition, but added grafts may be suggested over the years since the original grafting.

This patient was part of the group treated by external ultrasound only (XU). One of the objectives was to prove the theory that many of the fat cells easily extracted after XU were living cells that could be successfully regrafted. External ultrasound-assisted liposuction (XUAL) was used in the high hip rolls, the lower part of the buttock, and the banana roll area, and XU was used in the transition areas (see Figs. 9-5 and 9-6). Each individual depression marked with X's was pre-tunneled, and fat was placed both superficially and deeply as in the larger depression areas laterally. Two months postoperatively (see Figs. 9-7 and 9-8), the persistence of edema in the left and right banana fold areas will be addressed by infiltration, external ultrasound, and extraction of a small amount of fat with a small cannula. Regression in

the hip fold area and upper part of the back is complete. The regression in the upper back rolls was especially gratifying. This area was treated by ultrasound alone (areas marked in Fig. 9-5 by vertical lines).

For smaller buttock dimples, it is advisable to concentrate the fat either with a centrifuge or with the "Telfa pad drainage" technique and to inject these areas directly through the skin after undermining the area with the tip of a $1\frac{1}{2}$-inch, 16-gauge disposable needle attached to the injection gun. This direct freeing of attachments allows for overcorrection in the fat graft directly beneath the dermis. Additional fat is deposited in the deeper soft tissues, as well as the muscles directly beneath these areas, to produce an overcorrection of at least 30%. For the wider areas, fat that is extracted with syringe liposculpture is regrafted without removing the fat from the syringe. Because there is overcorrection in multiple layers and the area to be filled is a wide zone such as in this patient, it is not necessary to concentrate the fat. All the fat removed from this patient was regrafted. Results that we observed in patients such as this (see Figs. 9-9 to 9-12) at 3 and 4 months are the same results that are seen in this group at 4 and 5 years.

Case in point

In 1984, reports from Brazilian colleagues prompted many American surgeons to explore fat regrafting for the common buttock depressions, as in the patient in Figure 9-13 from another state. During the course of liposuction with "wet solution," a direct approach was made to each of the depressions with a Toledo "pickle fork" elevator. Concentrated fat was immediately transferred from the collection trap to these areas, with most placed in the subcutaneous area. Subsequent photographs show good resolution of the contour and retraction of the junction of the hip and buttock (see Fig. 9-14). This result was considered remarkably good

---

CLINICAL PEARL

In the August 1987 issue of *Technical Forum* I expressed disappointment with the longevity of Zyderm and Zyplast. Patients saw the glossy magazine ads and were infuriated when the results did not measure up and, worse, disappeared rapidly. Our original success with fat grafting in the buttock area in 1984 was soon followed by the pre-tunneling and withdrawal technique of fat grafting in the nasolabial areas. The early work of Dr. Adrien Aiache (Beverly Hills), Dr. Luiz Toledo (São Paulo), the Los Angeles surgeons, and others soon became accepted, with good results in each case. Concomitant liposuction of the nasolabial folds was a good suggestion and is now often used together with lipografts and soft tissue elevation in the nasolabial fold.

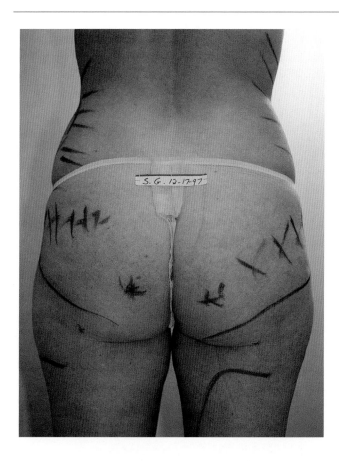

FIGURE 9-4 *Regrafting liposuctioned fat adds another positive element to body sculpture. Irregular defects, deep dimples, and XUAL zones are marked at the first interview and presurgically.*

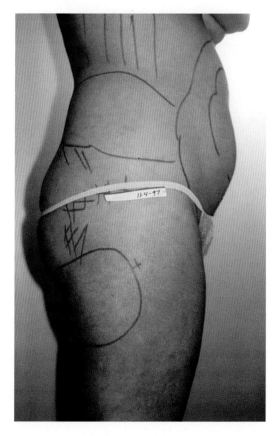

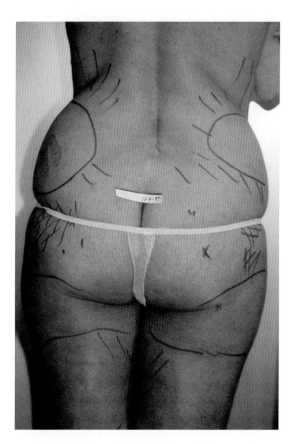

FIGURES 9-5 and 9-6 *In this patient, "high hip rolls" will be liposuctioned (XUAL) and not treated with ultrasound alone, as in Figure 9-4.*

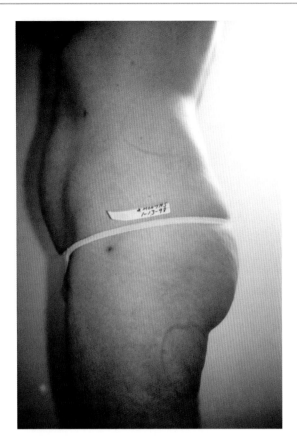
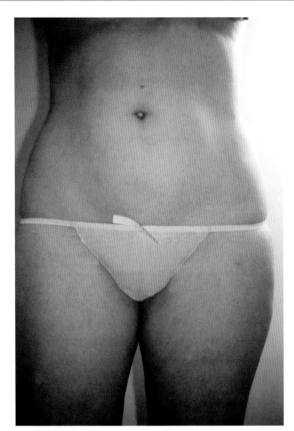

FIGURES 9-7 & 9-8   *At 2 months, contouring is almost complete.*

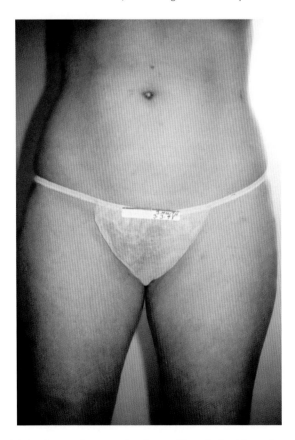
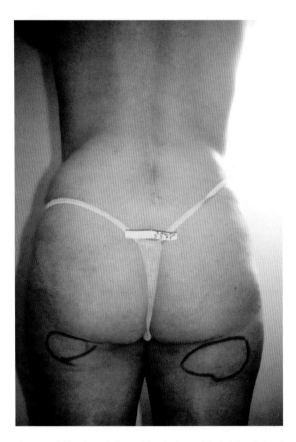

FIGURES 9-9 — 9-14   *Three months after grafting, the level buttock contours have stabilized, and the residual edema (circles) is minimal.*

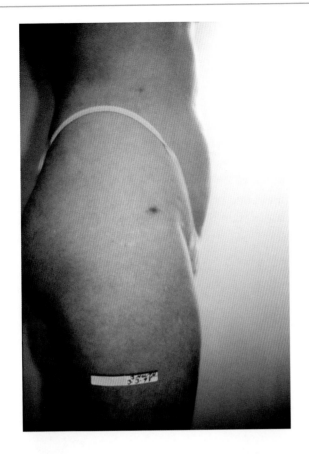
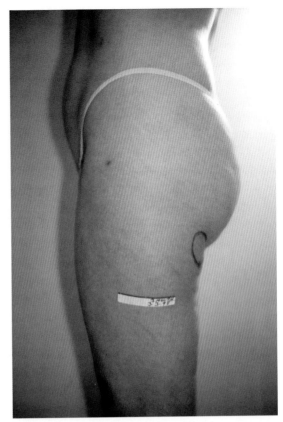
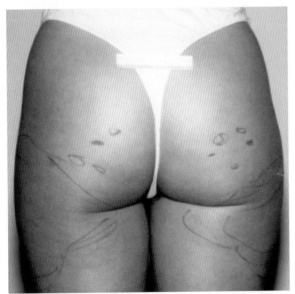
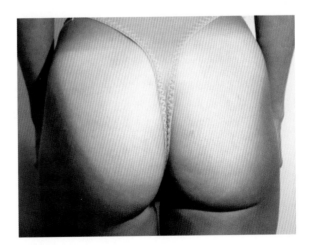

FIGURES 9-9 – 9-14   *Continued*

in 1984. The postoperative photograph is at 9 years. At that point, "super wet" infusions, ketamine-diazepam (Valium) dissociative anesthesia, and the syringe technique had supplanted the original procedures with more predictable results.

Case in point

Standard marking for liposuction consists of placing X's in areas to be grafted with fat in a multilayered technique (see Figs. 9-15 to 9-18). The striped lines indicated that XU will be used beyond the suction areas. Seven days after XUAL and liposuction with regrafting, differences from standard suction-assisted lipectomy (SAL) are apparent (see Figs. 9-19 to 9-22). Only the right outer hip area was not treated with XUAL. More bruising is evident in the SAL-treated right hip, as well as "run down" into the inner part of the thigh, which was liposuctioned as well. At 3 months, the green outline shows continued tissue edema in the right hip and, to a lesser degree, in the left (see Figs. 9-23 to 9-26). The inner thigh areas have already conformed and the fat grafting has stabilized. There is still a small amount of swelling on the inner aspect of the thighs and the mid-abdomen, a common occurrence even after meticulous liposuction. The interesting point is the retention of edema in the SAL-treated right hip. The patient reported that this area was still tender, in marked contrast to XUAL-treated areas.

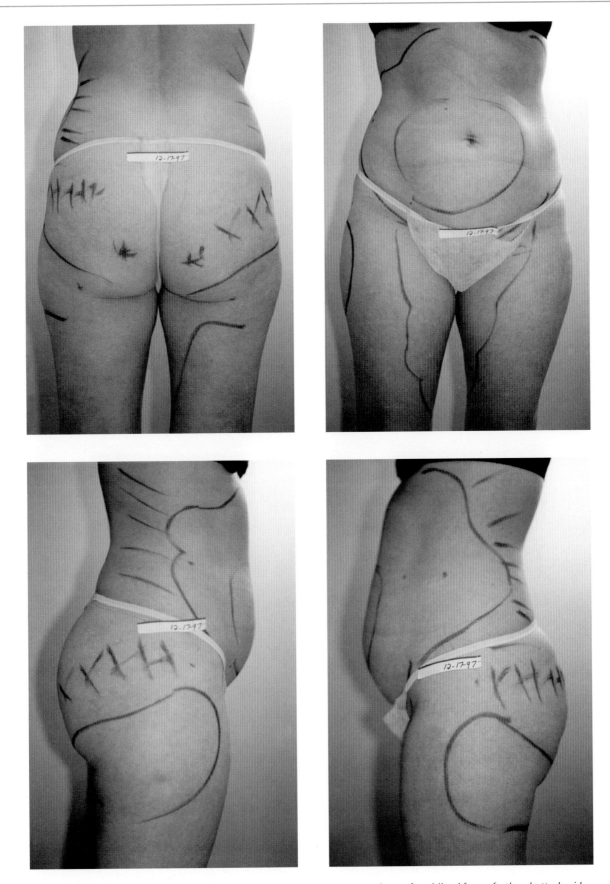

FIGURES 9-15 – 9-18 *Deeper sacral dimples at the pressure points require a greater volume of multilevel fat grafts than buttock-wide depressions and are thus designated in preoperative markings.*

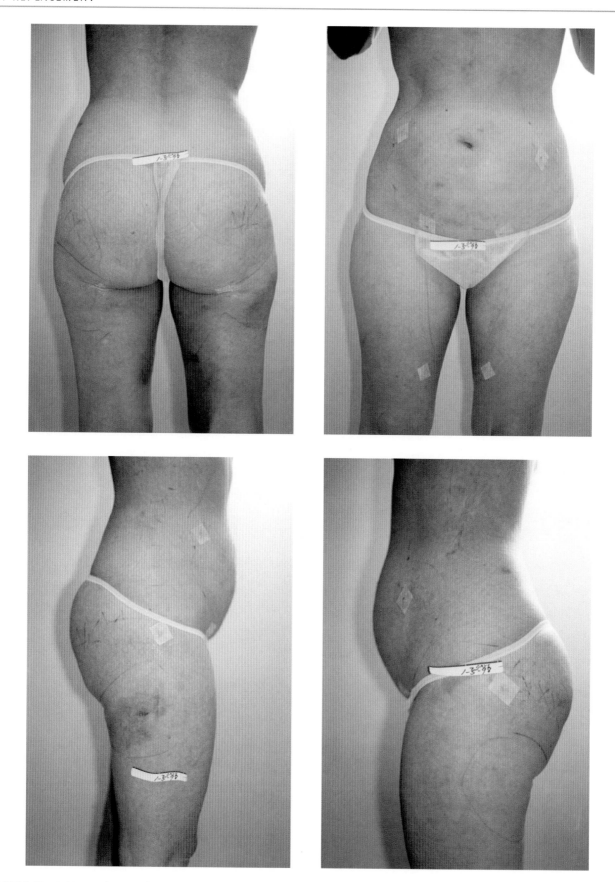

FIGURES 9-19 – 9-22 *Grafts are stable at 3 weeks. Note the persistent ecchymoses of the right (SAL) hip in comparison to the less edematous left hip (XUAL).*

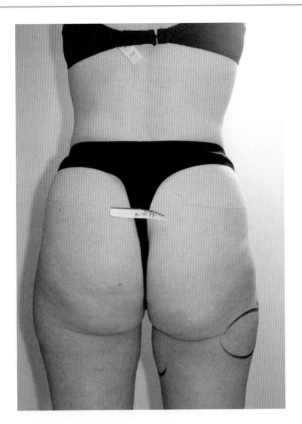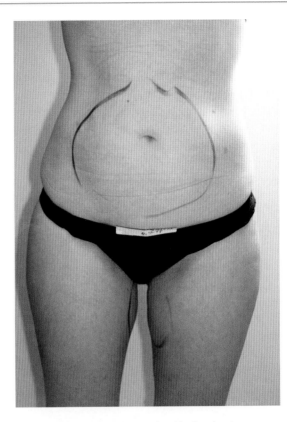

FIGURES 9-23 & 9-24 *In evaluating any new modality, the difference in diameter and fat content of opposite sides is taken into account. XUAL was used on the left hip, SAL on the right.*

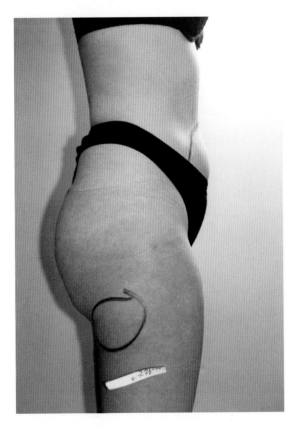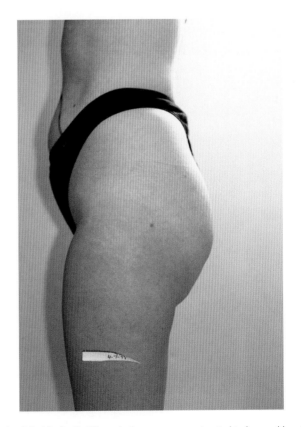

FIGURES 9-25 & 9-26 *The left hip (XUAL) has less residual edema than the right hip (SAL). All marked areas are now treated twice weekly with therapeutic ultrasound applications, obviously avoiding the mid-buttock fat replacement.*

Paying Attention to Cellulite

Fat regrafting into the buttock was pioneered by Brazilian surgeons, but little attention was paid to precise separation of the ligamentous bands in "cellulite" until 1989. The first fork V-tipped instrument with a cutting edge inside the V was described by Luiz Toledo and quickly adapted by other surgeons. These instruments are available with or without injection ports. See Figures 9-27 and 9-28.

MIDFACE

Fat Graft Augmentation of the Submalar Area

In this individual with "hollow cheeks," correction of the area beneath the malar prominence was requested. The equipment shown is the Byron Medical injection "gun" armed with a 12-inch, 16-gauge needle (see Fig. 9-29). This device allows penetration in a fan pattern with a lateral approach. With steady pressure, the fat graft is placed during withdrawal in the tunnels created by passage of the 16-gauge needle. Blunt and sharp techniques are equally effective. A second layer of fat grafts is placed several millimeters below the first and a third layer just above the facial musculature (see Fig. 9-30).

Fat Grafting of the Nasolabial Folds and Subcommissural Depressions

Photographs of this patient taken in 1996 were used in planning the facial procedure in 1998, which included blepharoplasty, submental repair, and elevation of the nasolabial area and subcommissure by fat grafting with minor augmentation of the lower lip (see Fig. 9-31). At 2 weeks, cheek smoothing is apparent (see Fig. 9-32). More important, the nasolabial folding has already receded after nonsurgical XU application to the mid-cheek and jowl. The changes that are apparent in this patient and others at 2 weeks appear to be permanent. There has been no recurrence of the nasolabial folding or any necessity for further fat grafting in the 5-year evaluation.

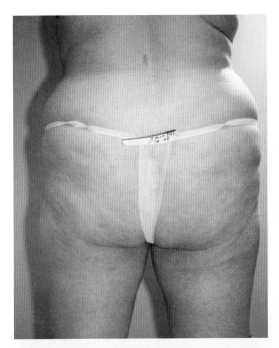
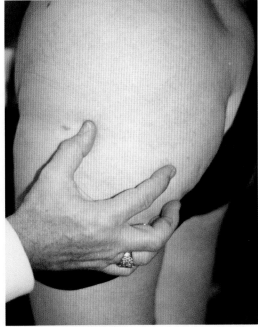

FIGURES 9-27 & 9-28
Spray-pattern intramuscular and subcutaneous fat grafting restored the lost contour of the entire buttock.

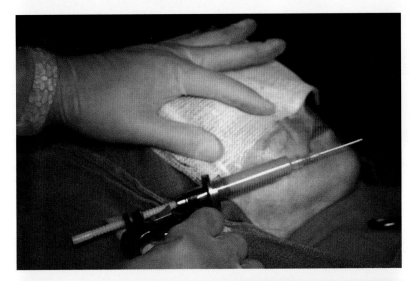

FIGURE 9-29 *Fat grafts for submalar depression. With minimal discrepancy in submalar fullness in comparison to the opposite cheek, a layered autologous fat graft is the treatment of choice.*

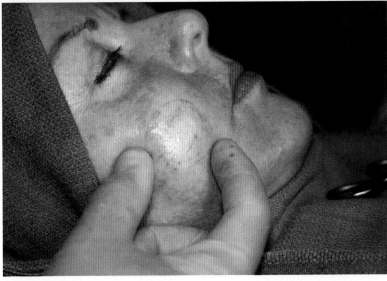

FIGURE 9-30 *Three layers of "spray pattern" tunnels filled with fat are used centrally for the highest elevation and lesser amounts peripherally.*

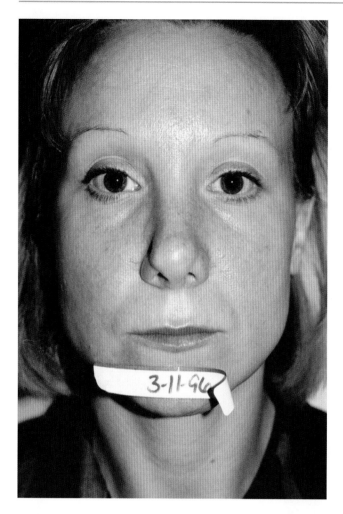

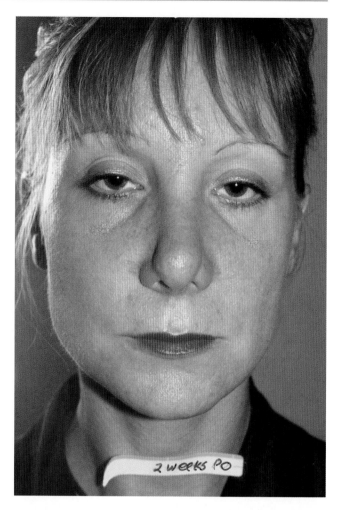

FIGURE 9-31 *Despite deep nasolabial folds from facial cheek descent, a less intrusive correction by fat grafting and cheek/jowl ultrasound was chosen.*

FIGURE 9-32 *Not surprisingly, cheek retraction and fold regression from ultrasound treatment reveal contouring as early as 2 weeks.*

LIPS

A primary question in lip enhancement is the preferred maximum size to be achieved. One way to help this discussion is to have patients bring in photographs of lips from magazines. They are instructed concerning lips that are too large, too full, too prominent, or "just right."

CLINICAL PEARL

Of all the techniques of lip enhancement with foreign materials, the most success has been achieved with AlloDerm in the hands of Dr. Rod Rohrich (Dallas). Long-term follow-up reveals that resorption is almost universal, but there has been no evidence of immune reactions. We have seen linear scar contracture, tenderness, and other unforeseen complications. AlloDerm is somewhat softer than other materials such as tendon sheath, Gore-Tex, or "SoftForm," which are palpable rolls of very firm material that is not only unbending but aesthetically unnatural as well. Extrusion is the major complication.

Comparison of Autologous and Synthetic Grafts

Gore-Tex expanded polytetrafluoroethylene (ePTFE) suturing material may well be useful in many areas, but it is *totally incorrect* to state that *only* Gore-Tex, liquid silicone, and polymethylmethacrylate (PMMA) injections can provide lip enhancement.

Although one is open to differences of opinion, it is difficult to accept an opinion that begins with the statement: "Thick lips are a symbol of youth and powerful character." Most physicians quickly become disenchanted with Gore-Tex. Attempts were made to minimize the problem of inflexible palpable strings by using a quadruple string of Gore-Tex threaded with a sharp needle into lip muscle. This is not a good idea, even if only 15% of the patients in one discussion had "poor results" *and* there was a "low rate" of infection, so wouldn't this make any prudent surgeon choose another method? Of course.[3]

In a letter to *Technical Forum*, which I edit, Dr. David Benvenuti (Newport Beach) had the following opinion: "I have recently seen several patients with lip and nasolabial augmentations with Gore-Tex. One patient's upper lip was contracted, stiff, irregular and pulled outward with large amounts of visible mucosa. The patients with nasolabial augmentation with Gore-Tex had visible ridges and irregularities. I have not seen these problems with soft tissue augmentation with dermal fat grafts or Alloderm. I feel that the implantation of the artificial material beneath thin facial skin results in a stiffness secondary to increased inflammation and scarring around the implant. I have not seen this problem in cadaveric grafts or autografts. I wonder if any of your readers have similar observations?"[3] Yes—many of my readers, and trial attorneys.

Lip Roll

The operation of "lip roll" to increase the visible vermilion of the upper lip in conjunction with fat grafting of an adequate lower lip is a key component in balancing the facial appearance. An incision is made in the "wet" mucosa just past the frenulum with undermining from inside the lip all the way up to the white roll area. Advancement of the mucosa so that it can become edematous creates a permanently fuller "dry" vermilion. Fat grafts survive only if sufficient space for pressure-free tunneling exists. Fat grafts may be added to the orbicularis oris during the open phase of the procedure for additional contouring.

We have learned from experience that fat grafting alone will not create fullness in "thin-lipped" individuals who have almost no vermilion. On the other hand, fat grafts work extremely well in the atrophic lip of an elderly face-lift patient.

Case in point

The patient shown in Figure 9-33 has very little substance to her upper lip, so a "lip roll" is being considered to enhance its fullness. Because the lower lip has sufficient volume to accept fat grafts, fat grafts are planned for both the upper and lower lips (see Fig. 9-34).

In the 2-year postoperative evaluation, good symmetry had been obtained in the upper and lower lips, and the addition of malar implants has changed the contour of her face acceptably. Not surprisingly, she asked for additional fullness of the upper and lower lips. At this point, fullness can be accomplished by multilayered fat grafting, which gave the result shown in Figure 9-35 after the secondary graft. This contour, 16 months after the second procedure, has persisted and gives good balance in this "full-lip" patient category. The permanence of multilayered fat grafting is definitely operator dependent.

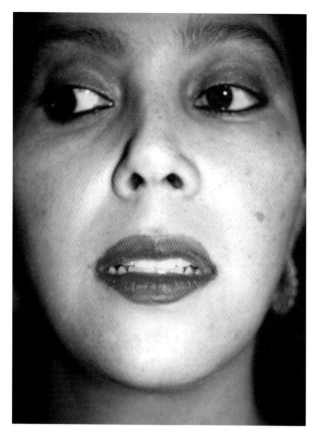

FIGURE 9-33 *Persons who desire moderate lip enhancement and who have adequate vermilion are treated with fat grafts. Those who desire maximum lip enlargement must have a combination of "lip roll" and grafts.*

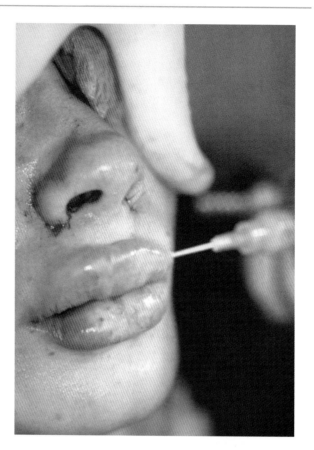

FIGURE 9-34 *After filling the exposed orbicularis muscle with pre-tunneled grafts and securing the advanced vermilion of the upper and lower lips, additional percutaneous tunnels for fat grafts may be required for symmetry.*

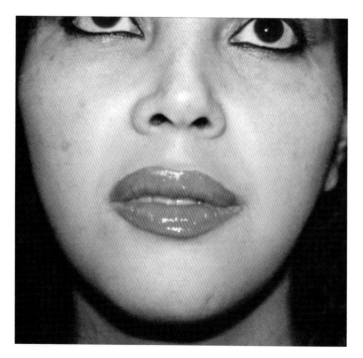

FIGURE 9-35 *This 4-year result met the patient's desire for the "fullest lips."*

Fat Grafting of the Lip

Selective fat grafting in younger individuals can accentuate the central "cupid's bow," as well as augment small deficiencies. In this individual, fat grafting was used to enhance the lower lip, for which she requested a small amount of augmentation (see Figs. 9-36 to 9-38). The additional fat grafts were placed in the central portion of the upper lip to accentuate the "cupid's bow" and laterally to fill in a flattened area. With minor fat grafts of this nature placed in the three-tunneled multilayered technique, edema is completely resolved in 3 weeks. If the recipient then decides that the lips are too large, "pressure crushing" of the lip will remove the graft. This two-finger compression is ineffective at 4 weeks. The grafts are then permanent.

Fat Grafting for a Full Lip

Concentrated fat is placed in a series of withdrawal tunnels beginning at the white roll and ending at the dry vermilion with steady pressure so that each tunnel is filled with 0.1 to 0.5 cc of concentrated fat, in this case delivered through a $1^1/_2$-inch, 16-gauge needle. For patients desiring complete filling to match a photograph, a second and third level of infiltration into the deeper soft tissue and into muscle tissue is required (see Fig. 9-39). The resulting fullness (see Fig. 9-40) is then checked for uniformity. Gentle manipulation is often required to determine that uniform deposition of fat throughout the lip has been achieved. The distance between the nose and white roll decreases, which is an added advantage.

Fat Grafting for Fuller Lips

Many patients request a greater degree of fullness and yet already have the lip shape that is often the maximum desired by others (see Figs. 9-41 to 9-43). For such patients, multilevel fat grafting is the ideal treatment. It is reversible and adjustable in the initial 2-week recovery period. At 2 months (see Figs. 9-44 to 9-46), the shape that is obtained will persist with little if any change until age atrophy appears. Individuals with this type of enhancement in which grafts are added to an already generous lip have been monitored since 1984. The soft and pliable results of multilevel autologous fat grafting is preferable to the often woody, unnatural appearance of grafts with other materials. At this point, she changed her mind and asked for even more lip volume. The second fat graft produced the result shown in Figures 9-47 to 9-49.

Fat Grafting beyond Lip Enhancement

Readers who may have attended our 1997 XUAL introductory seminar in San Antonio saw patients who volunteered to undergo fat grafting, as well as the first volunteers for XU. This 40-year-old woman shows the typical mid-life atrophy of the upper and lower lip and freely admits that she had always desired fuller lips than she had when she was a younger woman. In addition, there is evidence of early atrophy in the area beneath the commissures of her mouth and deep nasolabial folds (see Figs. 9-50 to 9-52).

With intravenous sedation and an abdominal donor site, 30 cc of fat was concentrated by the drainage–Telfa pad method and then placed into previously undermined areas. Entry into the nasolabial fold and subcommissure is through the nose with a "rhytid dissector." Once the flat areas have been elevated, direct placement of fat that has been concentrated covers the entire area in multiple subcutaneous tunnels without overlying tension. A second tunnel is created in the deeper layer, and in the nasolabial fold, a third layer may be needed several millimeters beneath, with impingement onto the facial musculature.

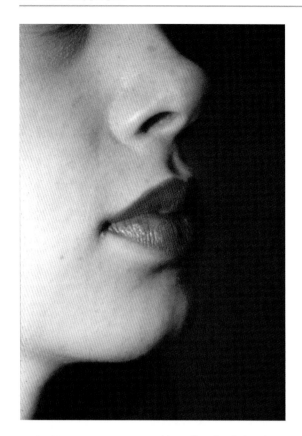

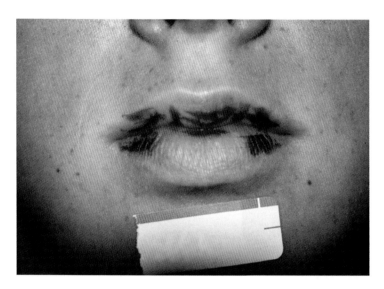

FIGURES 9-36 & 9-37   *Fat grafting offers the choice of spot enhancement for precise placement. Non-autologous devices do not.*

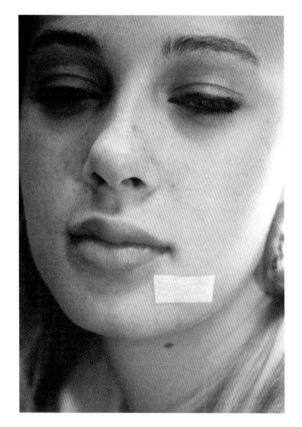

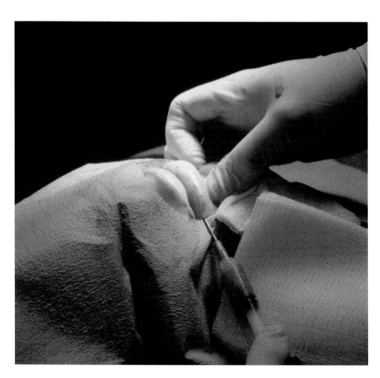

FIGURE 9-38   *Result of precise enlargement to accommodate the patient's choices.*

FIGURE 9-39   *With control by fingertip palpation, unidirectional pre-tunneling is the method of choice.*

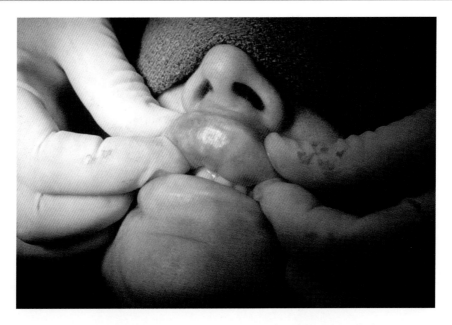

FIGURE 9-40 *Fat grafts are deposited in the tunnels during withdrawal. A final manipulation for uniformity may be required.*

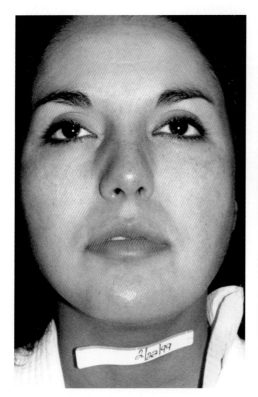
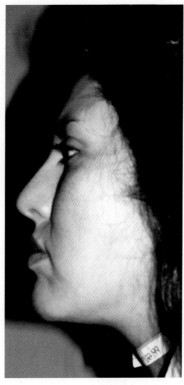
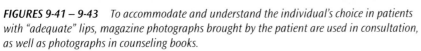
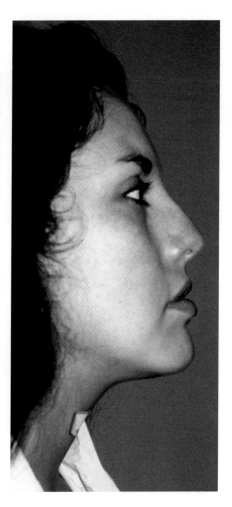

FIGURES 9-41 – 9-43 *To accommodate and understand the individual's choice in patients with "adequate" lips, magazine photographs brought by the patient are used in consultation, as well as photographs in counseling books.*

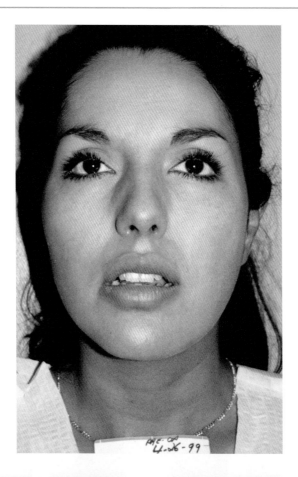

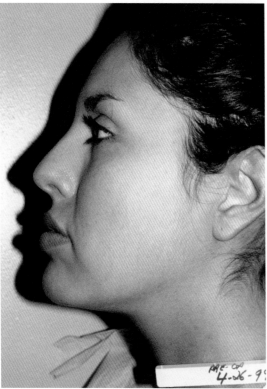
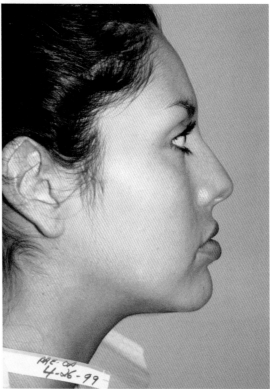

FIGURES 9-44 – 9-46   *This "above average" enhancement matched this patient's initial choice. After a period, further enlargement was requested.*

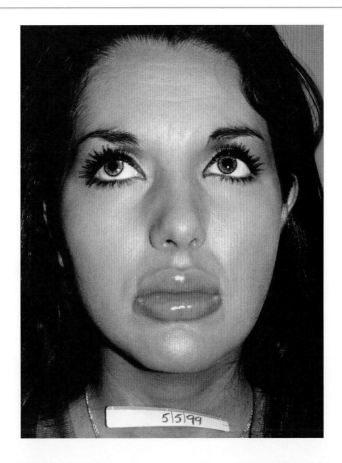

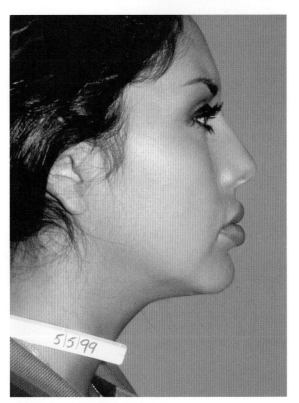

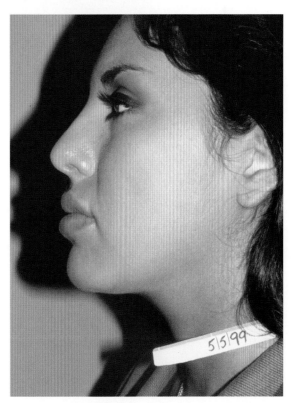

FIGURES 9-47 — 9-49   *Permanent enhancement to this degree by means of a secondary grafting procedure is still to her liking, as noted in a chance encounter 3 years after these photographs.*

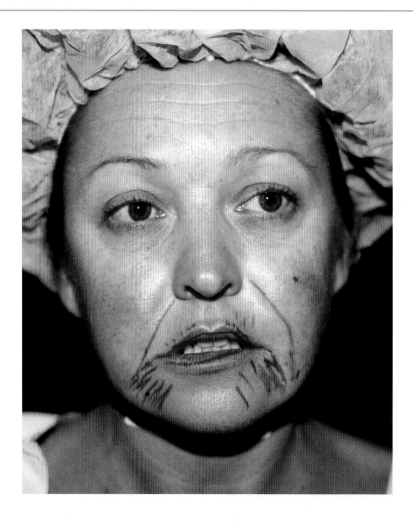

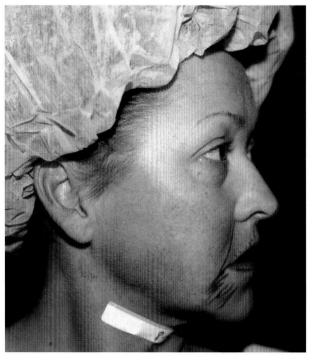
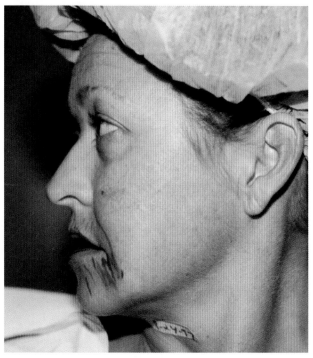

FIGURES 9-50 – 9-52 *With careful placement, fat grafts for the nasolabial lines, subcommissure, and lips were planned for this desired "full lip."*

The appearance of her face at 1 month is an indicator of the degree of correction that will be maintained (see Figs. 9-53 to 9-55). Note that she has adequate lip vermilion to allow this degree of enhancement by multi-level fat grafting alone. Correction of the commissures and softening of the nasolabial fold were accomplished by fat grafting, even though she would be considered a candidate for a mid-face–lift for better correction of aging changes. Note the uptilting of the upper lip.

Certain patients can benefit from either a lip roll alone or fat grafting with the tunnel technique alone or, to make an extremely full lip, a combination of the two. Fat grafting is easier than grafting dermis or fascia, but face-lifts provide a source of SMAS, which is useful in certain lip roll procedures. When the lip roll advancement mucosa is tacked into place (which leaves an exposed area of orbicularis muscle between the frenulum and the edge of the advancement, usually 1 cm or so), one may then place fat in tunnels within the muscle. The edema of the repositioned vermilion provides additional bulking. Avoid excision of the white roll to uptilt the lip. It looks unnatural.

Lip Roll Techniques

The rule of thumb is based on the patient's wishes. If the patient wants to have a fuller lip, do a full 1-cm or more advancement. If only a small amount is desired, do the same undermining but only advance 0.5 cm. Do not forget that transient postsurgical edema will develop in some of these people just below the nose. They benefit from the "reverse tennis headband" idea. A thin tennis headband worn taut across the upper lip provides pressure that will help resolve the edema problems more rapidly. Others may require judicious steroid injections. The same applies to "lumpy" or overgrafted vermilion.

Mucosal blistering is a rarity. I personally have not seen any mucosal losses. Prevention is achieved by careful dissection with blunt scissors just at the muscle-mucosa junction. If one injects 5 to 10 cc of Xylocaine with epinephrine under the mucosa, it is an easier procedure because the planes are more clearly defined.

The Search for Non-autologous Injectables

As expected, lip injection of Bioplastique, or textured silicone particles suspended in a gel carrier, was performed via a technique of multiple pre-tunneling and implantation. This was soon discontinued because of lumpiness, firmness, and irregularities. Polyacrylamide gel, a jelly-like transparent substance, did remain in place and was unchanged at an 18-month follow-up. SoftForm, the expanded form of Gore-Tex, could be palpated even 1 year after implantation and was more complicated to implant. Drawbacks included detectable scars. [**Editor's Note:** In the American experience, most of these implants were removed at the patient's request because of palpability, the "rolling log" problem, and discomfort. Medicolegally, injection of these materials, including Zyderm, Dermalogen, Cosmoplast (human collagen), and Restylane, is indefensible. They have a history of embolism and mucosal sloughing, plus Food and Drug Administration disapproval.]

In many individuals, advancement of the vermilion by the V-Y or my lip roll procedure is the only choice (see Figs. 9-56 to 9-58). Because only modest improvement is afforded patients by V-Y lip advancement techniques, I prefer the horizontal lip roll procedure, which I first presented over 30 years ago. In Figure 9-59, an excellent example of the preoperative view is shown, and the 3-year postoperative view is presented in Figure 9-60.

CLINICAL PEARL

The term "cow collagen" has been applied to purified bovine collagen that is used for soft tissue augmentation, with its only disadvantage being a short life and allergic reactions. Despite experimental studies showing anaphylactic shock in animals reacting to bovine collagen, this problem has not been seen in humans. Jack Friedland (Phoenix) thinks that collagen injections are "a good addition to our armamentarium especially if patients understand that it lasts no longer than three months."[4] Cosmoderm and Cosmoplast, the newest injectables of this sort, last slightly longer and do not require skin testing. Skin testing, as many individuals have noted with bovine collagen, is often misleading. Reports of granulomas after repeated collagen injections, glabellar sloughing, rashes, and irritation at the injection site were often overlooked in presentations to physicians.

Granulomas, early or late, are reported in European work with "Sculptra," "Perlane," and especially "Artecoll," and "Artefill." Any permanent foreign material will have sequelae. Other injectables, such as "Fascian" and "Cymetra" are in disfavor for other reasons.

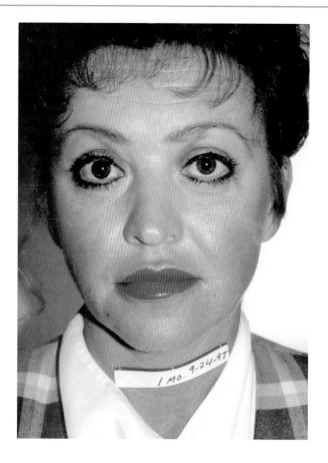

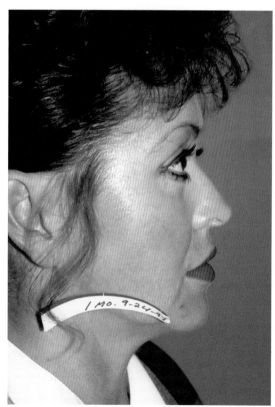

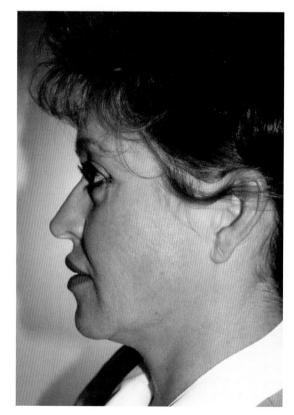

FIGURES 9-53 – 9-55   *Grafts are stabilized at 30 days. If she had desired reduction, crushing of the grafts manually would have been effective only between the 14th and 21st day.*

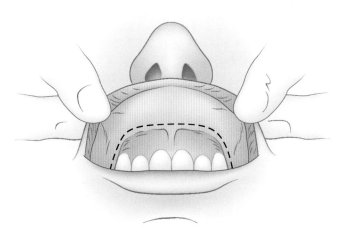
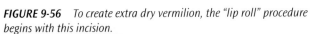

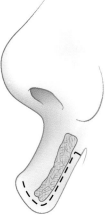
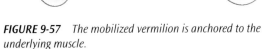

FIGURE 9-56 *To create extra dry vermilion, the "lip roll" procedure begins with this incision.*

FIGURE 9-57 *The mobilized vermilion is anchored to the underlying muscle.*

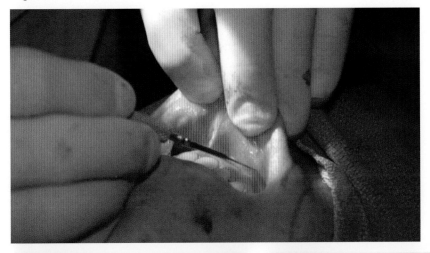

FIGURE 9-58 *After local infiltration of Xylocaine with epinephrine, the cut to the muscle layer is easily controlled.*

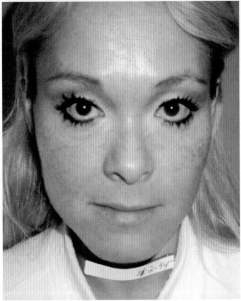

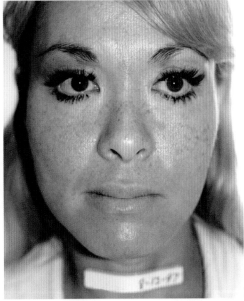

FIGURE 9-59 *Fat graft enhancement will be adequate for the lower lip in this case, but a "lip roll" is required to produce a matching upper lip.*

FIGURE 9-60 *Matching lips compared closely with the photographs she brought to the preoperative counseling sessions.*

Correction of the Aging Lip

In most patients, aging atrophy in the lips involves not only the surface but also the subdermal elements. Fat grafting plays a role in restoring the contour of the lip. My current technique involves undermining from within the nose and in a lateral-to-medial direction as shown in Figure 9-61. By freeing either the grooves or the entire lip, fat grafts carefully placed in these areas will produce the smoothness and require lesser resurfacing with abrasion or peel (see Fig. 9-62). As experienced surgeons know, the use of heavy dermabrasion laser obliteration results in loss of color in the upper lip. Deeper chemical peels have the same complication. By elevating the deep rhytids and performing preliminary light scalpel abrasion, restoration of the lip can be accomplished with little "downtime." My

preference is this procedure with a light application of 35% trichloracetic acid (TCA) first vertically in the rhytids and then across the entire area. TCA penetrates according to the amount applied. It is far wiser to do a secondary touchup with TCA than to have skin sloughing or loss of color (see Figs. 9-63 and 9-64).

Case in point

In these young women (see Figs. 9-65 to 9-68), rhinoplasty, lip roll, and chin reduction were the first priorities. To enhance the appearance of the eyes, we reduce the nasal prominence. There is insufficient upper lip vermilion to accept fat grafting. The long-term effect of the lip roll shown in these 3- and 5-year follow-up photographs is a more balanced face without a trace of artificiality.

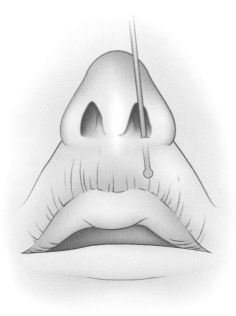

FIGURE 9-61 *Deeper rhytids are elevated with the transnasal blunt tip "rhytid dissector" (Byron Medical).*

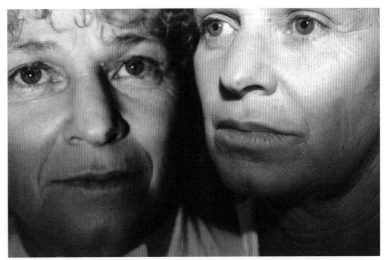

FIGURE 9-62 *A less problematic and quicker recovery (than with laser resurfacing) is achieved with a combination of "light" scalpel abrasion, rhytid elevation with autologous fat, and 35% TCA peels for aging atrophic lip rejuvenation.*

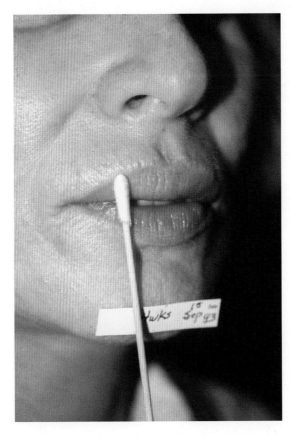

FIGURE 9-63 *Erasing lip wrinkles by dermabrasion, Baker formula phenol peels, or laser resurfacing is less desirable than a graduated quick-recovery approach. After light scalpel abrasion, fat grafting, and 35% TCA peel, any residual rhytids are identified and spot retreated.*

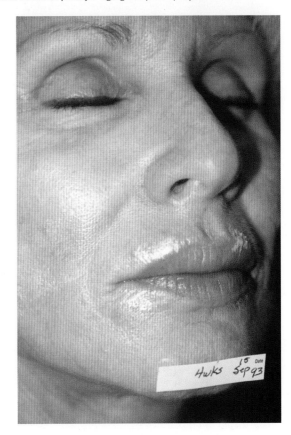

FIGURE 9-64 *The frosting of a "retreatment" is as transitory as erythema.*

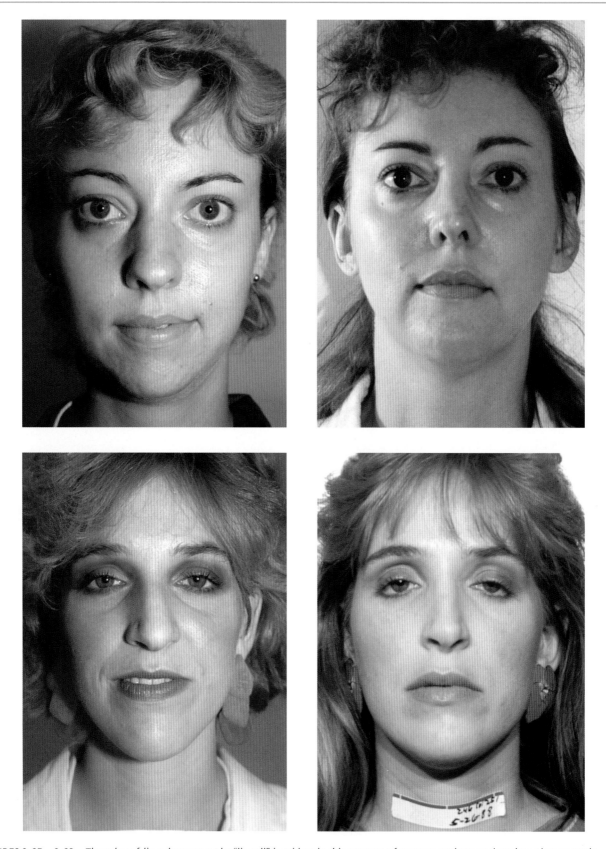

FIGURES 9-65 – 9-68   *The value of lip enhancement by "lip roll" is evident in this category of younger patients undergoing other cosmetic surgeries.*

RECOVERY FROM PERIORAL ENHANCEMENT

Although there is certainly individual variation and variation according to the degree of correction, in general, recovery from augmentation of the "wasting away" of the perioral area and lips is rapid unless, of course, deep laser resurfacing or deep abrasion is used. If the surgeon chooses fat grafting into the vertical lines as well as the lip vermillion and depressions at the edges of the oral commissure, the swelling recedes within 10 to 12 days. If, however, a patient requests a very large lip enhancement with or without the "lip roll" procedure, 3 to 4 weeks will elapse before the final result is achieved. During that time, one has a "Planet of the Apes" unsightly protuberance, especially in the first 10 days. If non-autologous materials such as SoftForm or Gore-Tex are used, recovery time may be somewhat less, but a major drawback is the firmness of the implant. As our Mexican and Canadian colleagues have told us so often, they remove more Gore-Tex and Gore-Tex analogues such as SoftForm from the lips than they put in.

The lips are unique in that any implant that is thicker than lip tissue is palpable. Patients describe feeling a "roll of something" inside the lip, whether it's a dermis graft, Gore-Tex, or any other form of augmentation. The same is true to a lesser degree in augmentation of the nasolabial fold.

The true disasters in plastic surgery are lip enhancements performed with silicone or solid-sphere injectables. Anecdotal reports of problems with injections of Bioplastique and Artecoll describe lumps and hard immobile lips that are practically impossible to correct. Gore-Tex often produces the same scarring and deformity. Remember, one advantage of fat grafting is that it is *reversible* by applying pressure after 10 days, when the edema of application has receded. Fat grafts are quite sensitive to pressure, and intermittent compression will result in total or partial resorption as desired. In general, the enhancement obtained at 30 days will persist, based on my observations over the past 17 years.

EXTREMITY LIPOSUCTION AND BUTTOCK FAT REGRAFTING: COMPARING SAL AND XUAL

In the trials of XUAL, one area was left for standard liposuction and all other areas were treated by XUAL before the beginning of the procedure.

Case in Point

The patient in Figures 9-69 to 9-72 shows the typical inner thigh thickness that would ordinarily be left untouched for fear that rippling would occur. In the 3-week comparison, it was readily apparent that the right hip "saddlebag" area was more bruised than the left. The records revealed that only the right hip had been treated with SAL (see Figs. 9-73 and 9-74), the rest with XUAL and XU. This area remained tender for some time thereafter. Note the pinpoint entry points for regrafting into the buttocks, which has completed the contour, and for entry into the banana roll area from the frontal approach.

Final photographs show good contouring of the banana rolls, the inner aspect of the thighs, and the knees, as well as recontouring of the mid-buttock depression with fat grafting (see Figs. 9-75 to 9-78). The end result with SAL and XUAL is equal, but the degree of contracture in the banana roll and the smoothness of the resultant contouring of the inner portion of the thigh in our opinion were superior to what we could obtain with standard liposuction alone. Postoperative ultrasound was used in all areas except the right hip to aid this contouring.

> **CLINICAL PEARL**
>
> Although Teimourian and others did not hesitate to inject significant quantities of fat into the ankles and calf, this procedure has largely been abandoned because of the significantly high complication rate, which includes not only swelling and ulceration but also irregularities and unpredictable absorption.

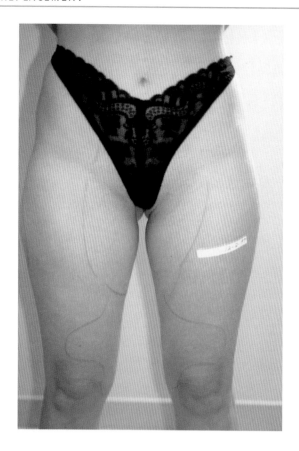
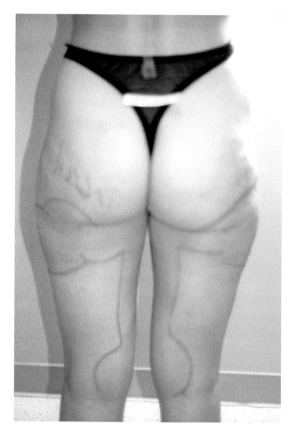
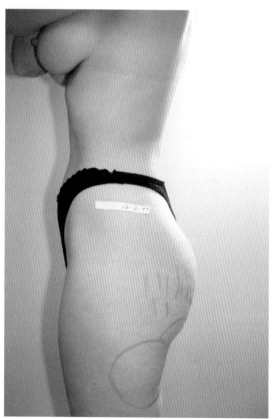
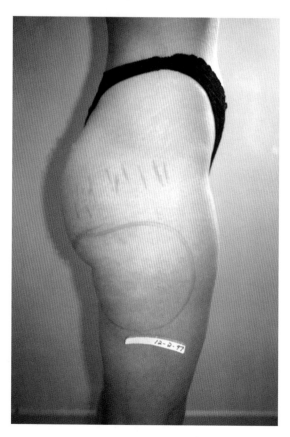

9-69 – 9-72   *Enhancement of the dimpled and flat buttock areas is an overall improvement. Areas are marked for XUAL with an improved result, especially in the inner aspect of the thighs.*

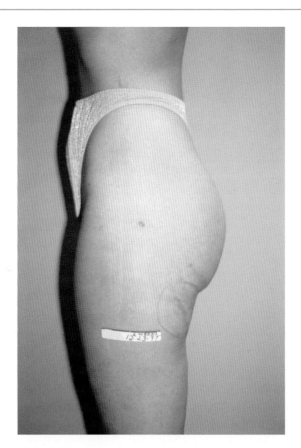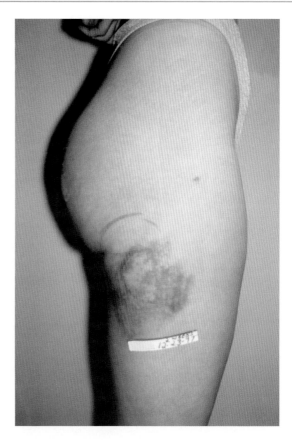

FIGURES 9-73 & 9-74   *Contrast of the XUAL left hip and the edematous ecchymotic SAL right hip.*

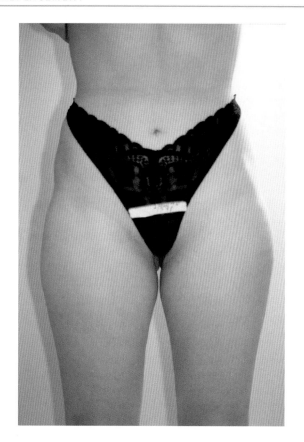
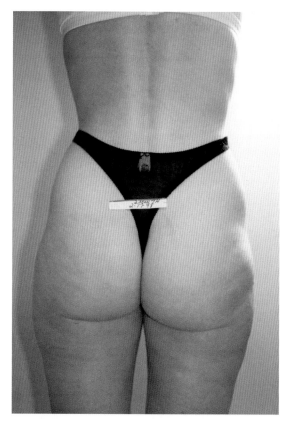
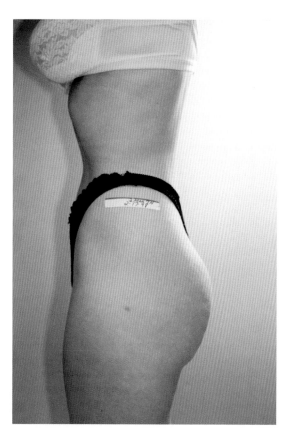
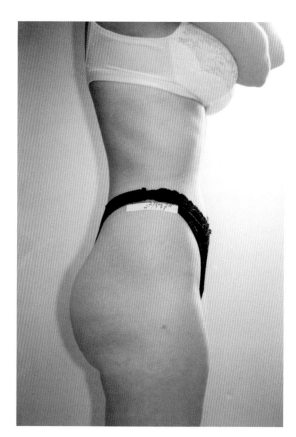

FIGURES 9-75 – 9-78   *The identical end result, with ongoing skin shrinkage in all areas except the right hip.*

PREVENTABLE PROBLEMS IN FAT GRAFTING— RICHARD ELLENBOGEN, M.D., F.A.C.S. (PLASTIC SURGEON, LOS ANGELES)

Preventing problems in fat grafting is quite simple. I reduced them to their most basic forms, as follows:

1. Be careful to not remove too much fat from the donor area or you will be fat-grafting this area to correct it in the future.

2. Fat is injected with 1-cc syringes with many passes. I do not use as many passes as Coleman does, and I do not use as much fat. I rarely use more than 40 g of fat on the face. Sidney uses sometimes five times that. I rarely make more than four or five passes per milliliter. Dr. Coleman uses four or five times that.

3. I use a Medrol Dosepak (methylprednisolone) in the postoperative period. I do not think that this decreases the take of fat. Dr. Coleman does not use steroids.

4. I believe that other preventable situations, such as lumpiness, are not generally problems if you move your depositing syringe quickly and mold the fat by pressure on the skin.

5. Do not use too much fat. You cannot count on it disappearing. Maintain a minimal overcorrection in almost all areas.

6. Symmetry is important and is very easy to achieve while injecting the fat. Watch it carefully.

7. Do not take out the fat, spin it, and leave it. Use it as quickly as you possibly can. I have noticed the difference between a tremendous amount of take and minimal take if I wait until the end of my face-lift to inject the fat. My happiest patients have been those who have had fat injected at the same time as their face-lift. The youthful restorative qualities of both are quite extraordinary. I now even prefer this when rebuilding the mid-face rather than lifting the malar fat pads or performing a mid-face–lift, which takes forever to heal. A patient who experiences the least pain and has the shortest recovery will be the happiest patient. We know that we can be better surgeons if we do not have worries about our previous patients.

8. I do my fat grafting with the patient under general anesthesia because I can re-inject into minimally anesthetized areas where no adrenaline is used. With the new anesthetic techniques and propofol, it is a relatively short procedure—perhaps 20 minutes to take the fat, 5 minutes to spin it, and about another 10 to 15 minutes to inject it.

9. Fat grafting in the body must be grossly overcorrected in numerous planes, close to the skin, deeper, and so forth, when correcting a bad liposuction. This is the only instance in which I do not use 1-cc syringes. I use 10 cc. You need so much more fat to correct a defect in the body than you do in the face itself.

10. If you penetrate the oral mucosa by mistake, take the injector off the table immediately; do not use it again. The danger of putting mouth bacteria into the cheek is high, and a less than optimal outcome will result. When larger amounts of fat are needed, rather than using Coleman's extractor, I use a small-diameter cannula with a Lukey collection tube, which allows small parcels of fat to be gathered in large amounts.

11. I use no bandages or tape over areas that are fat-grafted. I like the area to swell. Because I have placed the toothpicks of fat in multiple layers, there is no chance for them to shift, as there would be if I injected them with needles and created lakes of fat.

CONCLUSION

Fat grafting plays an important role in facial rejuvenation, body repair, and correction of post liposuction deformity. In contrast to dermis fat, pure fat grafts are fragile, living tissue.

The technical aspects are paramount, as shown in the excellent 20-year results obtained by many surgeons. Analysis of aging and beauty shows that volume restoration is the key factor. Fat grafting fills this need.

References

1. Finch L: Fresh faced: Fat grafting. *Plastic Surgery Products*, 2002;45-48.
2. Saylan Z: Liposhifting: Treatment of postliposuction irregularities. *International Journal of Cosmetic Surgery*, 1999;7:71-73.
3. Benvenuti D: Letter to the editor. *Technical Forum*, 2000;26(6):10.
4. Friedland J: Personal communication.

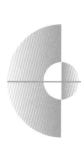

CHAPTER TEN

Aftercare

Plastic surgeons slowly became aware of the benefits of hand- and machine-assisted massage, lymph drainage, hydrotherapy, and skin care in body sculpture patients. We knew massage had a beneficial effect on scar resolution. Various combinations of topical oils and skin creams were soon developed and marketed with an improvement in patient comfort as well as smoothing of the results of liposuction. In the early days of liposuction, such aftercare was extremely important because of the relatively primitive equipment. Now that we have progressed to more sophisticated methods, aftercare is still important. An in-office spa is not only appreciated by patients for its privacy, comfort, and personal attention but can also be structured to include marketing of approved products. This concept was greeted with derision when my wife and I initially proposed it in the early 1980s. Her booth was the only one dedicated to skin care and postoperative cosmetics (*Wilkinson, Suzanne: GlamouR Prescribed Skin Care*). It has now become universally accepted as proper and is encouraged as a means of personal contact and improvement of the results of liposuction, abdomino-plasty, breast surgery, and facial surgery.

It is still debated whether aftercare garment compression is as important as originally believed. Yet common sense and logic dictate that reduction of edema by compression will not only reduce recovery time by preventing flow of tissue fluid into damaged areas but will certainly also play a role in the ultimate contouring. It is believed that damaged fat cells remain on site after liposuction but slowly dissolve from the trauma. This fat with its resultant breakdown products may influence the smoothness of the results. Compression should prevent "clumping."

In the early years of liposuction, massage therapy, either mechanical or physical, was not believed to be as important as it is today. My clinic has always incorporated a spa with massage therapy, lymph drainage, and now external ultrasound (XU) to speed recovery and decrease bruising.

The choice of compression garments is endless. In my experience, male patients were uncomfortable with the jackets designed for gynecomastia. Men preferred to use a simpler form of compression: a 6-inch elastic wrap that could be removed and reapplied. Various compression bands are used for facial surgery and gynecomastia. With poorer skin quality, as in arm reduction, compression is essential to promote the greatest degree of skin shrinkage possible.

With the advent of power-assisted liposuction (PAL), ultrasound-assisted liposuction (UAL), and external ultrasound-assisted liposuction (XUAL), compression time is no longer as extensive. In our experience, early physical activity with treadmill or bicycle exercise, hydrotherapy, and self-massage play a greater role. In abdominoplasty, it is certainly true that a compressive girdle or binder prevents inadvertent tearing of plication sutures, and yet failure to release the pressure of a girdle or binder over anesthetized areas may result in a difficult complication: "girdle burns." This compressive necrosis may occur in the upper part of the abdomen, the vulnerable area of abdominoplasty in the center of the repair, and liposuctioned areas also covered by a brassiere.

A number of skin care products are designed for aftercare, including aloe vera/vitamin E oil combinations. The massage creams and other preparations certainly have an advantage: patients are involved in their aftercare. The use of these products reduces skin trauma from the massage and promotes comfort.

TECHNIQUES AND TREATMENT

Case in Point—Rapid Recovery Enhanced by Postoperative XU

This patient, an active white male older than 60 years, illustrates that the use of XUAL and postoperative XU with "super wet" infusion, which promotes early pain-free physical activity, has the advantage of early resolution after liposuction.

With taut musculature, skin excision would have been considered before the advent of XUAL with its inherent skin contracture (see Figs. 10-1 to 10-4). Deep and superficial liposuction after the application of XU for 12 minutes to the typical male "love handle" mid-abdomen fatty deposits was combined with abdominal "etching." The imprint of abdominal etching is becoming visible in the 3-week postoperative photographs (see Figs. 10-5 to 10-8). "Etching" is not affected by the postoperative use of XU.

Using various ultrasound systems at "full power" (30 W), XU is applied to all the areas that have undergone liposuction, beginning 24 hours after the initial application of XU in the operating room (see Fig. 10-9). Although tissue edema is still present, the increased vascularity and dispersion of tissue fluid induced by XU result in quicker elimination of the edema of liposuction. Dermal collagen is increased, as well as the essential skin contracture that allows surgeons to achieve a flat abdomen without folds by XUAL and without skin excision in this group of individuals. This patient, who resumed full activity on the evening after surgery and did not require pain medication, seconds the premise that XU disperses the lidocaine (Xylocaine) and epinephrine into tissues. A compressive binder was used for 7 days and then "bicycle pants" compression garments occasionally during his workouts, which were gradually increased in intensity on the third and fourth postoperative days.

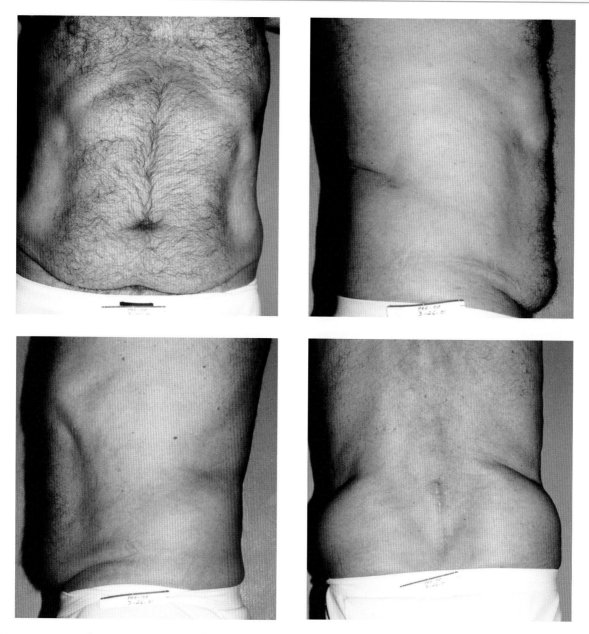

FIGURES 10-1 – 10-4 *At first glance, the preferred treatment for this middle-aged active man would be some form of abdominoplasty. We chose XUAL and postoperative XU treatments.*

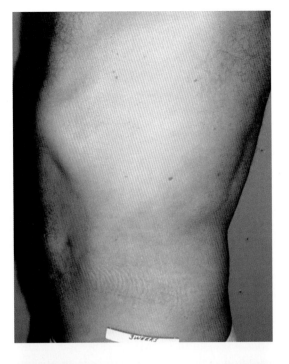
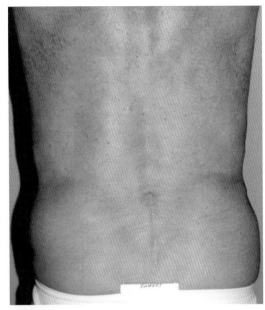
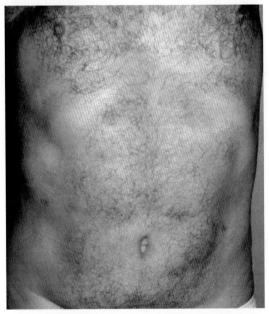
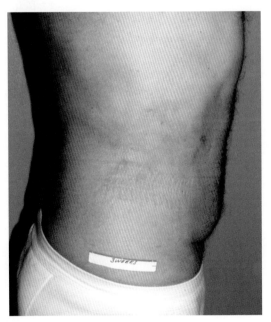

FIGURES 10-5 – 10-8 *Pain free, this patient "cleaned the whole house" 8 hours after surgery, resumed rigorous daily exercise, and at 3 weeks showed rapid shrinkage of the panniculus. Note that "etching" lines are beginning to emerge.*

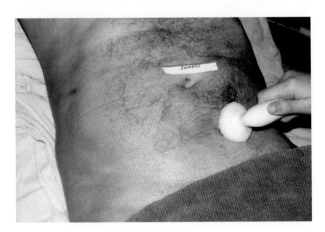

FIGURE 10-9 *Postoperative ultrasound is repeated until the edema has resolved and may contribute to a greater degree of shrinkage. Massage and hydrotherapy courses are completed by 10 days.*

Case in Point—Nonsurgical Massage Techniques for Extremity Reduction

Correspondents to *Technical Forum* initially expressed skepticism over claims of massage therapy using *machines that were purported to permanently reduce "cellulite."* Detailed analysis shows a temporary improvement, similar to that obtained with continuous hand massage by a skilled masseuse. Although the devices are popular in beauty salons, many plastic surgeons have relegated their use to postoperative post-liposuction massage as a means of reducing edema. They are very careful to not promise patients that these procedures alone will make a difference. The cost of the machine, plus the wages of the skilled operator, require the patient to pay an amount considered excessive for minimal or negligible improvement. Similar early reports of "Thermage," the application of dermal heat, reach the same conclusion, but with the complication of deep tissue damage. Ultrasonic energy peaks subdermally and affects only infused tissues.

Conceding that continuous massage will have *some beneficial effect,* a series of patients volunteered to undergo machine massage therapy on one lower extremity and hand massage therapy on the opposite with the addition of a single fluid injection and the application of XU. The patient shown (see Figs. 10-10 and 10-11) has large fatty deposits in the hips, knees, and anterior, posterior, and inner aspect of the thighs and is loath to undergo surgery. Despite a continuous program of twice-weekly massage, at the end of 1 month there was minimal visible difference between the two sides but some measurable improvement (see Fig. 10-12) on the ultrasound/massage side. This result is not sufficient to warrant continuing the evaluation. This is not to belittle the importance of postoperative massage therapy, but it clearly indicated that there was no cost-worthy advantage to either modality.

Case in Point—Jaw Bra

Figure 10-13 shows the "Jaw Bra" for facial soft tissue support, which is provided in a colorful array by the PMT Corporation (1-800-626-5463). This material is softer than the standard postoperative facial compression garment. Compression is important to prevent edema from settling in the submental or jowl area or even to prevent blood deposits from accumulating, which would prolong recovery and perhaps require cortisone injections. The single-unit compression garment provided by Design-V is another comfortable compression device that patients readily accept. Our choices now are decided purely by cost because these devices are furnished "free" to patients.

Case in Point—Cellulite

The term *cellulite* is certainly not a scientific one, but plastic surgeons have gradually accepted its widespread use in the lay community as a description of the dimpling of skin that occurs in women with mild to moderate fat gain. The original therapy for this condition was undercutting of the connective bands with some form of "pickle fork" and fat grafting, as developed by Dr. Luiz Toledo (São Paulo) and Dr. Fred Grazer (Newport Beach).

It would seem logical that some form of manipulation would be helpful, especially a stretching rather than a rolling maneuver. In a brief trial, I combined local infiltration XUAL with manual massage or mechanical massage. The practice of lymphatic drainage in our clinic did produce a beneficial effect postoperatively without surgical procedures; massage alone was of little help in resolving cellulite. If the effect is temporary removal of lymphatic fluid from swollen fat cells, would it be worth the expense?

External ultrasound affects the integrity of fibrous tissue, a common indication for ultrasound in the treatment of injuries. In liposuction, cells separate into small viable groups. XUAL plus massage can affect "cellulite," to a degree.

The patient in Figures 10-10 to 10-12 had a decrease in the circumference of her legs, though not a dramatic one. The measurements confirmed the patient's impression that multiple treatments with the Symedex MD-2000 were pleasant and "somewhat" effective. Unfortunately, this minimal reduction would not have been acceptable if we had charged for this treatment. Nevertheless, if a surgeon does not have access to a massage therapist, the use of a designer massage device should be considered for postoperative therapy.

> **CLINICAL PEARL**
>
> A good summary of postoperative therapy is that it soothes the patient emotionally and helps the physician from the standpoint of postoperative handholding, especially if caregivers include diet and exercise programs, as well as counseling programs to guide these patients into a definitive procedure: liposuction. Some patients are able to trim and tone themselves to the point that they do not need liposuction. This is certainly the case when one consults a personal training and massage therapist, so it is not an expected result of a mechanical massage device. Wellness programs combined with all modalities are certainly a valued adjunct to liposuction patients, but in all honesty, these programs must be viewed as no more than a helpful maneuver and not a substitute.

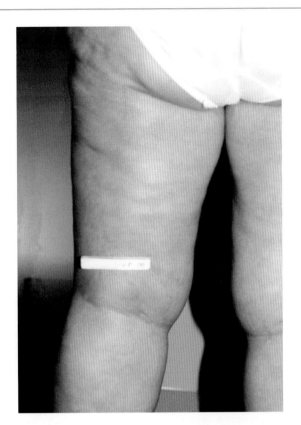
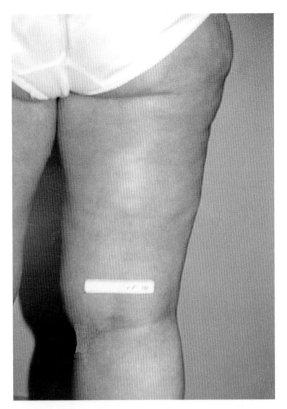
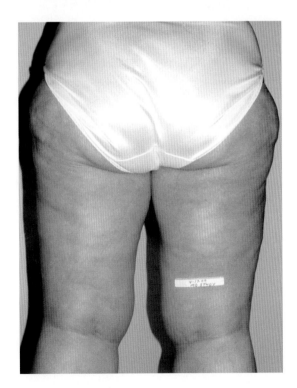

FIGURES 10-10 – 10-12 *A comparison of repeated mechanical massage with external ultrasound (single treatment) versus hand massage with ultrasound therapy shows little improvement on either side to warrant the expense.*

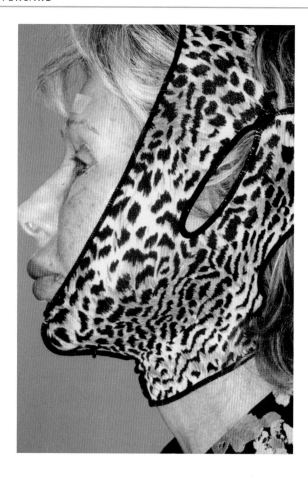

FIGURE 10-13 *A "kinder-gentler" compression device for XU-treated faces is the "Jaw Bra," which is available in many colors and designs. Compression is continued for 3 weeks.*

Case in Point— Girdle Burns

Preoperative evaluation of this patient showed taut upper abdominal musculature but a post-pregnancy diastasis from just above the umbilicus to the mons. In addition, she had considerable surface irregularity and large high hip and flank rolls. These "dents, divots, and depressions" were present across the entire lower half of the buttock area (see Figs. 10-14 to 10-16).

In this volunteer for the first abdominoplasty series performed with XUAL, limited abdominoplasty was performed with a "float" of the umbilicus to allow plication above the original umbilical position. External ultrasound resulted in excellent shrinkage of the upper part of the abdomen, as well as rapid recovery and good contouring in the buttock and hip rolls (see Figs. 10-17 to 10-19). On the fifth postoperative day, the panniculus had normal color and the drains were removed. However, the patient related *that she had worn the girdle without loosening it for 8 hours before falling asleep.* A 3 × 3-cm skin slough appeared the next morning in the midline despite tension-free closure, despite careful tailoring of the fat without liposuctioning below the umbilicus, and

without invasion of the lateral portion of the abdomen with liposuction cannulas.

One of the advantages of limited abdominoplasty is that tissue can be mobilized from the entire abdominal wall for secondary closure. Immediate excision of the sloughed area is preferable to prolonged recovery with a risk for further spread of infection. As shown in Figure 10-20, the flap has been elevated, the umbilicus relocated to allow expansion, and closure performed with minimal tacking sutures. Complete healing ensued. External ultrasound was used in the areas of flap thickening above the mons and resulted in softening 3 months after the original surgery (see Fig. 10-21).

Had this patient undergone standard abdominoplasty with resection of the entire panniculus below the umbilicus rather than a limited resection as shown in Figure 10-22, repair would have been difficult, if not impossible. Although flap mobilization is not difficult in the early postoperative period, the alternative of waiting for complete healing is not the best choice. External ultrasound certainly assisted in softening the predictably thickened panniculus resulting from surgical manipulation. No further revisions were required as of 7 years after this repair.

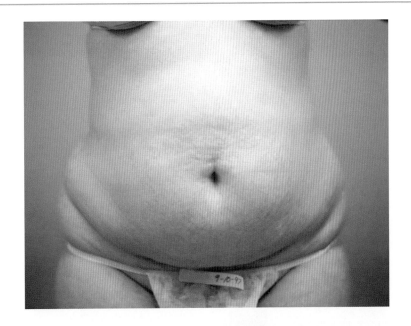

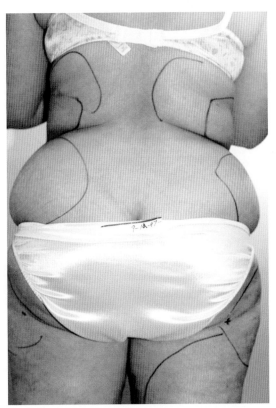
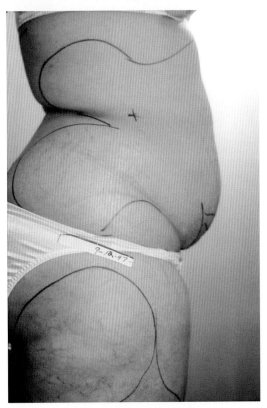

FIGURES 10-14 – 10-16 *Ordinarily, this body habitus designates such patients as "poor candidates" for body sculpture.*

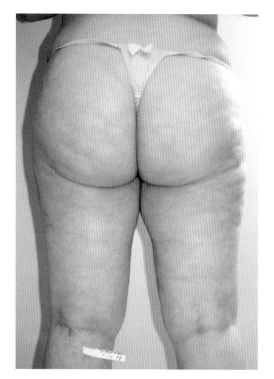

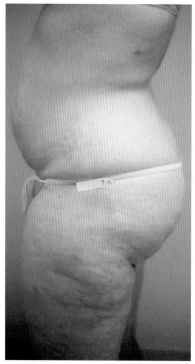

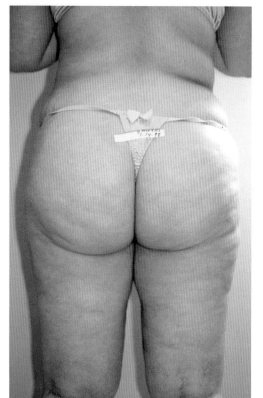

FIGURES 10-17 – 10-19 *Four-month views show unexpectedly good contouring despite the complication of a "girdle burn" (see text).*

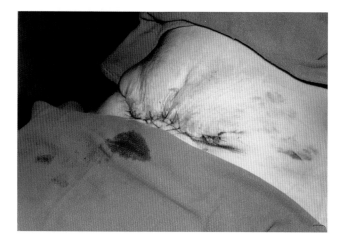

FIGURE 10-20 *Excision of the off-center necrosis and flap advancement for coverage.*

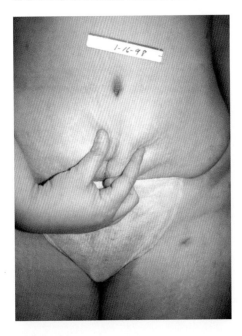

FIGURE 10-21 *Softening of the T-scar closure was accelerated by postoperative hydrotherapy, massage, and XU.*

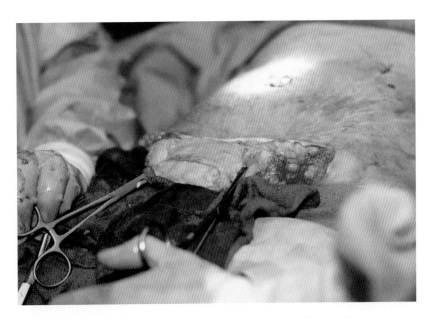

FIGURE 10-22 *Repair would have been difficult, if not impossible had this patient undergone standard abdominoplasty with resection of the entire panniculus below the umbilicus rather than a limited resection as shown.*

Case in Point—Postoperative Ultrasound Therapy to Improve the Limitations of Liposuction

This 67-year-old active woman would not consider an abdominoplasty or a more extensive procedure, but she did want to improve the appearance of her legs and body so that she could exercise in shorts without embarrassment. Photographs show the typical irregularity in skin texture together with moderate deposits in her ankles, large deposits in the inner aspect of her thighs, and a very high hip roll deformity that she thought was unimportant (see Figs. 10-23 to 10-26). Our plan was to treat this with XU alone and to use only XU on the front of her legs, as shown in the markings. As part of the initial study, she agreed that standard liposuction (suction-assisted lipectomy [SAL]) would be performed on the right thigh anteriorly and primarily in the posterior folds and that other areas would be treated with XUAL.

Ten days after the external liposuction procedure, bruising was evident on both inner thighs, but to a lesser degree on the left upper thigh and banana roll area in comparison to the ultrasound-treated opposite side. She reported that this area was not only more bruised but also more tender during the close follow-up period. *External ultrasound was used during the recovery phase in all areas.* She reported no pain postoperatively, even with walking at 24 hours, and only tenderness in the

SAL-treated area. She was able to resume full activities within 3 days and soon changed from her compressive girdle to spandex on the eighth postoperative day. A vigorous program of walking, exercise, soft massage, and hydrotherapy resulted in rapid shrinkage, totally unexpected for her age group and cellulite deformity.

At 1 month she reported that her congenitally larger right hip was still more swollen and tender after SAL than the opposite side treated with XUAL (see Figs. 10-27 to 10-30), although this did not limit her activity.

The fatty deposits in the posterior of the ankle were approached in the manner described by Mladick, with two entry points on either side of the Achilles tendon (see Fig. 10-31). To our surprise, equally rapid resolution occurred in the ankles, as shown in Figure 10-32 (10 days postoperatively), and was virtually complete at 3 weeks. Five months postoperatively, this patient requested a secondary touchup procedure in the mid-abdomen, which yielded 25 cc of fat removed and made a visible improvement. The inner thigh area continued to improve, however, and was not treated.

This patient illustrates the benefits that can be achieved in older active patients by liposuction as a lesser alternative to abdominal repair. The quick recovery suited her financially and accommodated her busy social schedule. With patients in this age group, motivation is extremely important, and they must be advised that secondary procedures are more common in their age group.

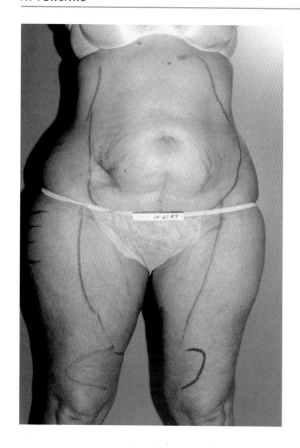
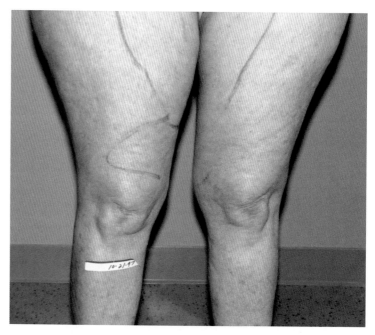
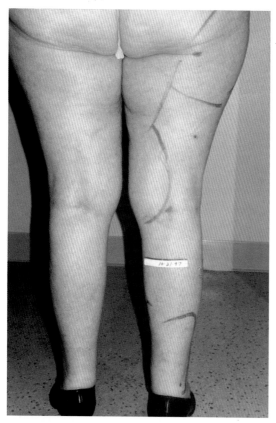
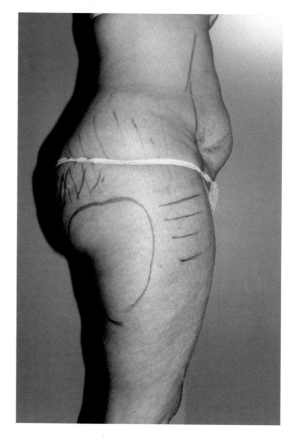

FIGURES 10-23 – 10-26 *Limiting objectives according to patient priorities. Extensive liposculpture and complete abdominoplasty are rejected by patients who simply want "less luggage" to promote an active lifestyle.*

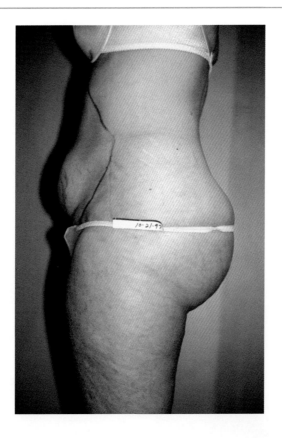

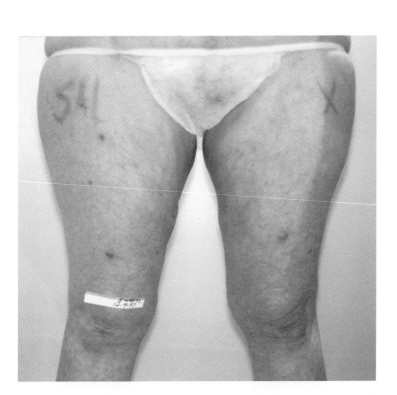

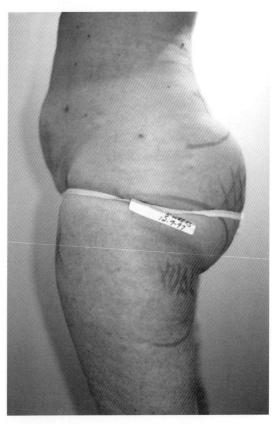

FIGURES 10-27 – 10-30 *With little difference except discomfort in the SAL- versus XUAL-treated areas, modest improvement without abdominoplasty was exactly what this older lady received.*

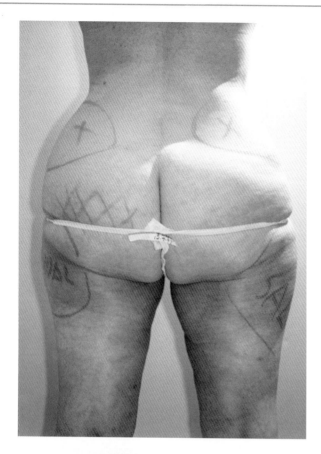

FIGURE 10-30   *Continued*

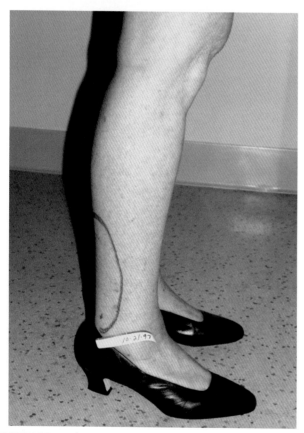

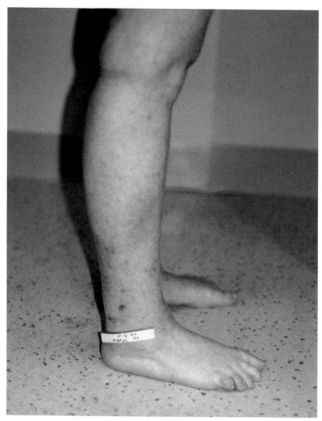

FIGURES 10-31 and 10-32   *As an afterthought she scheduled calf and ankle XUAL, "the only thing people will ever see."*

Case in Point—XUAL to Reduce Midline Edema in Short-Incision Abdominoplasty

Figure 10-33 shows use of a hand-held XUAL device (Byron Medical) for rapid resolution of the inevitable postoperative edema that develops in the tissues trapped between the upturned limbs of the "French line incision abdominoplasty." Note also that an abrasion developed above the incision from failure to release the compression garment at regular intervals. In this instance, fortunately, healing progressed without a visible increase in scarring.

External ultrasound is applied to any areas of postsurgical edema in the 24 hours after liposuction or abdominoplasty surgery, except in the midline where compromise in circulation is suspected. Ultrasound stimulates blood flow, which reduces edema, but if the flap is damaged by elevation and repositioning, there is a theoretical risk of inducing ultrasonic injury externally until after 48 hours. In our experience, no instances of necrosis have resulted with this program.

WEIGHT LOSS AFTER ABDOMINOPLASTY AND LIPOSUCTION

In general, weight loss after liposuction and abdominoplasty improves the result. The remaining fat cells shrink with weight loss, thus providing a nicer contour, in contrast to weight gain. We always advise diet and exercise postoperatively.

In the past, patients were urged to lose weight before liposuction. The opposite is actually better. Weight loss on a crash diet will cause the fat cells in the relevant area to contract. A well-planned liposuction will then leave too many fat cells, and they will certainly rebound when the patient resumes a normal diet. This may explain the variations noted in this patient. XUAL with a short-incision "limited abdominoplasty" and plication from the pubic area to just above the umbilicus was planned for the defects shown in Figures 10-34 and 10-35. Resolution occurred rapidly, with scar fading aided by XU applied postoperatively (see Fig. 10-36). A preoperative

view (see Fig. 10-37) and views at 1 and 6 months postoperatively (see Figs. 10-38 and 10-39) show shrinkage of the high hip roll, the banana roll, and the lateral aspect of the hip; the transition areas anteriorly treated with ultrasound alone; and change in the shadow pattern with fat regrafting in the mid-buttock. The patient was concerned that the lower part of her abdomen had not flattened sufficiently. She acknowledged that she had gained weight between the first and sixth months. Posterior views confirm this change, with an increase in the high hip roll and a minor increase in the low hip "saddlebag" area (see Fig. 10-40). Fortunately, diet and exercise corrected these problems and revision has not been necessary. An unwanted side effect of the weight loss that ensued after the 6-month evaluation had a deleterious effect on her breasts. A simultaneous circumareolar mastopexy had been performed with a very pleasing result. When the weight loss occurred, however, the breast lost volume (see Figs. 10-41 and 10-42). At this point the patient had a change of heart and decided to add more fullness. This is easily accomplished with internal tightening of the lower portion of the breast and the addition of a breast prosthesis (see Figs. 10-43 to 10-45).[1]

POSTOPERATIVE DEHISCENCE AFTER ABDOMINOPLASTY

During an unexpectedly difficult recovery from general anesthesia, a suture above the umbilicus in this middle-aged man was heard to break, and a seroma cavity as well as a visible bulge was left. After a period of 3 months, persistence of the bulge indicated that both layers of the repair had dehisced.

The repair was accomplished by complete separation of the umbilical stalk for visualization and placement of No. 1 absorbable sutures in a figure-of-eight pattern after first freeing the soft tissues for 5 cm on either side of the umbilicus and 10 cm above. When the sutures are tied, the umbilical stalk is reattached. A small opening is left for drainage as shown in Figure 10-45. Although exposure is limited, good lighting and careful technique make this local anesthesia repair safe and simple.

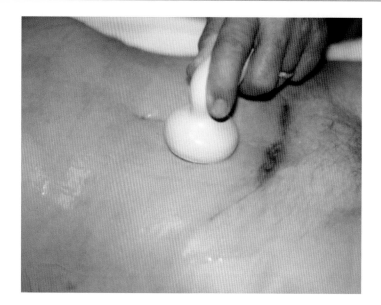

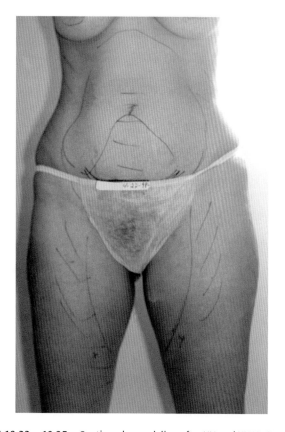
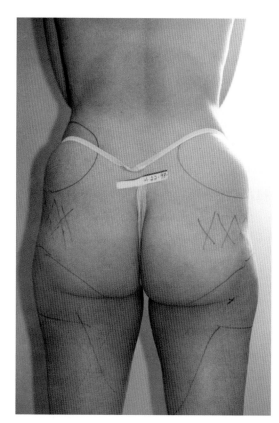

FIGURES 10-33 – 10-35 *Continued remodeling after XU and XUAL. Preoperative markings for limited abdominoplasty with XUAL; etching for vertical shadows; XUAL of the hips, "high hip area," and thighs; and mid-buttock fat grafts. The back, flanks, and anterior of the thighs were treated with XU alone, no fat extraction.*

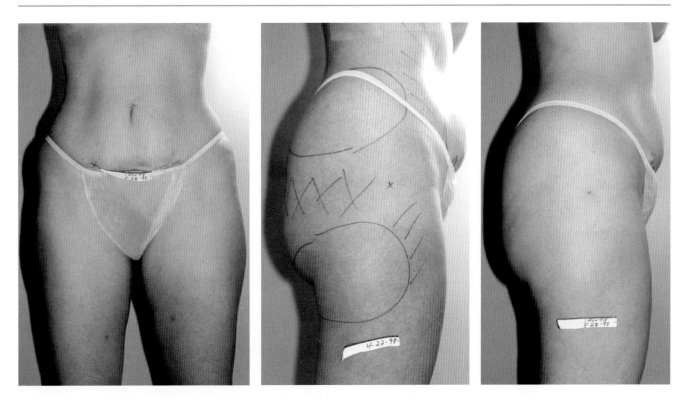

FIGURES 10-36 – 10-38   *Continued improvement of the limited abdominoplasty with XUAL.*

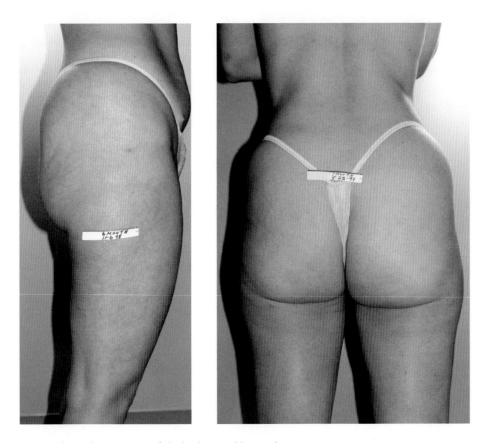

FIGURES 10-39 & 10-40   *Continued improvement of the back treated by XU alone.*

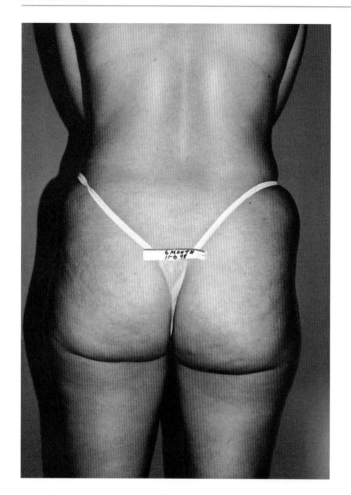 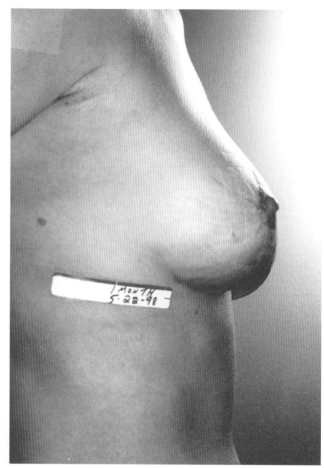

FIGURES 10-41 & 10-42   *Another "bloodless" procedure, circumareolar mastopexy was performed safely with this less than average contour chosen by the patient.*

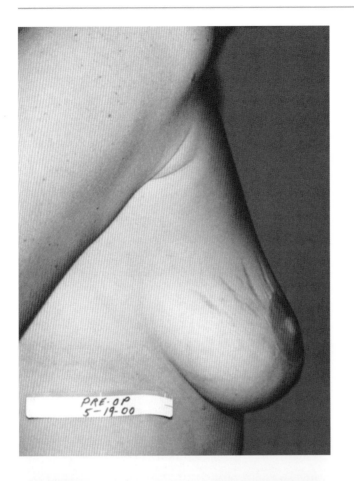

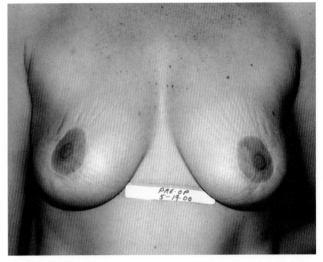

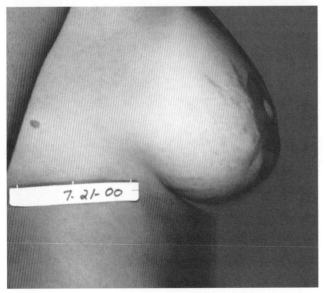

FIGURES 10-43 to 10-45 *Pleased with body shaping, many patients overcome their initial hesitation and request a further increase in breast volume. A textured gel prosthesis was placed for enhanced cleavage and elevation.*

"DOCTOR, I'M HAPPY, BUT . . ."

Ten Operations, Ten Traps—Alan Matarasso, M.D. (Plastic Surgeon, New York)

There are as many styles of patient consultation as there are surgeons who participate in them. Our training and experience, local community standards, and our own personality all factor into how we conduct our consultations with prospective patients. Professional societies and textbooks have done a credible job in teaching what should be conveyed about surgical complications, untoward sequelae, and appropriate informed consent for our operations. Moreover, many of our patients today arrive with preconceived expectations of what they think—and want—the procedures to accomplish.

Beyond these issues are the many unspoken gray zones of what the operation does *not* achieve. Consequently, I have found that over the years I spend as much or even more time discussing what surgery will not achieve as what it will achieve. Failure to do so results in the adage that if you didn't discuss it preoperatively, it is considered an excuse postoperatively.

In general, certain physiologic facts pertaining to postoperative recovery can expected in almost any surgical procedure. These concepts should be related to the prospective patient and include the following:
Skin will feel numb after surgery.

- Just because the bruising is gone does not mean that all the swelling is gone—it will take months or more to achieve the final result.
- How incisions heal is not entirely predictable, and much of their appearance is based on factors out of the surgeon's control. You can't have surgery without scars. The scars will fade and mature over time, but they will not disappear completely.
- It's impossible to tell exactly when one will be able to go back to work.
- It's impossible to predict whether an individual will be entirely satisfied with the results or the "percentage" that they will be improved.
- The surgeon has limited control over the body's immune response to implants.
- Avoiding procoagulants (such as aspirin) doesn't mean that you won't get a hematoma or that it's impossible for a hematoma to develop.

- Antibiotics don't prevent all infections.
- Though at lower risk, skin sloughing can also occur in non-smokers.
- Deep venous thrombosis and pulmonary embolism can occur—no matter what precautions are taken.
- Having local anesthesia versus general anesthesia does not eliminate all risks.
- Surgery improves the quantity, not the quality of skin.
- Genetics and anatomy are unique to a particular individual, who may not obtain the same results as a friend or relative.
- Having additional surgery isn't necessarily better.
- Everyone is asymmetric—no two sides of the body are the same.
- All surgery carries risks. There is no such thing as minor surgery.

These concepts represent general caveats. However, time and again, prolonged discussions seem to arise about specific operations. Here, then, are 10 operations and 10 "clubs" to keep you out of the sand trap of "Doctor, I'm happy, but . . ."

"Doctor, I'm happy, but . . .

1. (Upper eyelids) ". . . couldn't you have taken more skin? See, when I do this, it's better."

Patients who push their eyebrow up and state that this position is what they expected to achieve need to recognize the influence that a low brow position has on the appearance of upper eyelid skin. Preoperative discussion, one hopes, will circumvent postoperative inquiries about taking a "little bit more skin"—with the understanding that more excision will only pull the brow down further.

2. (Face-lifts) ". . . why didn't you make my face and neck tighter?"

An unaware patient who asks that the skin be pulled a little tighter doesn't realize that more tension won't restore the elasticity in a "chicken" neck and that after the edema subsides and normal activity returns, the diminished tone becomes evident and the wrinkling returns. Moreover, a lift won't improve lines (perioral) and minimally affects creases (marionette).

3. (Excisional surgery/dermatolipectomies) ". . . I still have loose skin."

There is no tissue like the original model. The best prevention is protection against undue deterioration by avoiding inciting factors beginning at a young age. Early intervention and maintenance procedures will remove excess loose skin, and such removal leaves permanent scars. However, no treatment can restore the elasticity in the remaining skin, which accounts for the residual laxity.

4. (Resurfacing) ". . . there are still some lines left."

A line is a permanent scar in the skin, like a crack in a piece of wood. Skin regenerates from below, so the deeper the wrinkle, the more likely that it will have some residual appearance after treatment. Resurfacing can go just so deep before it becomes unsafe. Fillers are temporary. Nothing, even the combination of filling, freezing, and smoothing, will restore entirely smooth skin.

5. (Abdomen) ". . . my waist isn't narrower."

The subcutaneous fat that can be accessed by liposuction accounts for only a portion of the abdominal girth. The intra-abdominal fat that accumulates with age won't be altered with liposuction or abdominoplasty. And even after abdominoplasty, the more intra-abdominal fat there is, the wider the waistline may appear postoperatively.

6. (SAL) ". . . there is more fat left."

"Rolls" that can be grabbed are composed of fat and loose skin. Liposuction only contours the fat. It does not remove or improve the excess skin, which when pulled and lifted, is what creates a smoother appearance. It's not necessarily residual fat.

7. (Lower lid blepharoplasty) ". . . my eyes are still loose."

Conventional eyelid surgery improves the fatty compartments know as "bags." In general, it does not remove a large amount of loose skin. Taking more skin will just cause the eyelid to pull down. Of the three crescents below the lower lid lash line observed preoperatively, the herniated fat is all that is routinely addressed—not the muscle roll or malar edema.

8. (Rhinoplasty) ". . . I am happy but the tip of my nose is still too thick."

What the surgeon can pinch and elevate off the nasal tip is skin. Rhinoplasty is not an operation on the skin but an operation that contours the bone and cartilage below the cutaneous cover. Even though the splint is off, healing continues for months. The final shape of the tip takes the longest time to achieve.

9. (Botox) ". . . see, I can move my eyebrows and there are still some lines."

It is normal, and expected, to be able to move one's eyebrows after Botox injection. Muscles in the surrounding area get recruited when one attempts to activate the treated site. In addition, temporarily "freezing" muscles won't improve all facial lines, such as static lines.

10. (Breast augmentation) ". . . I wanted to look like I do when I have my brassiere on."

Breast augmentation does not alter the inherent shape or position of the breast. Larger breasts won't necessarily have more cleavage and may still not look like models' breasts. Breasts that appear to be too high and hard probably have that appearance because of capsule formation.

I'm reminded of a hair stylist who conveyed her frustration to me about her customers' complaints. Exasperated after one particularly long session, she turned to the client and exclaimed, "This is a pair of scissors not a magic wand!" Similarly, a mentor let me know that he kept a conductor's baton in his treatment room for certain occasions. After the "umpteenth" explanation to a prospective patient, he would turn to his nurse and ask for his magic wand. Or the great plastic surgeon who had a crystal ball on his desk that he consulted when the patient asked him to predict what the ultimate appearance would be, or how long it would take to heal.

CONCLUSION

Aftercare is as important to the overall concept of care as is preoperative counseling. The availability of trained personnel and products allows us to provide "full service" to individuals who are seeking self-improvement.

Reference
1. Wilkinson TS, Aiache A, Toledo L: *Circumareolar Techniques for Breast Surgery.* New York, Springer-Verlag, 1995, pp 89-118.

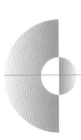

Index

Page numbers followed by f indicate figures.